Pharmacognosy - Medicinal Plants

Edited by Shagufta Perveen and Areej Al-Taweel

Published in London, United Kingdom

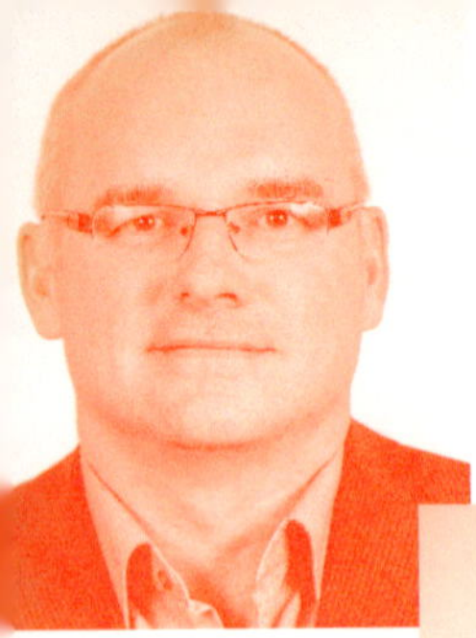
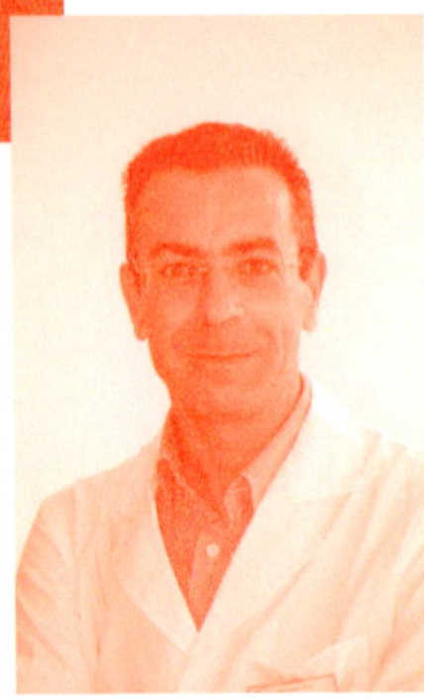
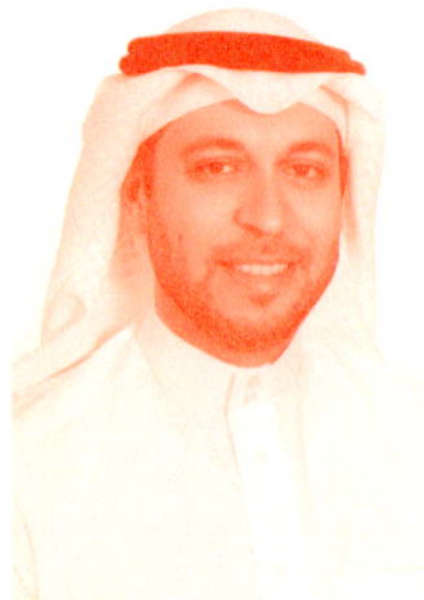
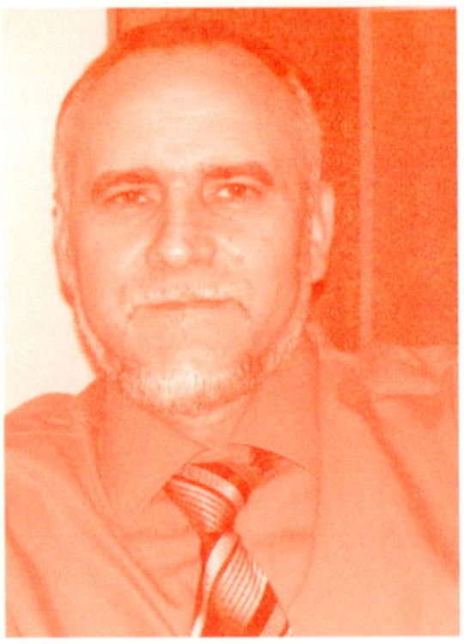
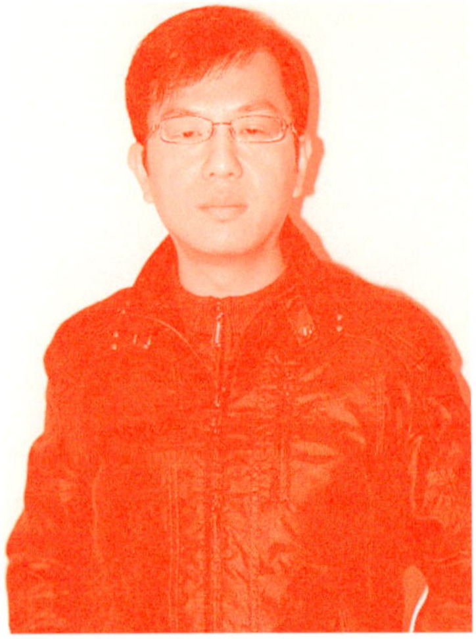
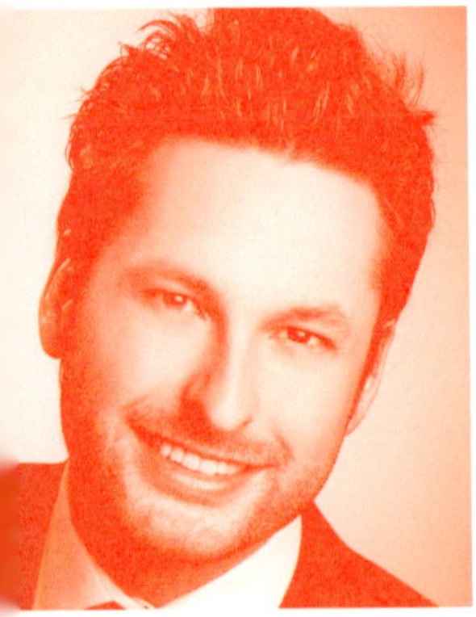
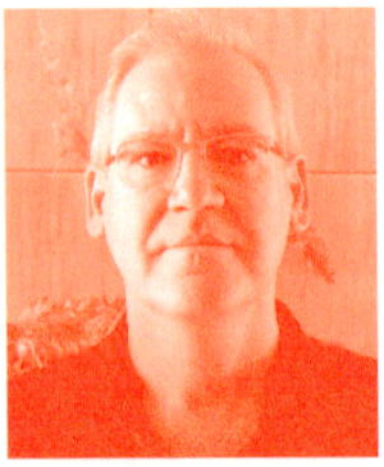

IntechOpen

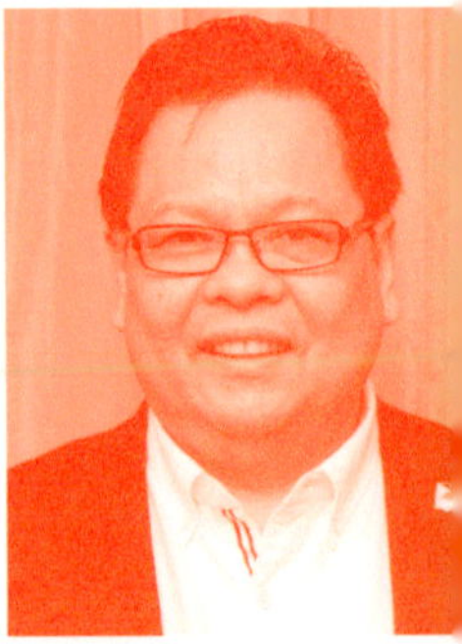
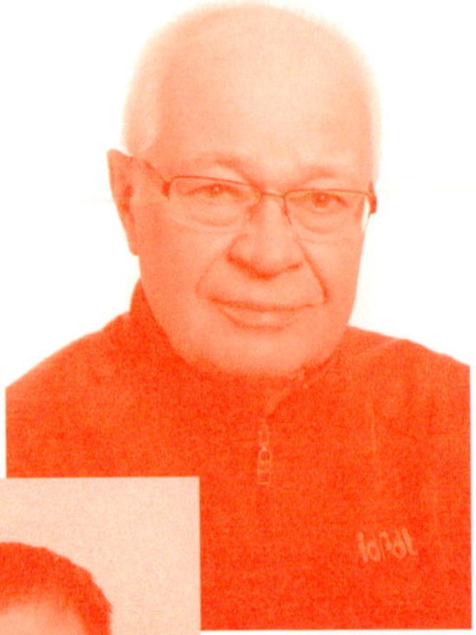
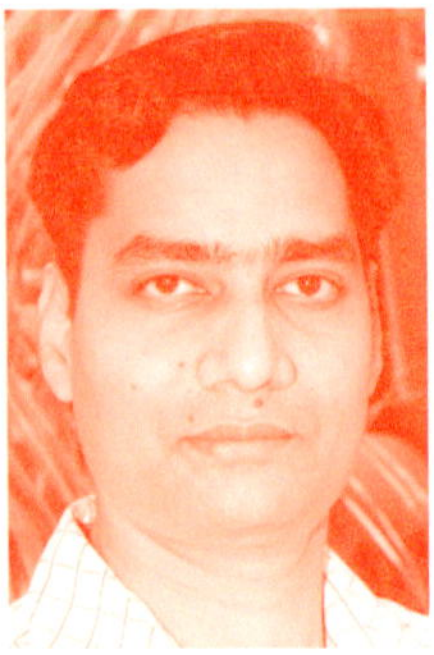
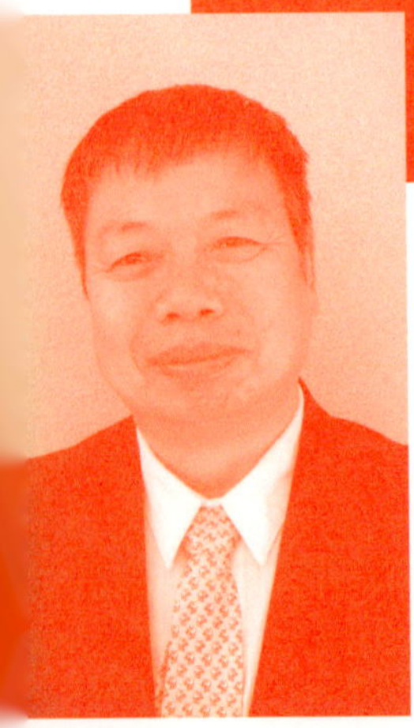
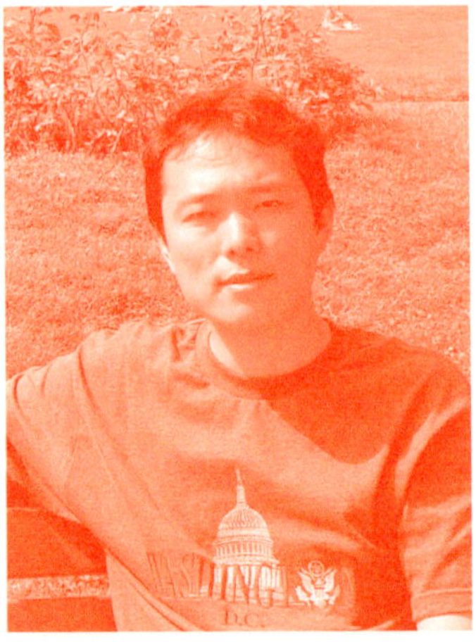
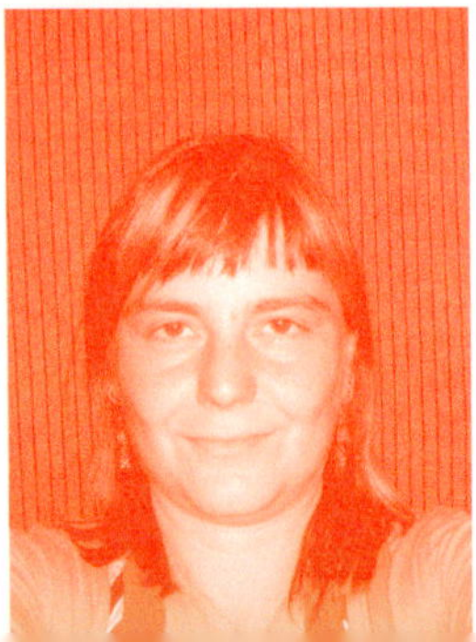

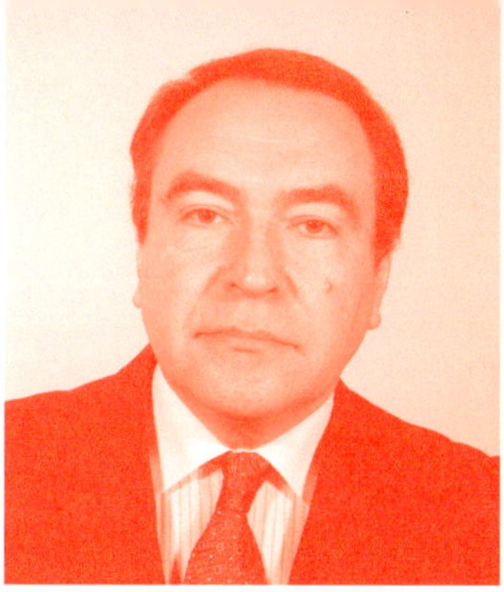

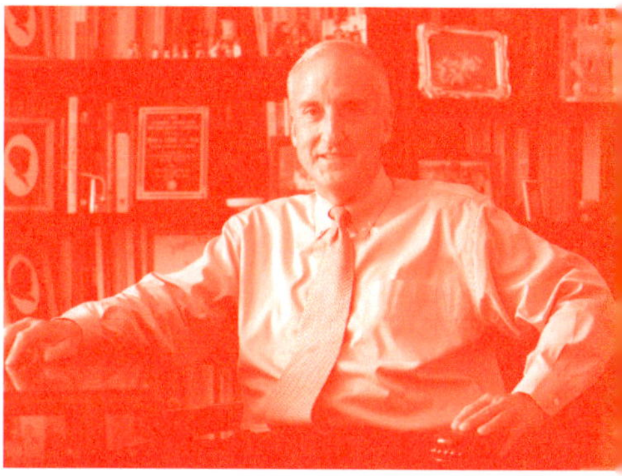

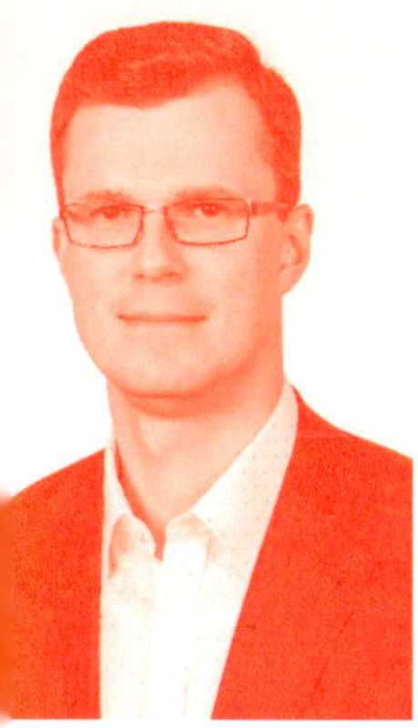

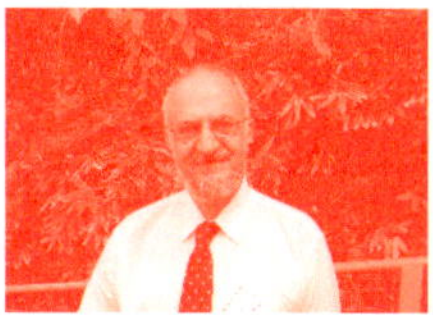

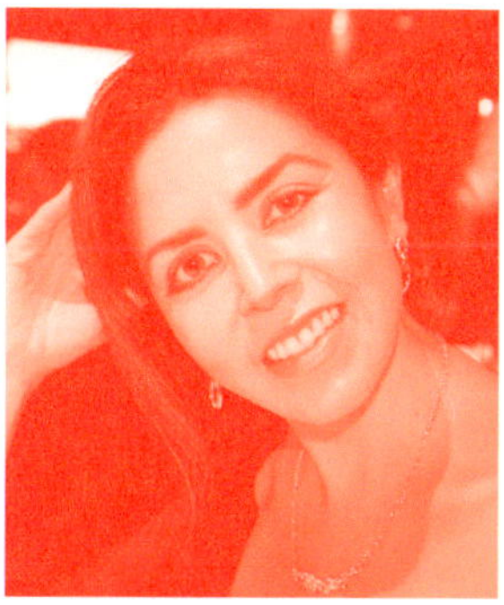

Supporting open minds since 2005

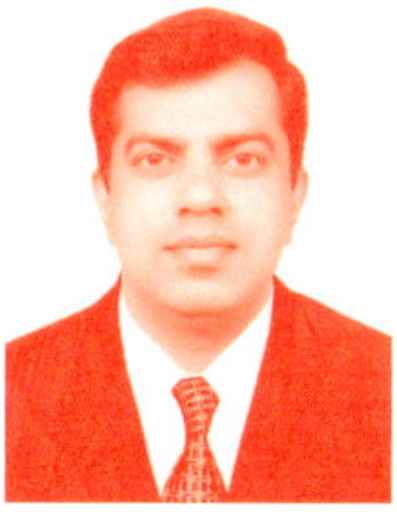

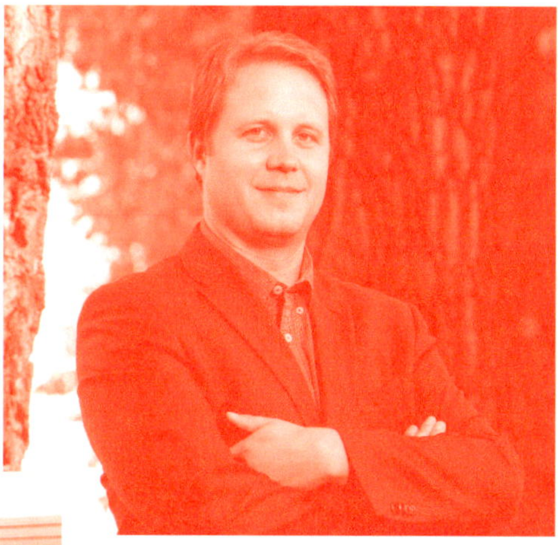

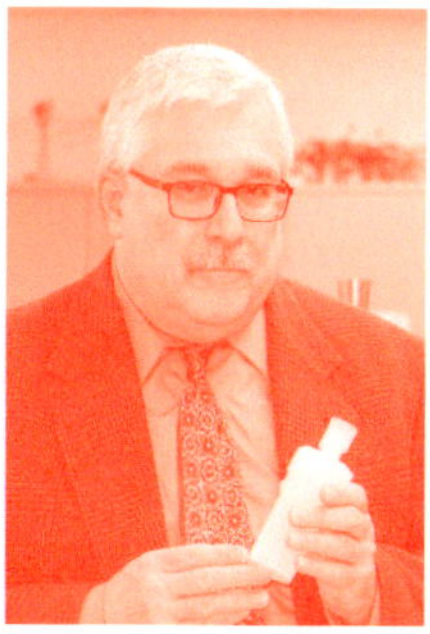

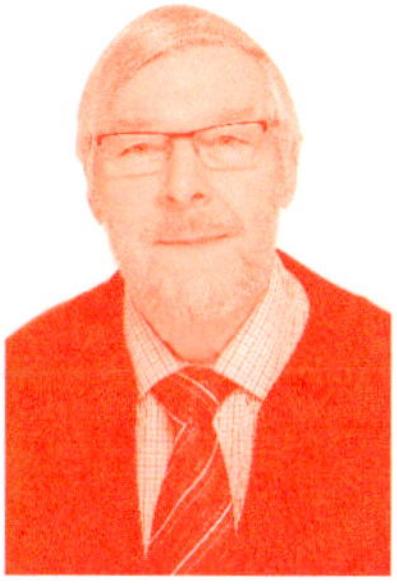

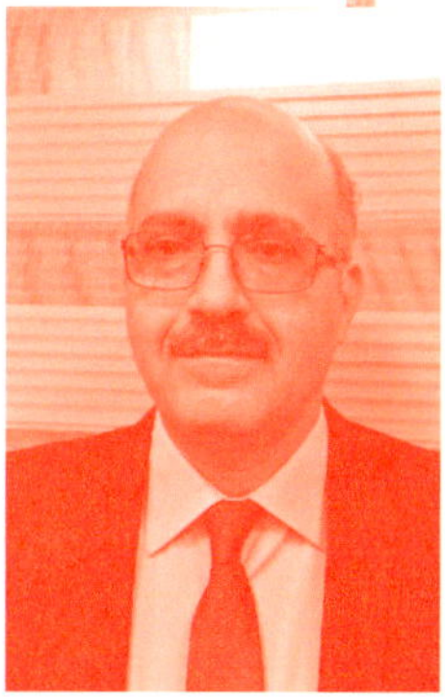

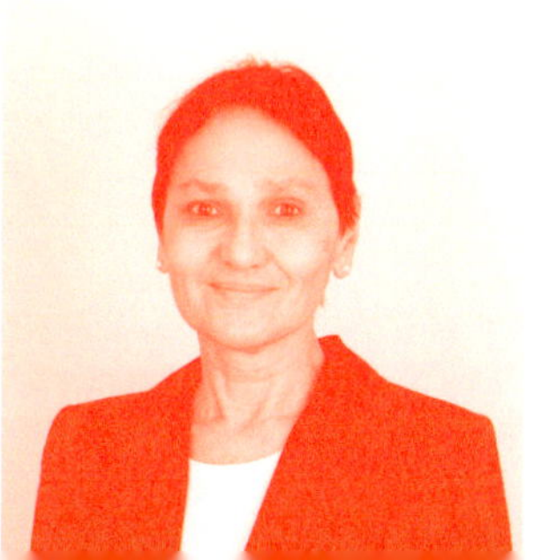

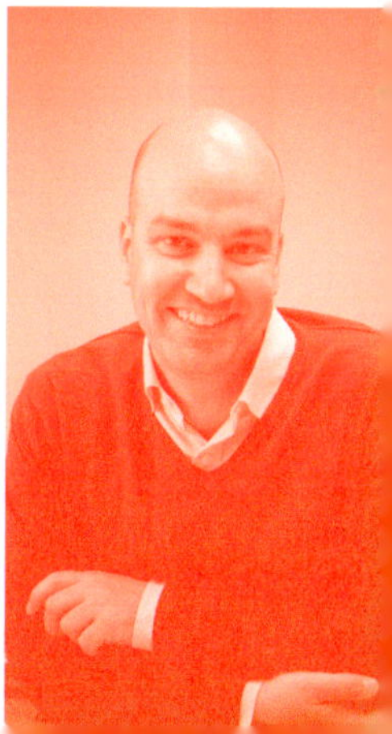

Pharmacognosy - Medicinal Plants
http://dx.doi.org/10.5772/intechopen.78419
Edited by Shagufta Perveen and Areej Al-Taweel

Contributors
Juan C. Castro, Marianela Cobos, J. Dylan Maddox, Gabriel Vargas-Arana, Anthony J. Fasabi, Jae D. Paredes, Jorge L. Marapara, Pedro M. Adrianzén, María Z. Casuso, Segundo L. Estela, Pranati Srivastava, Syed Abul Kalam, Fatai Oladunni Balogun, Ahmed Adedeji, Saheed Sabiu, Mutiu Idowu Kazeem, Abdulwakeel Ayokun-nun Ajao, Anofi Ashafa, Chella Perumal, Maiko Inoue, Shinichiro Hayashi, Lyle Craker, Susana Oteng Mintah, Mary-Ann Archer, Tonny Asafo-Agyei, Peter Atta-Adjei Junior, Daniel Boamah, Newman Osafo, Alfred Appiah, Augustine Ocloo, Yaw Duah Boakye, Christian Agyare, Akshada Koparde, Maxwell Egua, Adina-Elena Segneanu, Claudiu Cepan, Ioan Grozescu, Florentina Cziple, Sorin Olariu, Sonia Ratiu, Viorica Lazar, Silvia Velciov, Teodora Daniela Marti, Emelia Oppong Bekoe, Cindy Kitcher, Nana Ama Mireku-Gyimah, Mark Frimpong, Gladys Schwinger, Jesus Morlett, Raul Rodriguez-Herrera, Alberto Ascacio-Valdes, Mauricio Salinas-Santander, Patricia Alvarez-Ortiz, Alejandro Zugasti-Cruz, Ricardo Rangel-Zertuche, Victor Suarez-Valencia, Jose Luis Chavez-Servia, Mónica Lilian Pérez-Ochoa, Araceli Minerva Vera-Guzmán, Elia N. Aquino-Bolaños, José C. Carrillo-Rodríguez, Salud Perez, Katarzyna Barbara Wroblewska, Paulo Roberto H Moreno, Danielle C. S, Oliveira, Maria Tereza Grombone-Guratini, Dennis R. A. Mans, Euridice Irving, Shagufta Perveen

First published in London, United Kingdom, 2019 by IntechOpen
IntechOpen is the global imprint of INTECHOPEN LIMITED, registered in England and Wales, registration number: 11086078, The Shard, 25th floor, 32 London Bridge Street
London, SE19SG - United Kingdom
Printed in Croatia

British Library Cataloguing-in-Publication Data
A catalogue record for this book is available from the British Library

Additional hard and PDF copies can be obtained from orders@intechopen.com

Pharmacognosy - Medicinal Plants
Edited by Shagufta Perveen and Areej Al-Taweel
p. cm.
Print ISBN 978-1-83880-610-1
Online ISBN 978-1-83880-611-8
eBook (PDF) ISBN 978-1-83880-874-7

For EU product safety concerns:
IN TECH d.o.o., Prolaz Marije Krucifikse Kozulić 3, 51000 Rijeka, Croatia,
info@intechopen.com or visit our website at intechopen.com.

Meet the editors

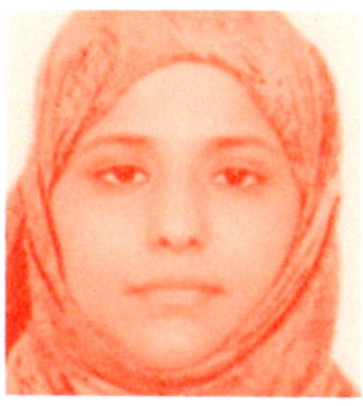

Shagufta Perveen is an associate professor at King Saud University in Saudi Arabia. She obtained her PhD from the H.E.J. Research Institute of Chemistry, University of Karachi, Pakistan, in 2009. Afterward, she joined King Saud University as an assistant professor, where she was promoted to associate professor in 2014. She began her research on natural product isolation and structure elucidation using different contemporary methods and techniques. She has published more than seventy original papers in different ISI-ranked journals, three chapters, and one book. She has collaborated with many researchers in Japan, the United Kingdom, the United States, Pakistan, and Italy. She is the editor of more than 10 journals and a reviewer of many others.

Prof. Dr. Areej Mohammad Al-Taweel obtained her PhD in the field of pharmacognosy from King Saud University in 2007. She then joined the same university as an assistant professor and was promoted to associate professor in 2013. She continues her research on the phytochemical investigation of different Saudi Arabian medicinal plants and has isolated many bioactive natural products. She has published more than 50 papers in ISI-ranked journals.

Contents

Preface

Pharmacognosy is a field of natural product chemistry that deals with secondary metabolites isolated from different natural sources, such as plants, animals, fungi, mushrooms, marine coral, sponges, and fish. Thousands of drugs have been isolated from these sources, including artemisinin from *Artemisia annua*, Taxol from the Pacific yew tree, morphine alkaloid from opium, ephedrine from *Ephedra*, quinine from *Cinchona*, and pilocarpine from *Pilocarpus*. The importance of natural product chemistry cannot be ignored because it has provided many active constituents throughout all periods of time, from the Stone Age to the present day. Many of the medicinal plants in different countries, especially in the Gulf region, have not yet been investigated, and their constituents need to be explored. According to the World Health Organization, 80% of people still rely on plant-based traditional medicines for primary health care and 80% of 122 plant-derived drugs are related to their original ethnopharmacological purpose. Therefore, secondary metabolites are good models for developing important drugs.

Shagufta Perveen and Areej Mohammad Al-Taweel
King Saud University,
Riad, Saudi Arabia

Section 1

Introduction

Chapter 1

Introductory Chapter: Pharmacognosy

Shagufta Perveen and Areej Mohammad Al-Taweel

1. Introduction

The word pharmacognosy consists of two Greek words, which mean drug and knowledge. In this field of science, researcher deals with the secondary metabolites found in many plants, animals, and microbial natural sources, for example, plant leaves, seeds, fruits, stem, roots, rhizosphere, herbs, spices, fungus, algae, corals, star fishes, jelly fishes, sponges, sea cucumber, sea urchins, sea weeds, snakes venom, frogs skin, cockroaches, and many more.

The American Society of Pharmacognosy (ASP) defines it as "the study of the physical, chemical, biochemical and biological properties of drugs, drug substances, or potential drugs or drug substances of natural origin as well as the search for new drugs from different natural sources" [1]. Most of the countries in South-East Asia Region of the WHO (World Health Organization) have a heritage of traditional medicine system. According to the recent WHO report, about 80% of world population is still using natural product for their primary healthcare needs. Pharmacognosy can provide safe and effective drugs in combination with modern medicine system.

2. Historical development

The history of herbal medication is as recent as human civilization. Herbal medicines, as the major remedy in ancient system of medicine, are employed in medical practices since antiquity [2, 3].

The early medicines of Pharaohs (3000 BC), the Greek (460–370 BC; Hippocratis), the Roman (37 BC; Disoscorides, a Greek physician of the first century AD was the writer of the first Materia Medica (78 AD). They described 600 medicinal plants and those of Middle Ages exemplified by the Arab Physicians (Rhazes 865–925; Avicenna 980–1037) relied mainly on plants for therapy [4].

India has renowned for practicing classical medicinal systems such as: Siddha, Buddha, Ayurveda, and Unani methods of medication and treatment. These medicinal systems are found even in the ancient Vedas and other ancient literatures and scriptures. The Ayurveda concept appeared and grew up between 500 and 2500 BC in India [5]. The authentic meaning of Ayurveda is "science of life," because ancient Indian system of health care focused on views of human and their sickness. It has been pointed out that the positive health means metabolically well-balanced human beings.

IntechOpen

3. Modern concept

Higher medicinal plants have a vital role in the development of new drugs. During the years 1950–1970, nearly hundreds of new drug-based plants were introduced into the USA drug markets, consisting on ricinin, derbipidine, reserbine (**Figure 1**), phenplastin, and phenicristine (**Figure 2**) derived from higher plants. From 1971 to 1990, new drugs, such as octoposide, teneboside, *E*- and *Z*-guggulsterone (**Figure 3**), nebulon, plonotol, and artemisinin (**Figure 4**), appeared all over the world.

About 2% of drugs were introduced from 1991 to 1995 including paciltaxel, toptecan, irinotecan (approved drug, FDA, USA), etc. Plant-based drugs provide outstanding contribution to modern therapeutics; for example, Vinblastine isolated from the *Catharanthus rosesus* [6] is used for the treatment of nature preceding: Hodgkin's chorio carcinoma, non-Hodgkin's lymphomas, leukemia in children, testicular, and neck cancer (**Figure 5**).

Vincristine is recommended for acute lymphocytic leukemia in childhood advanced stages of Hodgkin's lymophoma, small cell lung, cervical, and breast cancer [7]. Phophyllotoxin is isolated from *Phodophyllum emodi* (Berberidaceae), and used against small lung cancer cells and lymphomas (testicular cancer). An Asian indigenous tree *Nothapodytes nimmoniana* (Icacinaceae) is traditionally used in Japan for the women cervical cancer treatment (**Table 1**), and the main active compounds of this plant is Camptothecin (monoterpene indole alkaloid). Drugs derived from plants are used for solving many different health issues such as skin diseases, to cure mental sickness, lungs diseases, hypoglycemia, hyperglycemia, disorders of liver function, hypertension, heart problems, and cancer. These medicinal plants play a very important role in the development of potent therapeutic metabolites. Drugs isolated from plants came into human use in the modern way

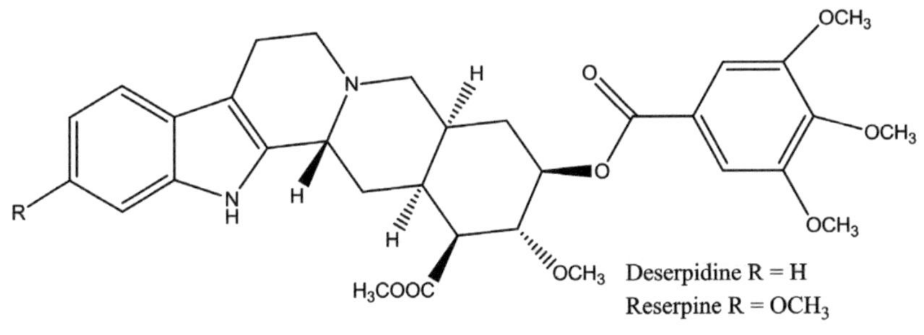

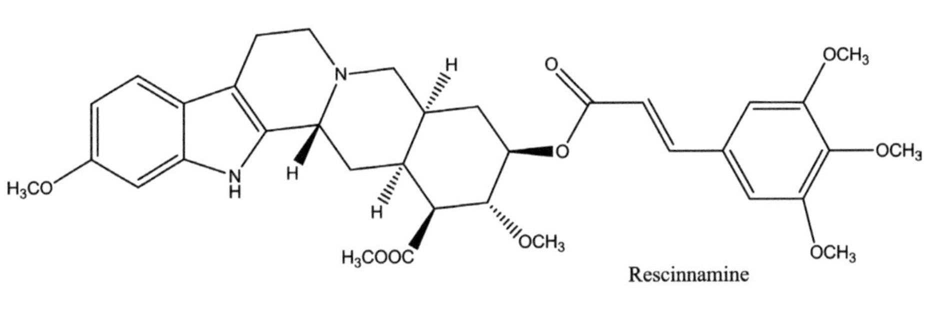

Figure 1.
Reserpine and its derivatives.

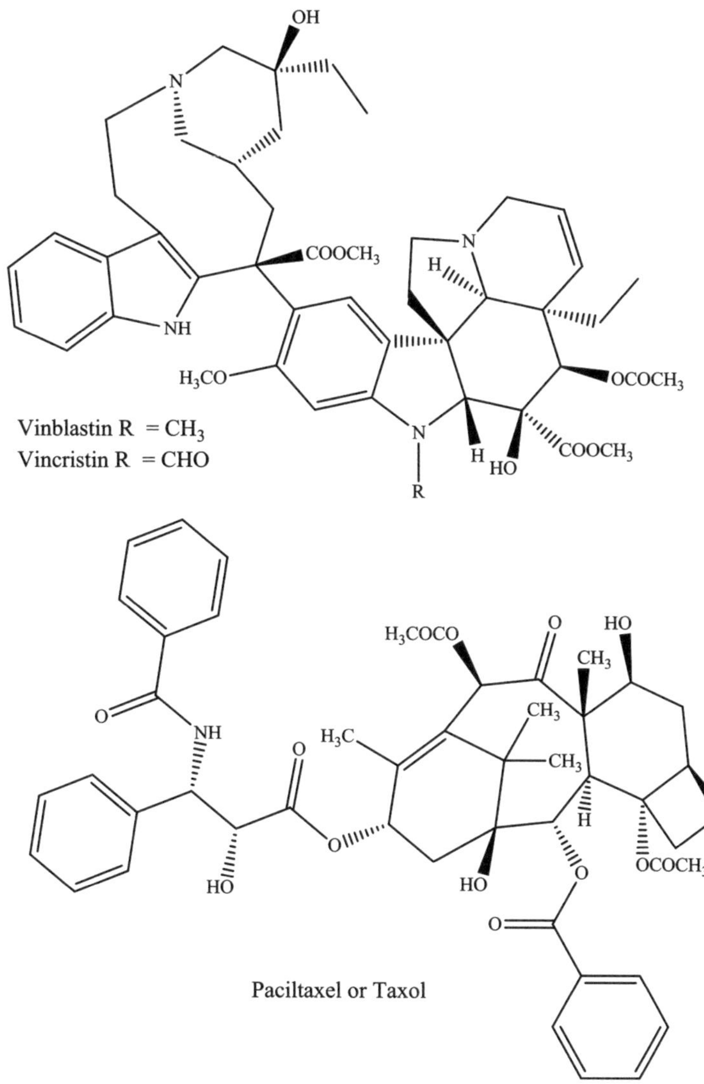

Figure 2.
Vinblastine and its derivatives.

of medicine through the uses of different plant material (leaves, roots stem, flower, stigma, bulb, and rhizosphere) as indigenous relieve in folk and conventional systems of medicine. More than hundred plants have been found to possess notable antibacterial activities; and many plants have been found to showed strong antidiabetic properties. Two compounds (etoposide and teniposide) isolated from one of the *Podophyllum* species were used for the treatment of testicular and lung cancer. Taxol, a well-known secondary metabolite from *Taxus brevifolius* (Taxaceae), is used for the treatment of lung cancer and ovarian cancer. The above-mentioned drugs came into use through the screening analysis of different medicinal plants, because they showed very little side and harmful effects, were profitable, and possessed good rapport. A racemic mixture (±1:1) of harringtonine and homo harringtonine isolated from *Cephalotaxus fortunei* (Cephalotaxaceae) has been used well in China for the treatment of acute chronic myelogenous leukemia and myelogenous leukemia [8]. Elliptinium, a *N*-methyl derivative of ellipticine isolated from *Bleekeria vitensis* (Apocynaceae), is marketed in different places in Europe (France) for the breast cancer treatment (**Table 1** and **Figure 1**) [9].

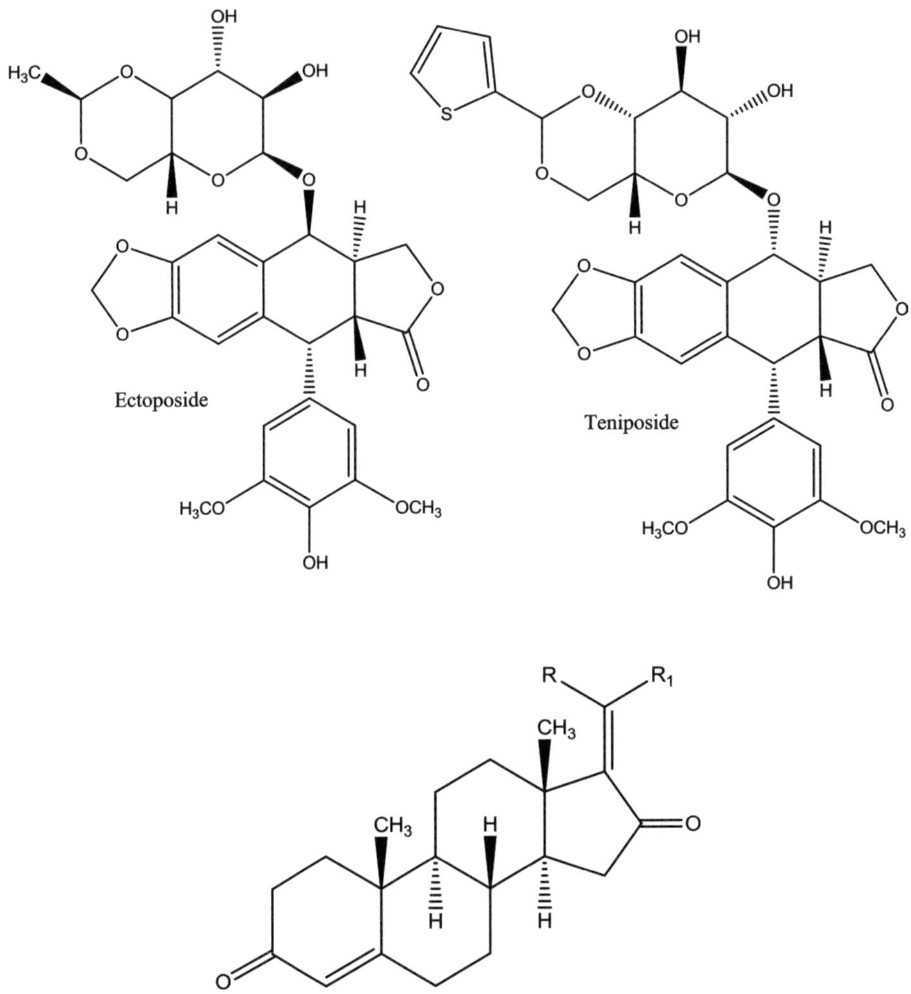

E-guggulsterone R = CH_3, R_1 = H
Z-guggulsterone R = H, R_1 = CH_3

Figure 3.
Ectoposide, teniposide, and E- and Z-guggulsterone.

4. Scope of pharmacognosy and phytochemistry

Pharmacognosy has always been a field of multidisciplinary science, and during the expansion of the orbit of this area, phytochemistry, phytomedicine, and phytochemical analysis have become important parts of this field.

Molecular biology field has become an extremely important area for medicinal plant drug discovery analysis through the determination and application of convenient screening assays directed physiologically related molecular targets, and modern pharmacognosy encapsulates all of these relevant new research areas into a distinct interdisciplinary natural product science.

The insistence and focus of research in pharmacognosy have alternated very significantly, from focusing on isolation and structure elucidation of drugs, including the information of active constituents, along with their biological activity as well as structure activity relationship (SAR) studies. Advanced researches in the field of ethnobiomedicine, ethnobotany, and ethnopharmacology has also become an essential

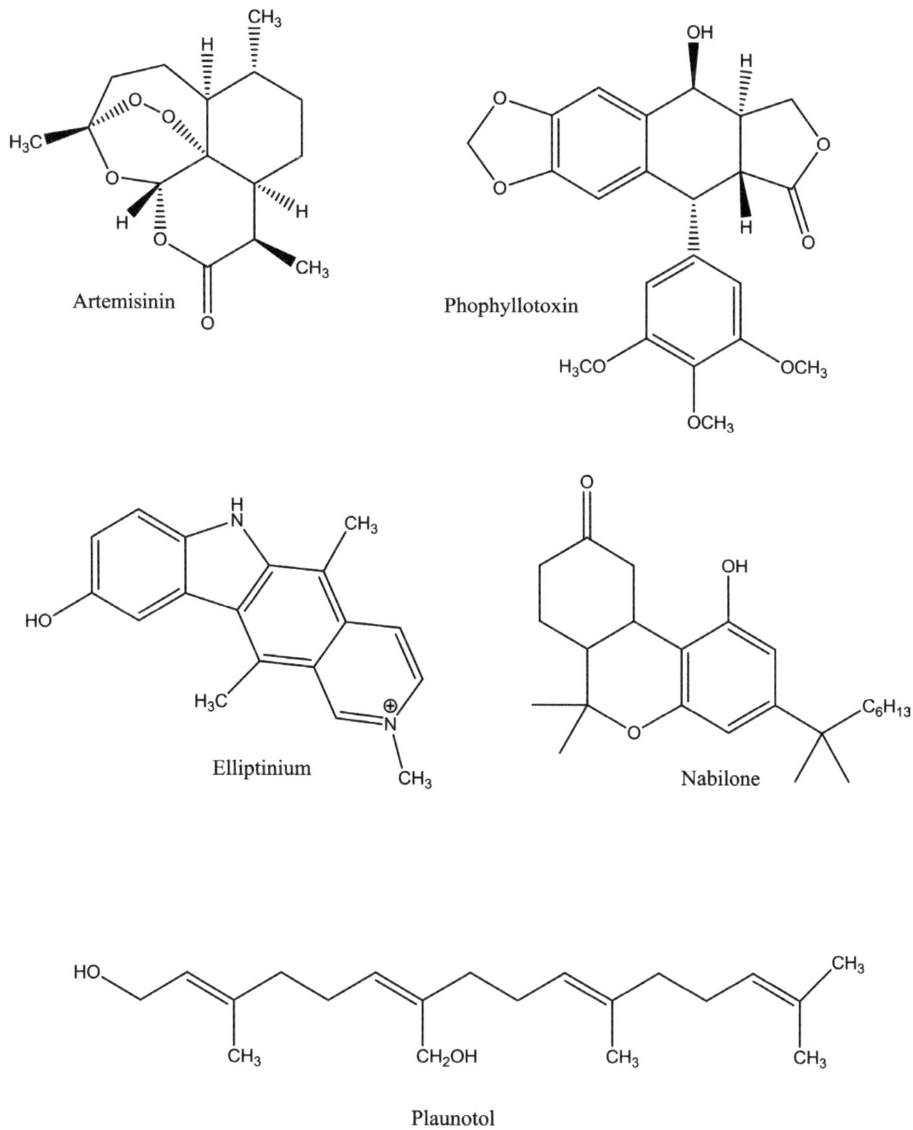

Figure 4.
Structures of few more anticancer drugs.

element in the orbit of pharmacognosy. Pharmacognosy deals an important association between medicinal chemistry and pharmacological studies (pharmaceutical chemistry) (**Table 2**). In recent years, as a result of fast development of advance phytochemistry and pharmacological testing ways and methods, new plant-derived drugs are finding their way into medicine as single phytochemical, rather than in the mixture form of traditional herbal preparations. The world is now moving toward the herbal medicine or phytomedicines that repair and strengthens bodily systems (especially the immune system, which can then properly fight foreign invaders) and help to destroy offending pathogens without toxic side effects.

However, presently, drug discoveries are increasing rapidly after adopting traditional/folk medicine-based uses/approaches to increase results and with safety concerns. Thus, different sub-branches of pharmacognosy, such as: analytical, industrial, and clinical, have been established as a modern and professional off shoots of specialized pharmacognosy to meet the most productive advancements and collaborations

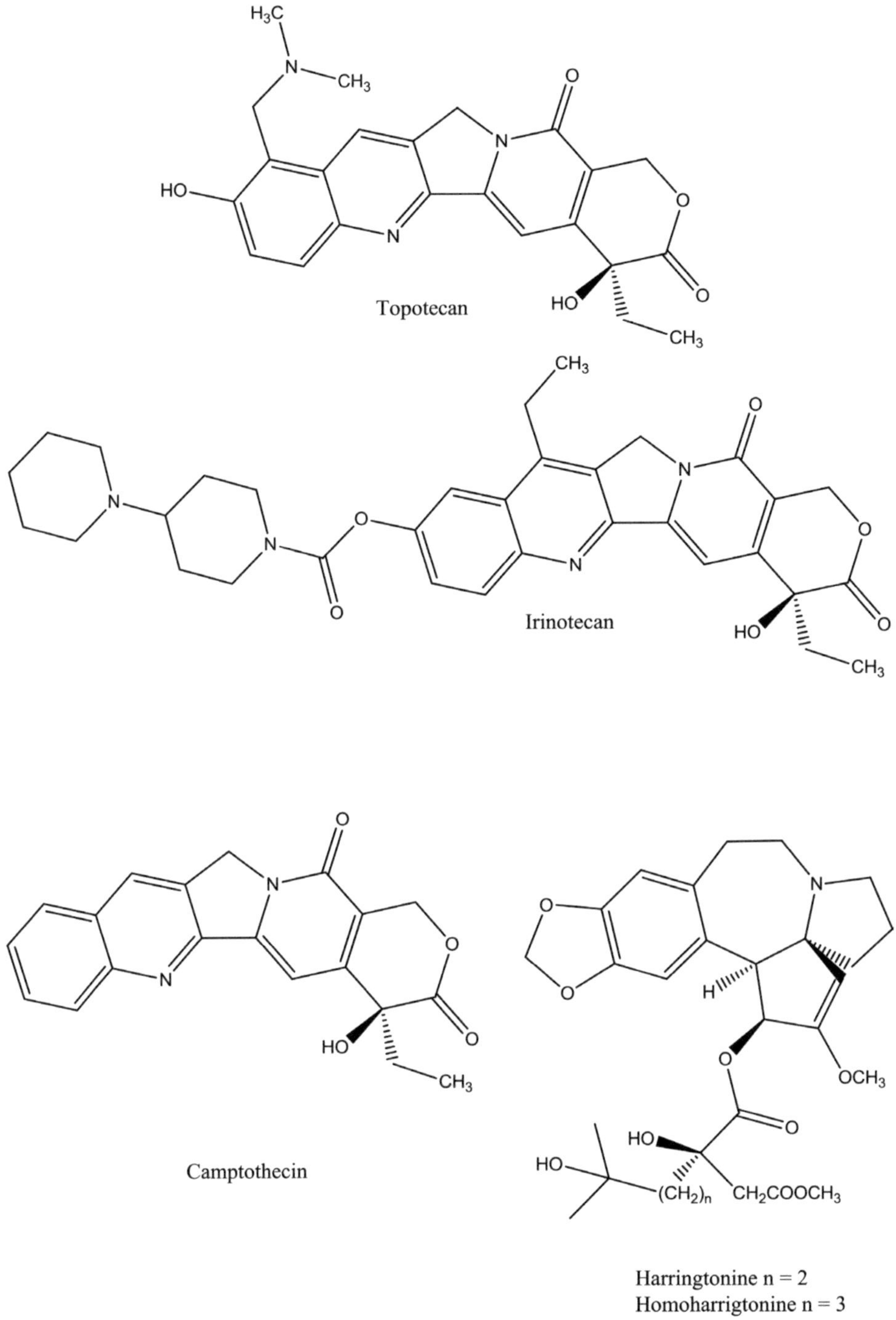

Figure 5.
Topotecan, irinotecan, camptothecin, harringtonine, and derivatives.

in this field. Furthermore, molecular, metabolomic, and genomic pharmacognosy have been introduced as the new and promising targets of research for accommodating future supply and demands in biomedicine, molecular biology, biotechnology, and analytical chemistry of traditional natural medicines and folk medicinal plants. Nevertheless, interdisciplinary combined and collaborative research work is very essential for optimizing the development of traditional biomedicines and pharmacognosy field of research, education, and techniques.

Plant name	Family	Drugs treatment
Cathranthus rosesus (Apocynaceae)	Vinblastine and Vincristine	Hodgkin's, Lymphoma, children leukemia, bladder, brain, and melanoma
Podophyllum emodi (Beriberidaceae)	Podophyllotaxin	Testicular cancer, lymphoma, and lungs cancer
Taxus brevifolius (Taxaceae)	Paciltaxel and Taxotere	Ovarian, malignant melanoma, breast, lungs, and pancreatic cancers
Mappia foetida (Icacinaceae)	Camptothecin, Irinotecan, and Topotecan	Lung, cervical, breast, and ovarian cancer
Comptotheca acuminate (Nyssaceae)	Quinoline and Camptothecin	Skin, lungs, and cervical cancer
Juniperus communis (Cupressaceae)	Teniposide and Etoposie	Lung cancer and lymphocytic leukemia in children

Table 1.
Few important medicinal plants used as modern drugs for cancer treatment.

Drug	Basic investigation
Digoxin	*Digitalis* leaves were being used in heart therapy in Europe during the eighteenth century
Emetine	Brazilian Indians and several others South American tribes used roots and rhizomes of *Cephaelis* sp. to induce vomiting and cure dysentery
Codeine, morphine	Opium, the latex of *Papaver somniferum* used by ancient Sumerians. Egyptians and Greeks for the treatment of headaches, arthritis and inducing sleep
Ephedrine	Crude drug (astringent yellow), derived from *Ephedra sinica*, had been used by Chinese for respiratory ailments since 2700 BC
Quinine	*Cinchona* sp. were used by Peruvian Indians for the treatment of fevers
Colchicine	Use of Colchicum in the treatment of gout has been known in Europe since 78 AD

Table 2.
Plant-derived ethnotherapeutics and traditional modern medicine.

Author details

Shagufta Perveen* and Areej Mohammad Al-Taweel
Department of Pharmacognosy, College of Pharmacy, King Saud University, Riyadh, Saudi Arabia

*Address all correspondence to: shagufta792000@yahoo.com

References

[1] https://en.wikipedia.org/wiki/Pharmacognosy

[2] Abdel NB, Ibrahim S. Medicinal & Aromatic Plants. 2012;**1**(2):1-109

[3] WHO. Guidelines on the Conservation of Medicinal Plants. Gland, Switzerland: IUCN; 1993. p. 52

[4] Subhose V, Srinivas P, Narayana A. Basic principles of pharmaceutical science in Ayurveda. Bulletin of the Indian Institute of History of Medicine. 2005;**35**(2):83-92

[5] Farnsworth NR, Blowster RN, Darmratoski D, Meer WA, Cammarato LV. Studies on *Catharanthus* alkaloids IV evaluation by means of TLC and ceric ammonium sulphate spray reagent. Lloydia. 1967;**27**:302-314

[6] Wagner H, Wolff P. New Natural Products and Plant Drugs with Pharmacological, Biological and Therapeutical Activity. Berlin: Springer Verlag; 1977

[7] Kantarjian HM, Brien SO, Anderlini P, Talpaz M. Treatment of chronic myelogenous leukemia: Current status and investigational options. Blood. 1996;**87**(8):3069-3081

[8] Cragg GM, Newman DJ. Plants as source of anti-cancer agents. Journal of Ethnopharmacology. 2005;**100**:72-79

[9] Taviad K, Vekariya S. The scope of pharmacognosy today & tomorrow. International Journal of Pharmacognosy and Chinese Medicine. 2018;**2**(1):1-2

Section 2

Medicinal Plants

Chapter 2

Role of Medicinal and Aromatic Plants: Past, Present, and Future

Maiko Inoue, Shinichiro Hayashi and Lyle E. Craker

Abstract

Before the concept of history began, humans undoubtedly acquired life benefits by discovering medicinal and aromatic plants that were food and medicine. As our early ancestors learned to recognize and consume selected plants, civilization and personal and group health could advance. Traditional medicine would become part of every civilization with medicinal and aromatic plants widely used and applied to maintain life. Undoubtedly, the variety of available plant materials would be tasted and tested to determine whether a plant was valuable as a food or medicine. Today, a variety of available herbs and spices are used and enjoyed throughout the world and continue to promote good health. As the benefits from medicinal and aromatic plants are recognized, these plants will have a special role for humans in the future.

Keywords: healing, pharmaceuticals, herbs, spices, remarkable constituents

1. Introduction

From the beginning, human life in prehistoric time was undoubtedly difficult. To survive, our ancestors needed food for energy and medicine to maintain health. While a high-energy food, such as meat, would be available by hunting animals, medicines to treat afflictions were undoubtedly more difficult to find. Although modern science has discovered plants and plant extracts that can treat and cure diseases, locating and identifying plants that contained health-promoting constituents during prehistoric time would be problematic.

The oldest available medicinal records, written in 5000–3000 BCE by Sumerians on clay tablets, demonstrate that humans understood diseases and that the use of medicine-containing plants could help maintain and restore good health. Medicinal plants discovered on the preserved body known as Ötzi, the Iceman that was accidently killed between 3400 and 3100 BCE in the cold, mountainous Alps, suggests that others were aware of medicinal plants. While the history of our early ancestors and medicines is incomplete, the value of medicinal plants in curing and maintaining health is fully recognized.

Plants, which are subject to destruction by foraging animals and insects, undoubtedly survived by producing repulsive, distasteful chemical constituents that repelled foraging animals. Humans could be selective in the parts of a plant they would eat, observing that consuming some plant tissues, such as fruit, leaves, or roots of some species, made people feel better. From these initial beginnings, gardens of desirable plants would be established for the food and the plant constituents that helped humans remain healthy.

Throughout time, medical care has continually progressed, moving from illnesses to vaccinations and new medicines along with improved health-care facilities that can more accurately diagnose and treat health problems. Advancements in modern medicine and medical care have enabled people to live longer and healthier lives. New medicines from plant materials and antibiotics from microflora have defeated most diseases. By using tissue and blood samples along with X-rays, and other materials, medical laboratories are able to diagnose the affliction, ensuring the physician can recommend the appropriate medicine in an appropriate amount.

Our prehistoric ancestors could only rely on their senses to test plants and plant constituents for taste and medicinal activity. From this beginning, however, medicinal and aromatic plants have brought many benefits, such as food flavoring, medicines, preservatives, decorations, beauty, and personal pleasure.

Accumulated knowledge of medicinal and aromatic plants from ancient history until today has passed from generation to generation, improving health and life. While the importance of medicinal and aromatic plants is not recognized by everyone, loss of species due to climate changes, plant diseases, or other plant attacks could eliminate several plant species along with the benefits to which we are accustomed.

Encouraging a lot of practices, the knowledge went down to later ages. On the other hand, various climates on earth have encouraged the selection of species, eventually many regional specific unique medicinal and aromatic plants exist in the whole world. Medicinal and aromatic plants and ethnobotany were used for an original medicine of each civilizations and cultures. The movement of human causes the spread of knowledge and distribution of materials.

Dramatic events of history were the discoveries of special plants and the chemical health constituents within the plants. Due to the scarcity of the plant materials, people ventured throughout the world to seek new spice plants and the habitat in which these plants grew (**Figure 1**) [1]. By the eighteenth century, spices were recognized as medicine, a preservative, and food flavoring. By the eighteenth century, important substances were discovered and invented important substances for human health (**Table 1**) [2]. Many synthesized medicines were patterned after plant extracts that provide outlines for new modern medicines.

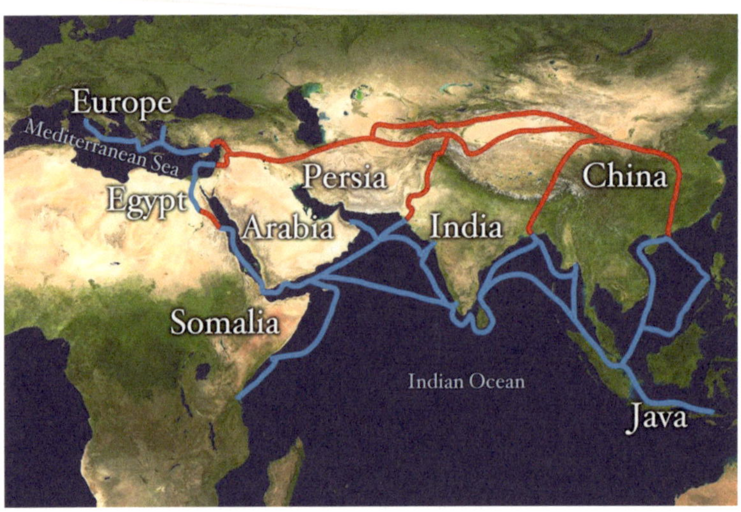

Figure 1.
Mail routes of the silk road [1].

Person	Achievements
C. W. Scheele (1742–1786)	Discovered chlorine, various organic acid, glycerol, tungsten, molybdenum
F. W. A. Sertürner (1783–1841)	Extracted morphine from opium for analgesics
P. J. Pelletier (1788–1842), J. B. Caventou (1795–1877)	Succeeded to extract quinine, specific remedy for malaria, from bark of cinchona
Friedrich Wöhler (1800–1882)	Created urea from an inorganic substance
Ludwig Knorr (1859–1921)	Created the first synthetic drug antipyrine during the try to synthesize quinine

Table 1.
The person who built organic chemistry [2].

Currently, a focus on integrated medicine provides plenty of plants and plant constituent choices for treatment of sickness. Not only in modern medicine, but also the use of plants, aromatherapy, crude drugs, and several other therapies have been adopted in the home and the hospital. Those natural drug and therapy are useful for preventive medicine too. Medicinal and aromatic plants are a good resource to develop new medicine and treat body and mind. The possibility of medicinal and aromatic plants is a hope continually for human live.

2. Past

2.1 Start of uses

Since the primitive ages, our ancestor ate plants and likely found medicines accidentally, and used for the treatments. The history related human and medicine is long, the oldest record was 5000–3000 BC in Alps from Ötzi, the Iceman used plant medicines [3]. Since then, for many centuries, human repeated trial and error and accumulate knowledge. At the same time, human likely thought to preserve the plants for a sudden health problem, such as dried plants, and started cultivations too. For example, Cannabis was cultivated in ancient Egypt [4], and opium poppy was cultivated in lower Mesopotamia and used in 3400 BC [5]. After human started to use language, they started recording medical information of plants and the records went down in later ages.

2.2 Brief history of traditional medicines

Before century, ancient civilizations were occurred around the four biggest rivers, the Nile, Tigris-Euphrates, Indus, and Yellow, which had own characteristic medicine. In China, 2800 BC to 1700 BC, Pen Ts'ao Shen Nung investigated about medicine and drug and established a foundation for traditional Chinese medicine. Later, Tao Hongjing (452–536) categorized medicinal plants to three phases: the first, second, and third. The first phase is harmlessness for long-term use, the second phase is mixed toxic and nontoxic one and as tonic, the third phase includes many toxic plants for curing disease and should not take for long term.

In Mesopotamia, the oldest medical text of around 2600 BC was found. The time, cypress oil, licorice, and opium were used frequently. A medicine of Egypt was started from 2900 BC, the knowledge of drugs were recorded on papyrus, especially Ebers' Papyrus which was written around 1500 BC showed 810 prescriptions, such as a collutorium, an inhalant, a suppository, a poultice, and a lotion. Greek Roma medicine was influenced of Egyptian medicine; Hippocrates (460–377 BC) used about 60 kinds of medicinal plants for medical treatments. De Materia Medica written by Dioscorides (40–90) was used as the world bible of medicine until sixteenth century. Galenus (130–201), called the greatest doctor in Roman era, developed many pharmaceutical preparations called galenical preparations now, the preparations are used even in present. The oldest pharmacy came into being at Baghdad in Islamic culture. The pharmacy carried Arabic spices, medicines of Persia, India, and China, camphor, clove, and musk. Avicenna (980–1037), called Galenus of Arab, had written Book of Healing and Canon of Medicine and invented steam distillation of essential oil extraction. Currently, an estimated 70,000 plant species are used in traditional medicine [6].

2.3 Spices

Early European medicine markets made use of spices coming from Asia via routes that followed the Silk Road and via crossing at the Isthmus of Suez located between the Red Sea and the Mediterranean Sea. Limited western trade with India and China occurred as early as 1600 BCE. The conquests of Alexander the Great into Northern India by 325 BCE undoubtedly introduced other European countries to spices as flavoring and medicines.

The Indonesian archipelago of the Moluccas (or Maluku Islands), commonly referred to as the Spice Islands, were the only or best sources of such spices as cloves, nutmeg, and mace until the 1700s. Arab traders introduced spices harvested in Moluccas to Europeans around the fourth century but sought to keep their sources secret. Monopoly by Arabian caused a big antipathy because of their absurd price of spices. European needs lots of spices to get epidemic away using the medicinal property of spices; therefore, some adventures tried to find a habitat and approached from a sea route which was supported by countries. Consequently, the monopoly by Arabian was broken by the Portuguese after Vasco da Gama's voyage to India around the Cape of Good Hope in 1497. The Portuguese strengthened their stranglehold on the spice trade during the sixteenth century, and in the seventeenth century, the Dutch took over control of the Moluccas which is known the Spice War. During the period, spices were worth more than their weight in gold. Finally, a nursery tree of spice was smuggled out of Moluccas, hence the Spice War was over, and the spice was cultivated in other places of the world. The occurrence leaded the reducing prices and making the commodity more available. If see the domestic dishes of each country, the diffusion of each spice could be seen as a spice route [3].

Action	Alkaloid compound
Analgesic, anesthesia	Morphine
Mydriasis	Atropine
Miosis	Pilocarpine
Blood-pressure increase	Ephedrine
Blood-pressure reduction	Reserpine
Bronchial expansion	Lobeline
Stimulus	Strychnine
Antimicrobial	Berberine
Antileukemia	Vinblastine

Table 2.
Actions of alkaloid compounds.

DOI: http://dx.doi.org/10.5772/intechopen.82497

2.4 Remarkable discovery of compound

Generally, alkaloid from the plant has a conspicuous influence upon the central nerve of human even if taking a small quantity alkaloid, very strong action is showed (**Table 2** and **Figure 2**) [7]. The plants which have an alkaloid have restriction of uses or on the list of poisonous plant. However, those alkaloids are used for

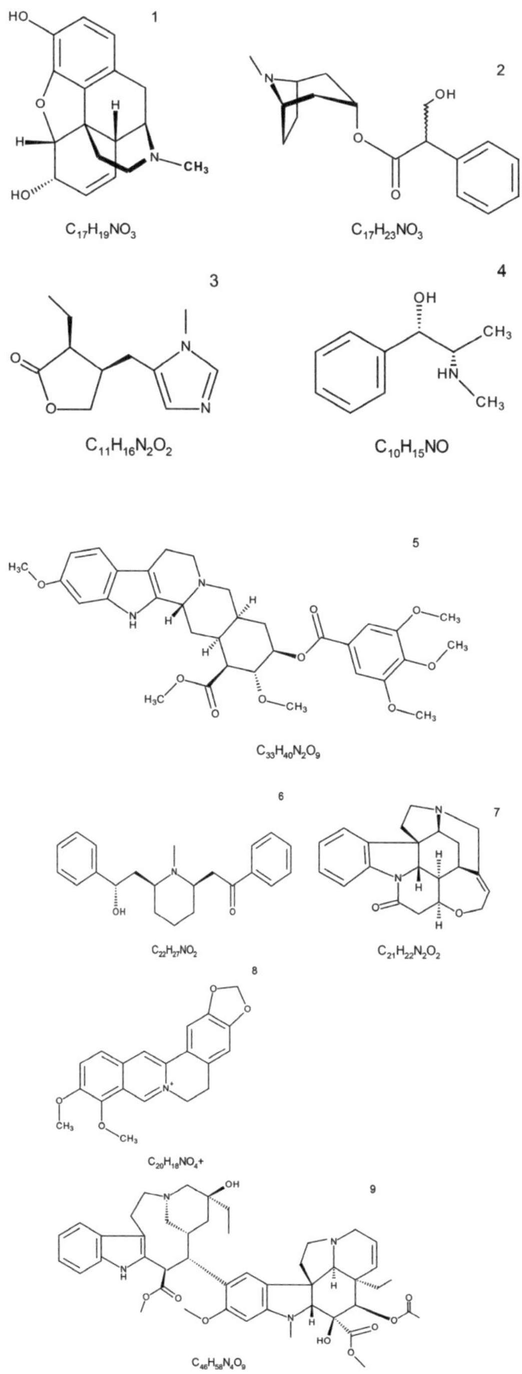

Figure 2.
Diagram of alkaloid compounds of **Table 2**. *(1) Morphine, (2) atropine, (3) pilocarpine, (4) ephedrine, (5) reserpine, (6) lobeline, (7) strychnine, (8) berberine and (9) vinblastine.*

materials of medical and pharmaceutical products widely. A lot of splendid studies to discover useful alkaloid were reported [8].

Examples of narcotic analgesics are (parentheses indicated trade name):

- Codeine
- Hydrocodone (Zohydro ER)
- Oxycodone (OxyContin, Roxicodone)
- Methadone
- Hydromorphone (Dilaudid, Exalgo)
- Morphine (Avinza, Kadian, MSIR, MS Contin)
- Fentanyl (Actiq, Duragesic)

3. Present

3.1 Medicinal and aromatic plants for human life

The magical compound of medicinal and aromatic plants keeps saving human until present, such as medicine, food, healing, and recreation. One of the huge benefits from medicinal and aromatic plants was to overcome many difficult illnesses, such as contagious disease, cancer, and AIDS/HIV. The National Cancer Institute (NCI) screens plants for the possibility of new drugs and active plant chemicals for cancer and AIDS/HIV in several ongoing collaborative programs [9]. **Table 3** indicated anticancer drugs which have received FDA approval for commercial production.

Drug name	Plant resource	Feature
Taxol/paclitaxel	Pacific yew tree	Now the first drug of choice in several tumorous cancers including breast cancer
Vinblastine	Madagascar periwinkle	The first drug of choice in many forms of leukemia, and since the 1950s. it has increased the survival rate of childhood leukemias by 80%
Vincristine	Madagascar periwinkle	Another antileukemic drug
Topotecan	*Camptotheca acuminata*	Has been approved by the FDA for the treatment of ovarian and small cell lung cancer
Irinotecan	Camptotheca acuminata	Has been approved by the FDA for the treatment of metastatic colorectal cancer
Etoposide	*Podophyllum peltatum*	A semisynthetic derivative of a plant chemical epipodophyllotoxin
Teniposide	Podophyllum peltatum	Another semisynthetic derivative of a plant chemical

Table 3.
Plant-derived anticancer drugs have received FDA approval for commercial production.

3.2 Integrated medicine

Integrated medicine is a medicine to perform a satisfiable living and improve the quality of life (QOL). Integrated medicine is accepted in not only the treatment of illness but also in the treatment of the presymptomatic state, prevention of illness, or maintenance of health. Integrated medicine includes, for example, western and eastern medicine and traditional medicines. Each medicine has strong and weak point, the advantage of western medicine is quick action by operation and medicine and examination, weak point is side effect. On the other hand, the advantage of eastern medicine is that it can make a balance of whole body, regarding inveterate and chronicity disease, and for infant, aged, and pregnant woman, and weak point might be the time consumption for cure. Patient chooses the most appropriate treatment depending on the circumstances; however, the most important thinking regarding "cure" is self-healing power that could cure yourself using medicinal help, not the drug that cures yourself.

3.3 Medicinal and aromatic plants in Asia

Recently, people concern health of body and mind, prevention diseases, detox, and longevity. Consequently, integrated medicine or preventive medicine is focused and accepted in modern medicine and daily life. Some medicinal and aromatic plant origins of Asia are daily used in the world because of the popularity and variety. Daily-use medicinal plants were enumerated bellow.

3.3.1 Japanese pepper (Zanthoxylum piperitum)

The origin is Japan and south of the Korean Peninsula (**Figure 3(1)**). Japanese pepper inhabit from north to south in Japan, half-shade, and humid are suited. Dioecism and 1–3 m height, a tiny green fruit matures in September and turns red including one black seed, the pungent peel is used as spice and crude drug. A fresh leaf is popular as condiment and garnish. According to a historic record in China, fruits are used as medicine in the tenth century in Japan. The constituents of essential oil include citronellal, linalool, isopulegol, geranyl acetate, and α-terpineol. The medical actions are antioxidation, stomachic, digestion promotion, and improvement of blood circulation. Japanese pepper symbolized the prosperity of posterity for the fecundity.

3.3.2 Kumazasa (Sasa veitchii)

The origin is Japan, the Korean Peninsula, the Kuril Islands, and Kamchatka (**Figure 3(2)**). Perennial and 1–2 m height, the rhizome propagation is shown a forest floor in mountains in Japan. The edge of leaf changes white in winter. The leaves are used for rapping of cooked rice because of the antimicrobial action. An herb tea of kumazasa leaves effects a breath-freshening for the deodorization. The constituents include chlorophyll, vitamin B1, B2, and K, calcium, magnesium, potassium, and benzoic acid. The dried leaves are crude drugs which effect for stanching, diuresis, antimicrobial, anti-inflammatory, detoxification, and intestinal.

3.3.3 Dokudami (Houttuynia cordata)

The origin is Japan, Southeast Asia, and China (**Figure 3(3)**). A cold resistance and perennial, 20–30 cm height, rhizome propagation, dokudami inhabit

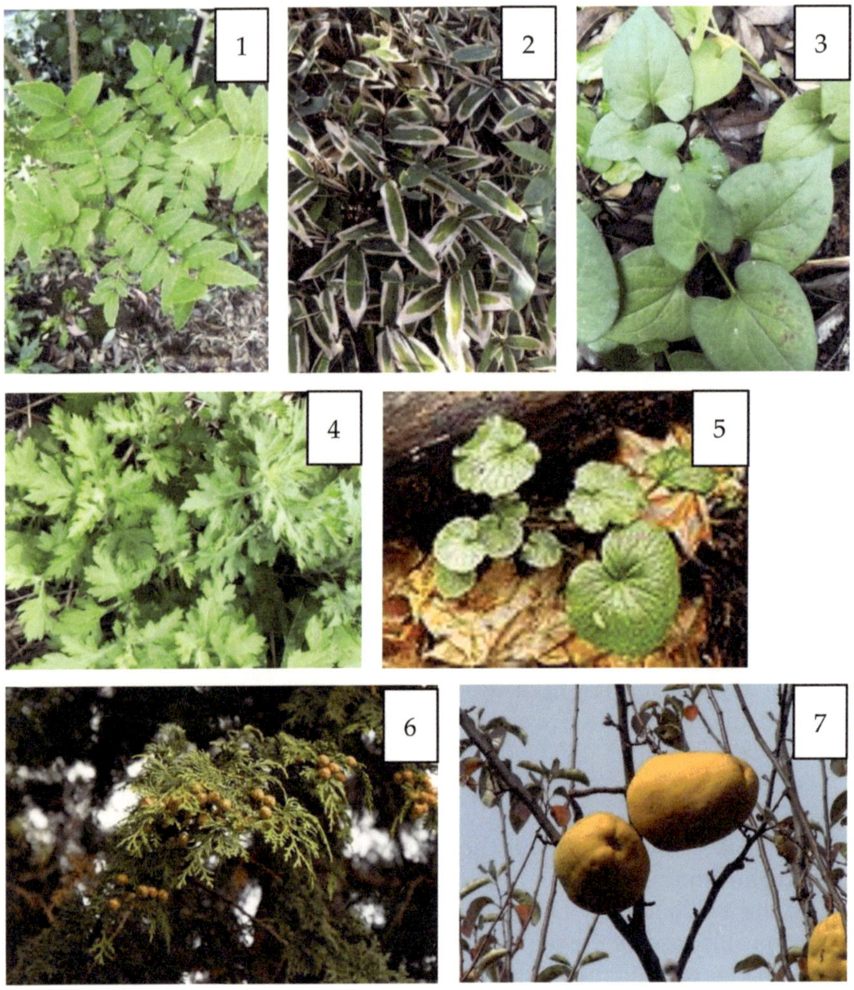

Figure 3.
Medicinal and aromatic plants in Asia. (1) Japanese pepper, (2) kumazasa, (3) dokudami, (4) Japanese mugwort, (5) wasabi, (6) hinoki cypress, and (7) Chinese quince.

throughout Japan, and the whole plant is used for cosmetics and cooking. The dried leaves have no offensive odor compared with flesh. The crude drug effects for diuresis, laxative, anti-inflammatory, detoxification, and the herb tea relieves a constipation, hypertension, and strengthen capillary. However, dokudami is inappropriate for weakening sufferer. A tincture is used as body lotion for skin care, and crushed flesh leaves are used for dermatological problem, for example, to put crushed flesh leaves on a rash. The constituents of dokudami are quercetin, quercitrin, potassium, and rutin.

3.3.4 Japanese mugwort (Artemisia indica)

The origin is Japan, perennial, 50–100 cm height, the back side of leaf has fluff, and Japanese mugwort is used as medicine for eczema, stanching, toothache, stomachic, and diarrhea since ninth century in Japan (**Figure 3(4)**). A collected fluff is used for moxa treatment and decoction of leaves effects eczema, heat rash, lumbago, and hemorrhoids. Japanese mugwort is used for side dishes and flavor of steamed rice cake and dye in daily life. The constituents are vitamin

B1, B2, C, D, β-carotene, chlorophyll, and minerals. The essential oil includes 1,8-cineole, thujone, β-caryophyllene, borneol, and camphor. The person who has an allergy of Asteraceae should be careful.

3.3.5 Wasabi (Eutrema japonicum)

The origin is Japan, one of the most famous spices of Asia, remarked the antibacterial power, perennial, 40 cm height, a radical leaf has 30 cm of petiole (**Figure 3(5)**). Wasabi could be cultivated in the water or field and the growth temperature is 10–17°C. The root is used for spice. The history of use is very old, in Edo era, wasabi became popular used for sushi. As crude drug, the root is used for an appetite stimulant, an obstipant, stomachic, and an analgesic. Especially, the antibacterial power is very powerful for an enteritis vibrio, O-157, a salmonella, and *Helicobacter pylori*. The constituents are sinigrin, sulfinyl, and potassium.

3.3.6 Hinoki cypress (Chamaecyparis obtusa)

The origin is Japan, evergreen, monoecism, 10–30 m height, the xylem has aroma (**Figure 3(6)**). The hinoki cypress is superior timber of Japan from ancient times; Horyuji temple, which is the oldest wooden building in the world, was built using hinoki cypress, which proves the great quarity. It is said there are no ticks and less mosquitos in a house made by hinoki cypress. In recent Japan, essential oil of hinoki cypress is getting popular because of the tranquilize effect and sleep-promoting derived from α-pinene, γ-cadinene, and hinokinin. The essential oil is used for cosmetics and bath salts.

3.3.7 Chinese quince (Chaenomeles sinensis)

The origin is China, 6–10 m height, flowering in spring and mature yellow fruit has great aroma in autumn (**Figure 3(7)**). In China, more than 2000 years ago, the fruits were used as a medicine for cough and recovering from fatigue and an aromatic. The fresh fruit is very solid and astringent; therefore, it needs to be cooked or steeped in liquor or sugar and used for cough, sore throat, tonic, diuresis, analgesic, obstipant, and calming intestinal. The constituents are malic acid, citric acid, tartaric acid, saponin, tannin, sucrose, and fructose.

4. Future

4.1 Expect role—medical Marijuana

Marijuana, *Cannabis sativa*, a plant frequently referred to as cannabis or pot, is a psychoactive, medicinal drug plant (**Figure 4(1)**). The plant tissues synthesize cannabinoid acids that under warm temperatures are converted to two major constituents: tetrahydrocannabinol, abbreviated as THC (**Figure 4(2)**), and cannabidiol, abbreviated as CBD (**Figure 4(3)**). THC is an intoxicating plant constituent that activates a brain receptor that initiates the intoxication and activates a pleasurable reward system in the brain. CBD, a nonpsychoactive constituent in marijuana, is considered to have therapeutic applications, especially for seizures.

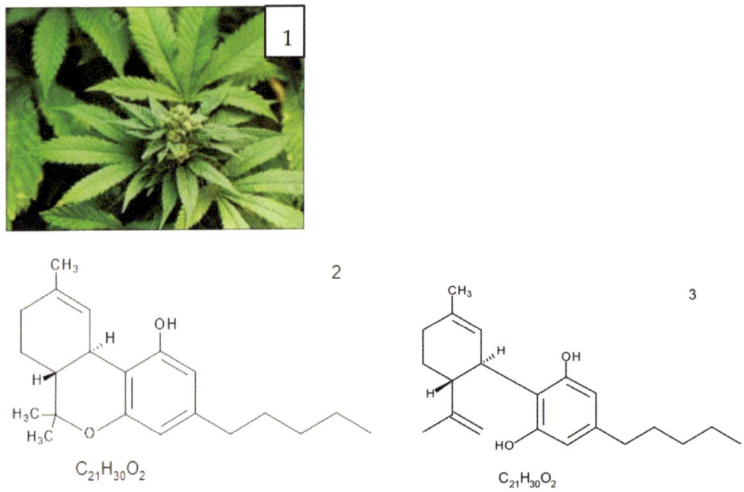

Figure 4.
(1) Marijuana (Cannabis sativa), (2) diagram of THC, tetrahydrocannabinol, (3) diagram of CBD, cannabidiol.

4.2 Development of new drug, progress of research

Pharmaceutical industry is growing every year, especially the industry in United States added an estimated $790 billion to the economy in 2014 [10]. Organic chemical of plant materials will give a hint to create a new drug including the level of family, plant species, and cultivars. Today, at least 120 distinct chemical substances derived from plants are considered as important drugs [9]. The structure of compound and constituent shows unique medicinal action (**Table 4**) [11] and knowledge and practices of traditional medicinal plants indicated the appropriate uses for the symptom. The information will become a signpost to develop a new drug. Traditional medicinal plants and ethnobotany have possibility to be great resources, such as artemisinin (discovered in *Artemisia annua*) and quinine (from *Cinchona*

Compound group	Typical constituent	Action
Hydrocarbon	Pinene, limonene	Stimulus, decongestant, antivirus, antitumor
Alcohol	Menthol, terpinen-4-ol, geraniol	Antimicrobial, sterilization, activation, spasmolysis
Aldehyde	Citral, citronellal	Spasmolysis, sedation, antivirus
Cyclicaldehyde	Cinnamaldehyde, vanillin	Spasmolysis
Ketone	Camphor, thujone	Mucolytic, cell regeneration, neurotoxin
Phenol	Thymol, eugenol, carvacrol	Antimicrobial, stimulus, immune function stimulus
Phenolether	Safrole, anethole, myristicin	
Oxide	Cineole, ascaridole	
Ester	Methyl salicylate, allyl isothiocyanate	Spasmolysis, sedation, antifungal

Table 4.
Compound groups included in essential oils and actions of the compound groups.

officinalis) [12]. Once single compound was identified, extraction or synthesis was possible, which is almost full-drug stage. After clinical trial indicated effectiveness, the compound will be a new drug [13].

4.3 Prospects

At least, 28,187 plant species are currently recorded as being of medicinal use in the world; however, only 4478 of the species used in plant-based medicines are cited in a medicinal regulatory publication [12]. It means a huge possibility to find new drug in the future. The global market of herbal medicines is glowing year by year with the interest in natural medicine. According to estimation of the World Health Organization in 2003, the annual global market for herbal medicines is reported to be worth US$60 billion and by 2012 the global industry in Traditional Chinese Medicine (TCM) alone was reported to be worth US$83 billion [12].

However, human surviving and development of new drugs is as a result of existence of medicinal and aromatic plants. Sustaining the plant species and conservation of genetic resources is the most priority role of human changing with the circumstances of earth. Climate change already causes a serious state for plants throughout the world. A research group assessed late twenty-first century distributions for 1350 European plants species under seven climate change scenarios. As a result, more than half of the species could be vulnerable or threatened by 2080 [14]. As is generally known, some countermeasures against climate change need an enduring cooperative effort from national and international interdisciplinary researchers.

5. Conclusions

Medicinal and aromatic plants still have unknown and uncountable potential, though there is a long history for use since prehistoric times. To loose genetic resources leads a weighty loss in the future; therefore, the coexistence balance among plants, animal, and human should not be upset. The role of medicinal and aromatic plants is changing continuously in accord to a period and the role expands such as cure of disease to prevention of disease. The accumulated massive knowledge, information, and materials should be shared in the whole world and go down to generation to generation. The blessings of medicinal and aromatic plants are treasures that belong to all lives.

Author details

Maiko Inoue[1*], Shinichiro Hayashi[2] and Lyle E. Craker[3]

1 Specified Nonprofit Corporation of Horticulture Therapy and Zen, Hamamatsu, Japan

2 GREEN FLASK Inc., Tokyo, Japan

3 University of Massachusetts, Amherst, MA, USA

*Address all correspondence to: den8mai@yahoo.co.jp

References

[1] Silk Road. Wikipedia [Internet]. 2018. Available from: https://en.wikipedia.org/wiki/Silk_Road [Accessed: October 25, 2018]

[2] Sashida Y. Partner Pharmacognosy (in Japanese). Tokyo: Nankodo; 2007. 394 p. ISBN-10: 4524402241

[3] Inoue M, Craker L. Medicinal and aromatic plants-uses and functions. In: Dixon G, Aldous D, editors. Horticulture: Plants for People and Places. Vol. 2. Dordrecht: Springer; 2014. pp. 645-669. DOI: 10.1007/978-94-017-8581-5

[4] Ibrahim V. Cannabis (Marijuana-Hemp) in Ancient Egypt [Internet]. 2017. Available from: https://www.researchgate.net/profile/Venice_Attia/publication/321420351_Cannabis_marijuana-_hemp_in_Ancient_Egypt/links/5a212c49aca272ab5a623bef/Cannabis-marijuana-hemp-in-Ancient-Egypt [Accessed: September 11, 2018]

[5] Drug Enforcement Administration Museum. Cannabis, Coca, & Poppy: Nature's Addictive Plants [Internet]. Available from: https://www.deamuseum.org/ccp/opium/history.html [Accessed: September 11, 2018]

[6] Farnsworth NR, Soejarto DD. Global importance of medicinal plants. In: Akereb O, Heywood V, Synge H, editors. Conservation of Medicinal Plants. Cambridge: Cambridge University Press; 1991

[7] Tyler V. Herbs affecting the central nervous system. In: Janick J, editor. Perspectives on New Crops and New Uses. Alexandria: ASHS Press; 1999. pp. 442-449

[8] Robinson T. The biochemical pharmacology of plant alkaloids. In: Craker L, Simon J, editors. Herbs, Spices, & Medicinal Plants. Vol. 1. Phoenix: Oryx Press; 1986. pp. 135-166

[9] Taylor L. Plant Based Drugs and Medicines [Internet]. 2000. Available from: http://www.rain-tree.com/plantdrugs.htm#.W6T0x2hKjIU [Accessed: September 21, 2018]

[10] U.S. Department of Commerce International Trade Administration Industry & Analysis. 2016 Top Markets Report Pharmaceuticals. 2016 ITA Pharmaceuticals Top Markets Report. Available from: https://www.trade.gov/topmarkets/pdf/Pharmaceuticals_Executive_Summary.pdf [Accessed: September 17, 2018]

[11] Pengelly A. The Constituents of Medicinal Plants: An Introduction to the Chemistry and Therapeutics of Herbal Medicine. 2nd ed. Wallingford: CABI; 2004. 184 p. ISBN-10: 0851998070

[12] Allkin B. Useful plants–medicines. At least 28,187 plant species are currently recorded as being of medicinal use. In: Willis KJ, editor. Royal Botanic Gardens, Kew. London: Royal Botanic Gardens, Kew; 2017. pp. 22-29. NBK464488

[13] Pan SY, Zhou SF, Gao SH, Yu ZL, Zhang SF, Tang MT, et al. New perspectives on how to discover drugs from herbal medicines: CAM's outstanding contribution to modern therapeutics. Evidence-Based Complementary and Alternative Medicine. Vol. 2013. Hindawi Publishing Corporation; 2013. p. 25. Article ID 627375. http://dx.doi.org/10.1155/2013/627375

[14] Thuiller W, Lavorel S, Araújo M, Sykes M, Prentice C. Climate change threats to plant diversity in Europe. PNAS. 2005;**102**(23):8245-8250. DOI: 10.1073/pnas.0409902102

Chapter 3

Medicinal Plants of the Peruvian Amazon: Bioactive Phytochemicals, Mechanisms of Action, and Biosynthetic Pathways

Juan Carlos Castro, Joseph Dylan Maddox, Marianela Cobos, Jae Diana Paredes, Anthony Jhoao Fasabi, Gabriel Vargas-Arana, Jorge Luis Marapara, Pedro Marcelino Adrianzen, María Zadith Casuso and Segundo Levi Estela

Abstract

The objective of this book chapter is to provide consolidated and updated scientific information about the medicinal plants of the Peruvian Amazon, which has a great richness of plants; many of these are used in folkloric medicine to treat several diseases. Recently, investigations have reported that these medicinal plants possess bioactive phytochemicals against several diseases such as diabetes, cancer, inflammation, infectious diseases, and several other health problems, thus corroborating some ethnopharmacological reports. The mechanism of action for selected bioactive phytochemicals was demonstrated at the molecular level as well as the metabolic pathways involved in their biosynthesis were described. Due to the large gap in scientific information revealed in this review, we formulated a series of strategies to close these scientific knowledge gaps and achieve a sustainable exploitation of medicinal plants in the Peruvian Amazon.

Keywords: cancer, diabetes, ethnopharmacological survey, folkloric medicine

1. Introduction

Peru is cataloged as a megadiverse country due to its great diversity of species, particularly in plants [1, 2]. This diversity is attributed to the large number of eco-regions present in our territory [3], which were originated by their particular geologic evolution [4]. The Peruvian Amazon includes a large proportion of this richness in plant species, and several are endemic to this region [5, 6]. The diversity, however, remains underestimated because until now a complete and updated inventory of plant species is lacking, but some estimates suggest that more than 50% of plant species are unknown to science [7, 8].

Similarly, there are many gaps in the scientific knowledge of medicinal plants of the Peruvian Amazon. These gaps are evident at various knowledge levels from the inventory of medicinal plants and their taxonomic identification, the bioactive phytochemicals produced, the mechanisms of action of the bioactive phytochemicals, and the metabolic pathways involved in the biosynthesis of bioactive phytochemicals. In part, these gaps in the scientific knowledge can be attributed to several factors: (1) the ethnopharmaceutical information has been obtained from few ethnic groups (probably <10%); (2) the majority of ethnopharmaceutical surveys have been focused on plant species to treat protozoal diseases, with particular emphasis on malaria and leishmania [9–12]; and (3) the research centers in the Peruvian Amazon generally lack trained scientist, laboratory equipment, and standard methods to perform bioassays for the discovery of bioactive phytochemicals against diabetes, inflammation, hypertension, cancer, infectious diseases (viral, bacterial, and fungal), and other health problems. Consequently, it is fundamental to implement strategies to surpass these limitations and to close these large knowledge gaps.

Parts of the problems mentioned are addressed in this book chapter that consists of six topics. The first topic "The diversity of plants in the Peruvian Amazon" describes the diversity of species reported for the country and the Peruvian Amazon and are mentioned the possible factors involved in light of current knowledge. The second topic "Medicinal plants and indigenous people in the Peruvian Amazon" highlights information about medicinal plants and ethnic groups. Relevant information of the recently elaborated partial database of medicinal plants is also discussed. The third topic "Some bioactive phytochemicals identified in medicinal plants" presents structures of bioactive phytochemicals against cancer, inflammation, diarrhea, malaria, and diabetes. The fourth topic "Mechanism of action of select bioactive phytochemicals" explains the molecular bases of the mechanisms of action of well-characterized phytochemicals such as taspine, crofelemer, mitraphylline, quercetin, linalool, and bixin. The fifth topic "Biosynthetic pathways for relevant bioactive phytochemicals" describes and provides graphically key metabolic pathways involved in the biosynthesis of quercetin, linalool, and bixin. The final topic "Strategies for the sustainable use of medicinal plants" recommends the adoption of strategies to accelerate the generation of scientific knowledge that permits a sustainable exploitation of the medicinal plants in the Peruvian Amazon.

2. The diversity of plants in the Peruvian Amazon

The plant diversity in the Amazonian lowland rain forest is astounding. This diversity was recently demonstrated with a large-scale taxonomic inventory, which identified 14,003 species; 1788 genera; and 188 families of seed plants, in which 50% of these species can reach ≥10 cm stem diameter at breast height (DBH). More than 52% of seed plant species diversity in this region include shrubs, small trees, lianas, vines, and herbs [1]. The Peruvian Amazon includes ~39% (5401 species) of these species. Also, a previous study showed that a forest near to Iquitos is the most species-rich in the world, with ~300 species ≥10 cm in DBH [2]. In addition, it is estimated that ~17,143 plant species are circumscribed within the national boundaries [13], and approximately 13% of these plant species are endemic to the Peruvian Amazon [5, 6]. It is speculated, however, that only 60% of the Peruvian flora has been identified [7]. Consequently, Peru is considered to be one of the 17 megadiverse countries, a global center for species richness of plants and other organisms [14]. This peculiarity is attributed to the most Holdridge life zones (containing 84 of the 107 eco-regions of the world) that possess our country [3], which was determined for their particular geologic evolution [4].

3. Medicinal plants and indigenous people in the Peruvian Amazon

The Amazon lowland rain forest provides multiple benefits to its inhabitants [15]. According to Schultes [16], rain forests have an incalculable value as an untapped emporium of germplasm for new commercial plants. For example, to the inhabitants of Mishana (a community near Iquitos), the tropical forest provides timber resources (e.g., sawlogs and pulpwood) and several forest products such as edible fruits, oils, latex, fiber, and medicines. The yield of these forest products is provided by 72 species (26.2%) that are sold in the Iquitos market [17]. In addition, it is estimated that ~4400 native plant species of the Peruvian flora are used by inhabitants for 49 different applications [18]. With reference to bioactive plants, it was reported that more than 1300 species are used by natives in the northwest Amazon as medicines, poisons, or narcotics [16]. To date, however, the list of medicinal plants useful for the discovery and development

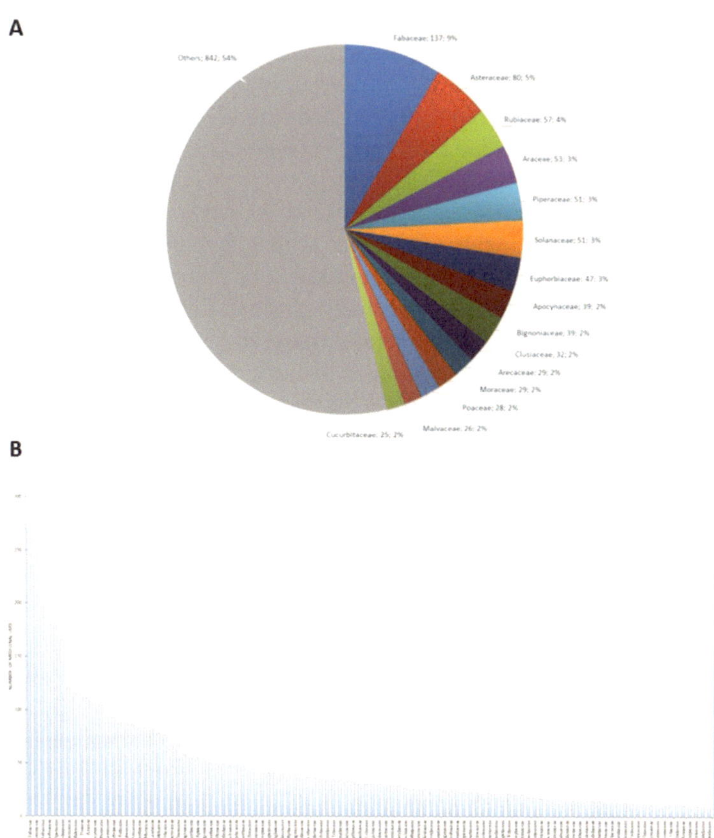

Figure 1.
Families of medicinal plants (A) and number of their uses (B) to treat diseases in the Peruvian Amazon.

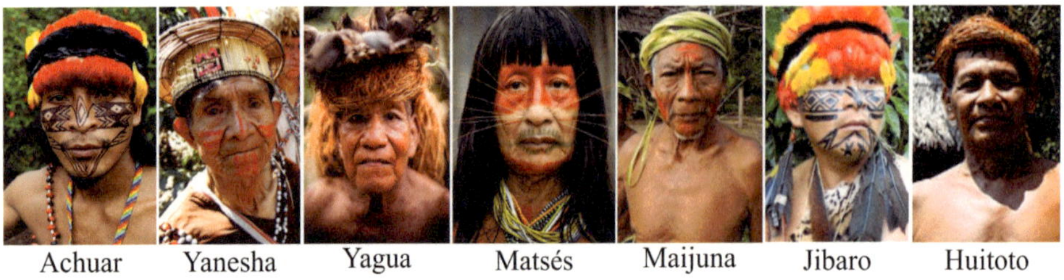

Figure 2.
Selected ethnic groups from the Peruvian Amazon.

of drugs is fragmentary and incomplete, because the ethnopharmacological surveys conducted in the Peruvian Amazon are sporadic and scarce. Recently, we elaborated a partial database of medicinal plants of the Peruvian Amazon, which is based on the few available ethnobotanical studies [9–12, 19–25], one list of the Research Institute of The Peruvian Amazon (IIAP) and surveys carried out by our research group in the *Pasaje Paquito* (the main center for commercialization of medicinal plants in the Loreto region, Iquitos). The medicinal plant database includes 1410 species belonging to 157 plant families; these taxonomic assignations were verified with the Plant List database (http://www.theplantlist.org/). Of these, the top 10 families by number of medicinal plant species are Fabaceae (137), Asteraceae (80), Rubiaceae (57), Araceae (53), Piperaceae (51), Solanaceae (51), Euphorbiaceae (47), Apocynaceae (39), Bignoniaceae (39), and Clusiaceae (32). In addition, this database reveals that the plant families with the highest number of medicinal uses are Fabaceae (272), Asteraceae (244), Rubiaceae (197), Euphorbiaceae (180), Piperaceae (179), and Solanaceae with 166 medicinal uses (**Figure 1**).

It is paradoxical that only some ethnic groups were evaluated to date for ethnopharmacological surveys, given the Peruvian Amazon's ethnic diversity (**Figure 2**). According to a recent national census, the indigenous population of the Peruvian Amazon consists of 332,975 inhabitants that include 13 linguistic families that are grouped into 51 ethnic groups. Of the total number of communities registered, 21 are polyethnic [26, 27]. In all these ethnic groups, the millenary knowledge of medicinal plants used to combat common diseases is a fundamental component within the indigenous health systems, which has been maintained from generation to generation. However, due to the transculturation by modernization and globalization, this ancestral knowledge is being lost [15]. Consequently, it is necessary to implement strategies to preserve this invaluable knowledge for the benefit of humankind.

4. Some bioactive phytochemicals identified in medicinal plants

Presently, the list of medicinal plants of the Peruvian Amazon is partial; in consequence, only for the most known plants were identified a few bioactive phytochemicals (**Figure 3**). There is no way to estimate how many new biochemical structures, probably of great value to humankind, remain undiscovered in the Peruvian Amazon. Some of the phytochemicals isolated and with corroborated bioactivity against cancer [28], inflammation [29], diarrhea [30], malaria [31], diabetes [32], and several other diseases were determined [33].

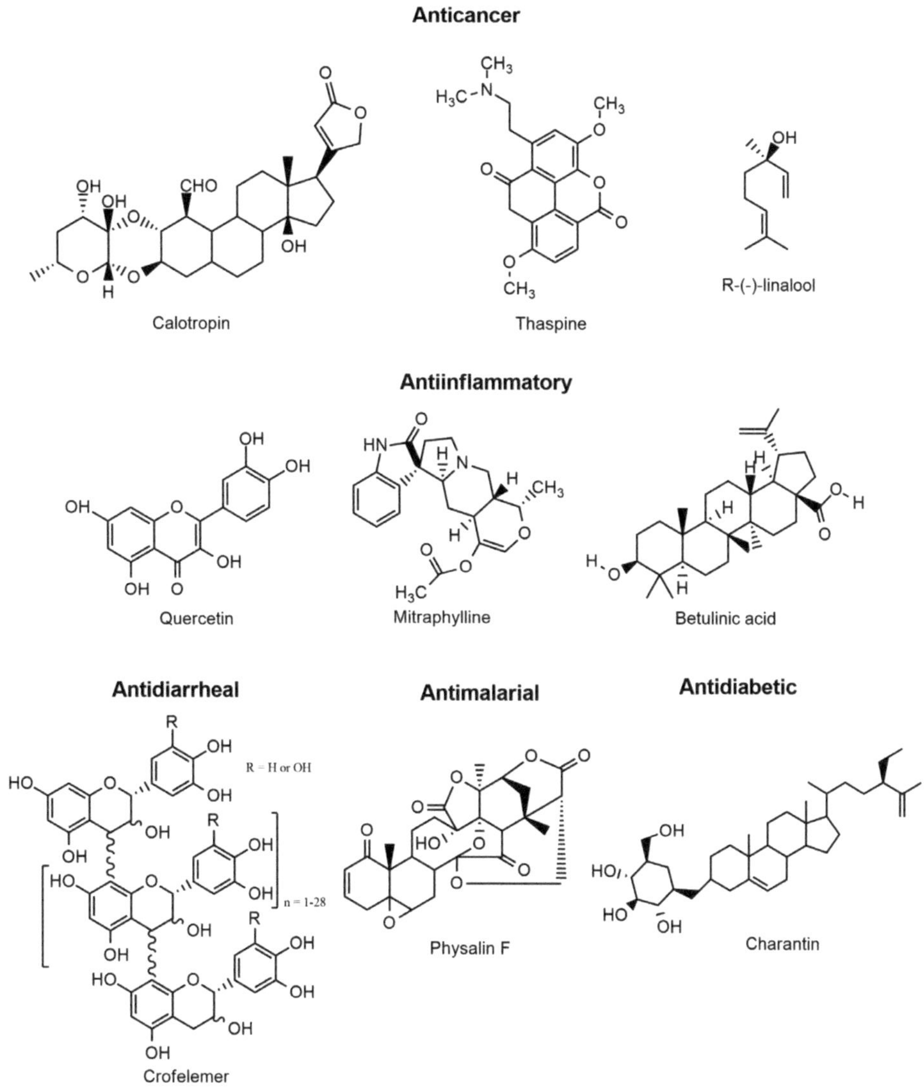

Figure 3.
A small selection of bioactive phytochemicals identified in medicinal plants of the Peruvian Amazon.

5. Mechanism of action of select bioactive phytochemicals

5.1 Bixin

Bixin constitutes the main pigment of the industrial annatto obtained from the seed coat of *Bixa orellana* [34]. This phytochemical belongs to the relatively small family of apocarotenoids; it was the first cis-carotenoid to be isolated from natural sources [35]. However, it was not until 1961 that its chemical structure and stereochemistry were determined through nuclear magnetic resonance spectroscopy studies [36].

This phytochemical compound shows pleiotropic bioactivities with health-promoting properties. It was recently demonstrated that bixin caused arrest of Hep3B cell line at G2/M checkpoint of the cell cycle and the molecular mechanism of action was demonstrated by a modeling study, which was based in the favorable binding of bixin to domains of Bax BH3 and FasL proteins [37]. Consequently, bixin should be used for developing agents to combat human hepatocellular carcinoma. Bixin is also a potent activator of the transcription factor nuclear factor erythroid 2-related factor 2 (NRF2), which is the master regulator of the cellular antioxidant response protecting the skin against various environmental stressors including UV radiation and electrophilic pollutants [38–40]. The protective effects against solar UV-induced skin damage are due to the NRF2-dependence of bixin-induced antioxidant and anti-inflammatory effects [39]. In addition, bixin displays molecular activities as antioxidant, excited-state quencher, peroxisome proliferator-activated receptor α/γ agonist, and Toll-like receptor 4/nuclear factor kappa-light-chain-enhancer of activated B-cell antagonist. Together, these bioactivities may be important to the improvement of skin barrier function and environmental stress protection [40].

5.2 Crofelemer

Crofelemer previously known as SP-303 is a large proanthocyanidin oligomer isolated from the bark latex of the plant *Croton lechleri* Müll. Arg. [41]. Initial studies have demonstrated the immense antiviral activity of crofelemer against a gamma of DNA and RNA viruses such as respiratory syncytial virus, influenza A virus, parainfluenza virus, herpesvirus types 1 and 2, and hepatitis A and B viruses. The antiviral mechanism implies the direct interaction of crofelemer to components of the viral envelope, blocking both the viral attachment and the cell invasion [41]. More recently, crofelemer is used as a first-in-class antidiarrheal medication, and its efficacy has been investigated *in vivo* assays [42] and in patients with HIV-associated diarrhea, diarrhea of various infectious etiologies, as well as diarrhea-predominant irritable bowel syndrome [43]. Crofelemer was recently approved by the FDA to treat diarrhea in HIV/AIDS patients on antiretroviral therapy [44].

The mechanism of action as antidiarrheal of this proanthocyanidin oligomer consists in the dual inhibitory action on two structurally unrelated prosecretory intestinal Cl– channels, which are responsible for chloride secretion and subsequent luminal hydration. The first target is an extracellular site of the cystic fibrosis transmembrane regulator (CFTR) Cl- channel (~60%, IC50 ~ 7 μM), which produces a voltage-independent block with stabilization of the channel closed state. The second target is the intestinal calcium-activated Cl- channel (CaCC) by a voltage-independent inhibition mechanism (>90%, IC50 ~ 6.5 μM) [45].

5.3 Linalool

An abundant (~90%) essential oil of the leaves of *Aniba rosaeodora* [46, 47] that is used in the traditional medicine of the Peruvian and Brazilian Amazon for its effects on the central nervous system, such as sedative, anticonvulsant, and antidepressant [19, 47, 48]. Additionally, linalool has anti-inflammatory [49], anticancer [50–52], antihyperlipidemic, antinociceptive, analgesic, anxiolytic, and neuroprotective properties [53]. Several studies have demonstrated a gamma of anti-infectious activity like antiviral [54], antibacterial [55–57], antifungal [58, 59], and antileishmanial [55, 60, 61].

The anticancer mechanisms of action of linalool in hepatocellular carcinoma (HCC) HepG2 cells were recently revealed by Rodenak-Kladniew et al. [50] (**Figure 4**). According to these researchers, linalool in a dose-dependently blocked cell proliferation by inducing G0/G1 cell cycle arrest, through Cdk4 and cyclin A downregulation, p21 and p27 upregulation, and apoptosis, characterized by

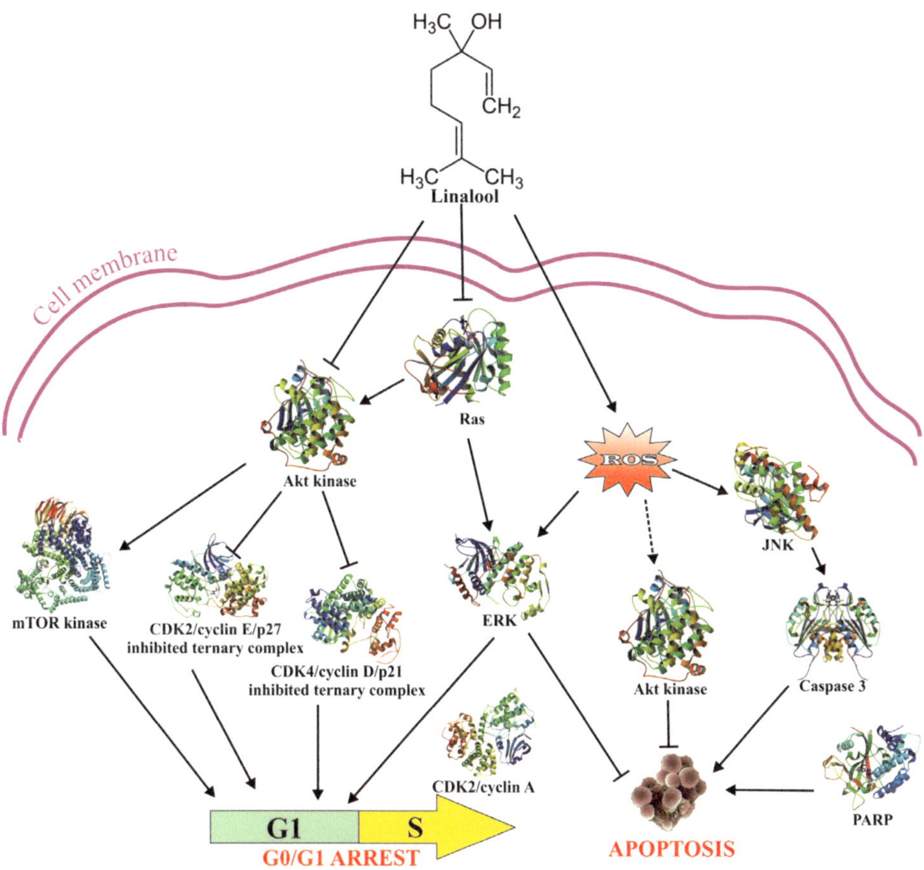

Figure 4.
Anticancer mechanisms of action of linalool in hepatocellular carcinoma (HCC) HepG2 cells.

mitochondrial membrane potential loss, caspase-3 activation, poly(ADP-ribose) polymerase cleavage, and DNA fragmentation

5.4 Mitraphylline

A pentacyclic oxindolic alkaloid that was isolated from the alkaloid fraction of the dried inner bark of *Uncaria tomentosa* (Willd. ex Schult.) DC; it represents the most abundant phytochemical (40%) of the alkaloid fraction [62]. Several investigations have demonstrated the immunoregulatory activity of this compound or the pentacyclic oxindolic alkaloid-enriched fraction [63–67].

The mechanism of action as immunoregulator of mitraphylline consists in both to protect cells against oxidative stress and to elicit a response via an NF-kβ-dependent mechanism. The first mechanism is based on the inhibition of the inducible nitric oxide synthase gene expression; consequently, nitrite formation and programmed cell death are avoided. Finally, in the second mechanism, the inhibition of NF-kβ signaling permits the abrogation of the release of pro-inflammatory cytokines such as TNFα, IL-6, IL-1 α, IL-1β, IL-4, IL-17, and IFN-α [63–67].

5.5 Quercetin

A polyphenol categorized as a flavonol, one of the five subclasses of flavonoid compounds. This bioactive phytochemical is biosynthesized and accumulated in tissues and organs of several medicinal plants of the Peruvian Amazon such as *Annona montana*, *Bauhinia longifolia*, *Bertholletia excelsa*, *Genipa americana*, *Inga edulis*, *Mauritia flexuosa*, *Myrciaria dubia*, *Oenocarpus bataua*, *Solanum sessiliflorum*, *Theobroma bicolor*, *T. cacao*, and *T. grandiflorum* [68–70]. Quercetin exhibits multifaceted therapeutic applications for multiplicity of unrelated acute and chronic human ailments like allergy, arthritis, asthma, bacterial and viral infections, cancer, cardiovascular diseases, inflammation, obesity, diabetes, mood disorders, neuropathologies, and other health problems [71–76].

This multiple health beneficial properties of quercetin are attributed to their particular mechanism of action based on inhibition of several key proteins and enzymes (**Figure 5**). For example, a recent research showed that this compound is a potent inhibitor of 25 human serine/threonine kinases [77]. The multitarget inhibitor explains its beneficial pleiotropic effects on humans. This flavonoid-type inhibitor is effective against xanthine oxidase, appropriate for the treatment of hyperuricemia, gout, and inflammatory disease states. The inhibitory mechanism is based on the favorable steric complementarity of the conjugated three-ring structure of quercetin with the active site of xanthine oxidase. The enzyme-quercetin binary complex is stabilized by van der Waals forces and hydrogen-bonding interactions with both binding and catalytic amino acid residues, respectively [78, 79]. Recently, Hamilton et al. [80] have demonstrated that quercetin is a competitive inhibitor of glucose uptake by GLUT1. These researchers showed that the inhibitory effect is simply by binding of quercetin to the surface of GLUT1 [80]. Finally, several structural studies by X-ray diffraction have corroborated the inhibitory complex of quercetin with several human protein kinases [81–83].

5.6 Taspine

An alkaloid isolated for the first time by Vaisberg et al. [84] from the bark latex of the plant species *Croton lechleri* Müll. Arg. Previous *in vitro* and *in vivo* investigations have demonstrated that taspine promotes early phases of wound healing in a dose-dependent manner [84, 85]. Taspine was also demonstrated to activate the pro-apoptotic cascade, which oligomerizes Bak/Bax into pores that result in the release of cytochrome c and consequently apoptosis in HCT116 colon carcinoma cells [86]. Similar results were reported for an *in vivo* study conducted with ZR-75-30 human breast cancer xenografts in athymic mice [87].

The mechanism of action of taspine as a topoisomerase inhibitor was revealed recently. Initially, using *in vitro* assays, Fayad et al. [86] observed the inhibition of both topoisomerases I and II by taspine. Castelli et al. [88] corroborated the

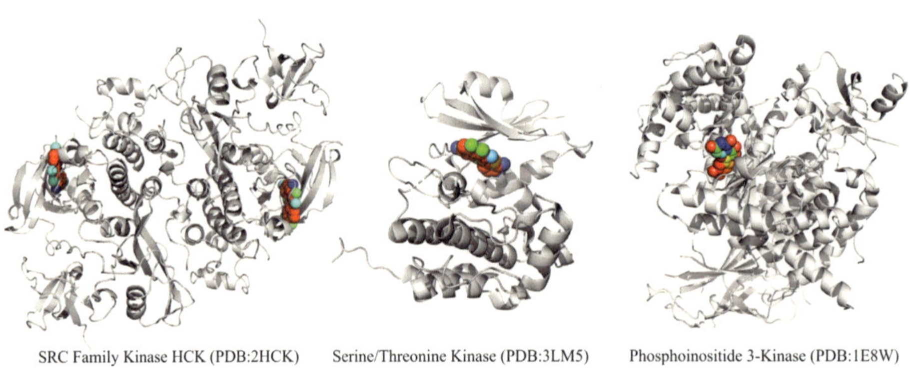

Figure 5.
Inhibitory complex of quercetin with selected human kinase targets.

inhibitory action of taspine on purified topoisomerase I and provided the molecular details of the inhibitory action. These researchers showed that taspine inhibits the catalytic process (cleavage and religation), and molecular docking simulations showed that the formation of the complex enzyme-taspine is accomplished by the interaction in the proximity of the active site preventing the cleavage reaction. While, that the religation inhibition is explained by DNA intercalation of the inhibitor with the enzyme-DNA-binary complex.

6. Biosynthetic pathways for relevant bioactive phytochemicals

6.1 Bixin biosynthesis

The biosynthesis of the apocarotenoid ester bixin from lycopene requires four enzymatic reactions (**Figure 6**). The first enzymatic reaction of bixin biosynthesis is the 5-6/5′-6′ oxidative cleavage of lycopene catalyzed by lycopene cleavage oxygenase to produce two sulcatone and one bixin aldehyde molecule. The second enzymatic reaction is the oxidative conversion of aldehyde into carboxylic acid groups in bixin aldehyde to produce norbixin by bixin aldehyde dehydrogenase. The third enzymatic reaction is the methylation of one norbixin carboxyl group to produce bixin by norbixin methyltransferase. This enzyme utilizes *S*-adenosyl-L-methionine as a methyl-group donor. Finally, the last biochemical reaction is the methylation of one bixin carboxyl group to produce bixin dimethyl ester by bixin methyltransferase, using *S*-adenosyl-L-methionine as methyl-group donor [89–91].

6.2 Linalool biosynthesis

The fundamental building blocks in plants for terpenoid production, i.e., isopentenyl diphosphate (IPP) and dimethylallyl diphosphate (DMAPP), are generated via two independent pathways, namely, 2-C-methyl-D-erythritol 4-phosphate (MEP) pathway and the mevalonate acid (MVA) pathway [92, 93]. The plastid terpenes are formed exclusively via the MEP pathway; however, sterols are biosynthesized via MVA pathway in the cytoplasm and mitochondria [94, 95]. Radiolabeling studies in the early 1970s showed that in *Cinnamomum camphora* the biosynthesis of linalool is accomplished via the MVA pathway [96]. Nevertheless, recent transcriptome analysis of leaves in two chemotypes of *C. camphora* showed that both pathways provide the biosynthetic precursors IPP and DMAPP for the main monoterpenes (i.e., linalool and borneol) synthesis [97]. The balance of IPP/DMAPP is controlled by type 1 and type 2 isopentenyl diphosphate:dimethylallyl diphosphate isomerase, which reversibly converts IPP to DMAPP [98, 99]. Further, IPP and DMAPP are condensed by geranyl diphosphate synthase and isopentenyl diphosphate to produce geranyl diphosphate by geranyl diphosphate synthase. Finally, geranyl diphosphate is transformed in linalool by the action of linalool synthase (**Figure 7**).

6.3 Quercetin biosynthesis

A bioactive phytochemical that is biosynthesized through the phenylpropanoid pathway [100]. The initial reactions transform phenylalanine into 4-coumaroyl-CoA, which enters into the flavonoid biosynthesis pathway (**Figure 8**). The first committed enzyme in the flavonoid pathway, chalcone synthase, uses malonyl-CoA and 4-coumaroyl-CoA as substrates to produce naringenin chalcone. This metabolic

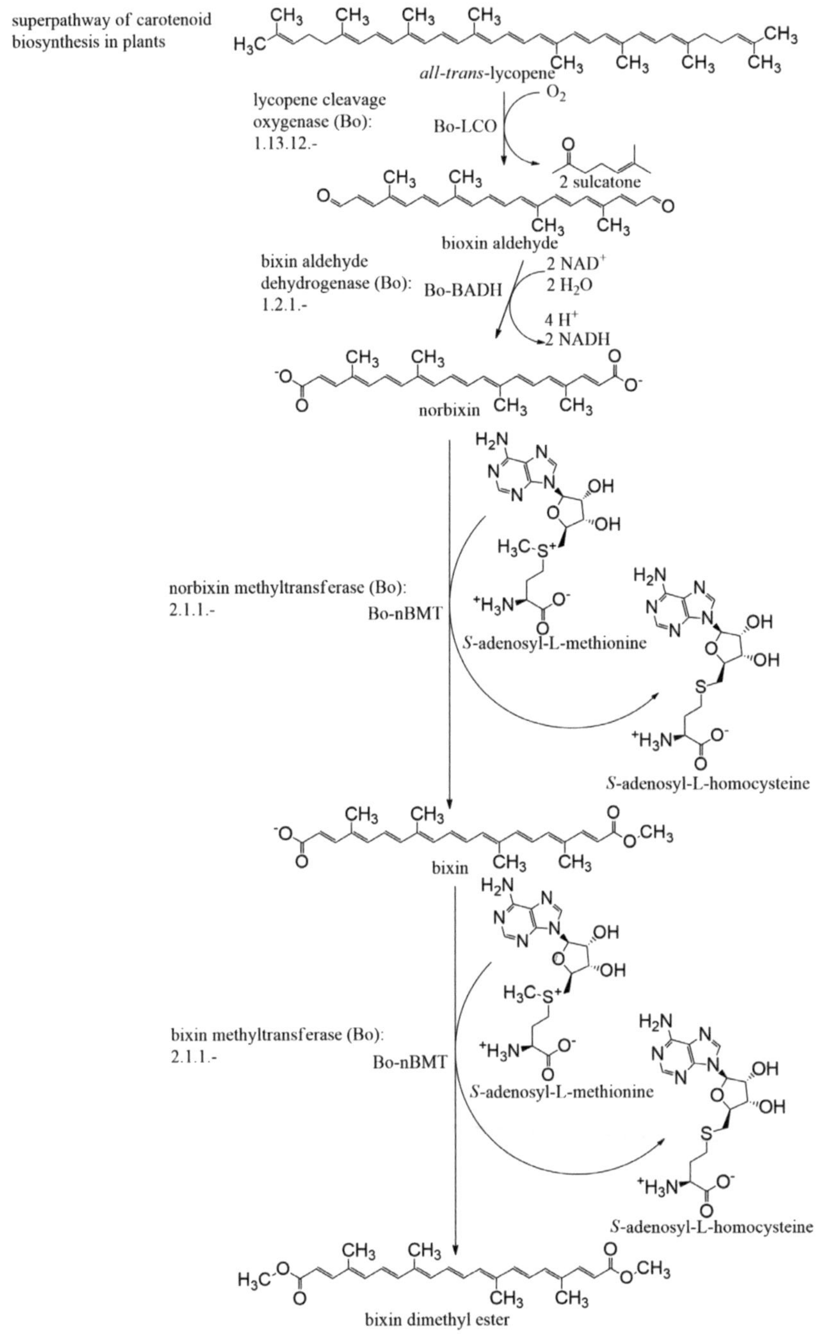

Figure 6.
Biosynthetic pathway for bixin.

intermediary is converted to (+)-dihydrokaempferol by the action of two enzymes, one isomerase and one dioxygenase, respectively. Next, (+)-dihydrokaempferol quercetin is biosynthesized by two alternative and consecutive enzymatic reactions: first, enzymes (+)-dihydrokaempferol 3′-hydroxylase and quercetin synthase produce (+)-taxifolin as a metabolic intermediary, and, second, enzymes dihydrokaempferol synthase and kaempferol monooxygenase produce kaempferol as a metabolic intermediary [101].

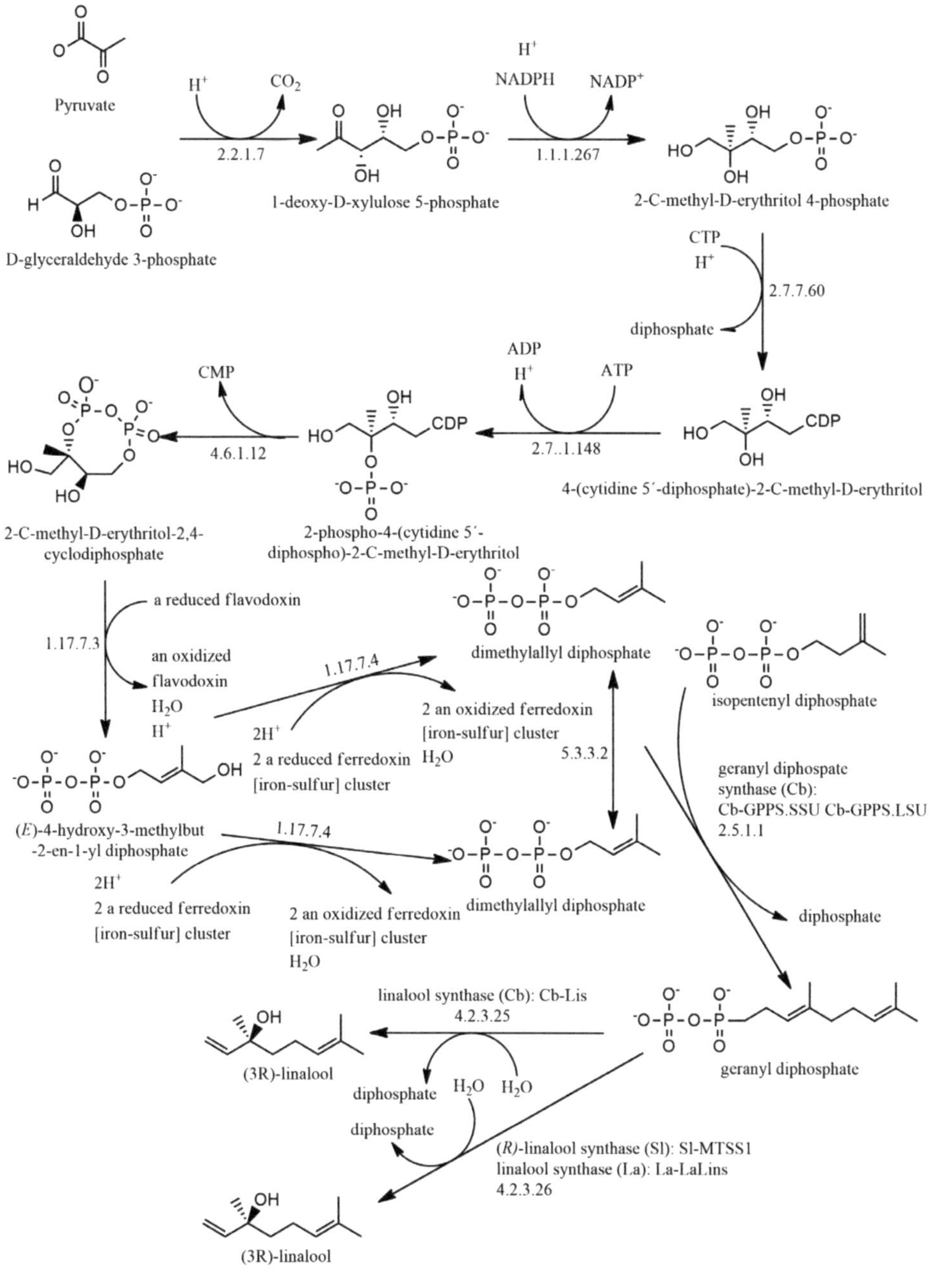

Figure 7.
Biosynthetic pathway for linalool through the MEP pathway.

7. Strategies for the sustainable use of medicinal plants

To date, the research contributions of the Peruvian Amazon to ethnopharmacology have been very limited, and data are still fragmentary and dispersed. Consequently, to ensure a sustainable economic development, we need to obtain a competitive advantage based on our medicinal plant resources. To achieve these goals, we must formulate appropriate strategies based on solid scientific knowledge. First, we need to record the millenary knowledge of folk medicine practiced by the total ethnic groups of the Peruvian Amazon. Second, based on this information, we

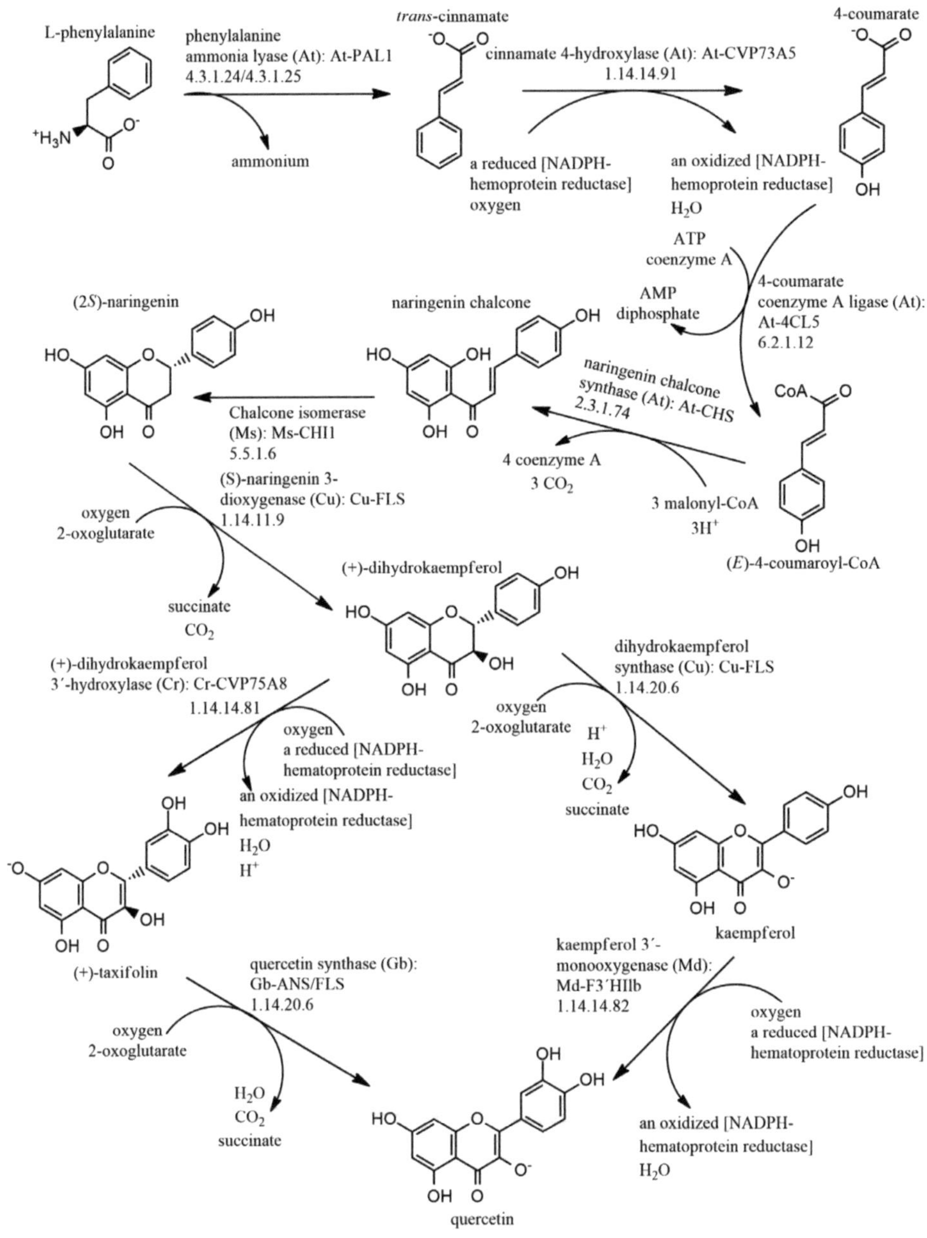

Figure 8.
Biosynthetic pathway for quercetin.

should construct a complete catalog of known medicinal plants with correct taxonomic identifications. Third, an enriched germplasm bank of medicinal plants should be established with accessions of several sites of the Peruvian Amazon. Fourth, the bioactivity of extracts/bio-guided isolated and purified phytochemicals with a battery of *in vitro* and *in vivo* standardized bioassays against multiple diseases (e.g., diabetes, cancer, bacterial infections, etc.) should be established. Fifth, multiomics approaches such as genomics, transcriptomics, proteomics, and metabolomics should be performed to identify key genes, enzymes, and metabolic pathways responsible for the biosynthesis of promising bioactive phytochemicals. Sixth, in the short term, a web-based computerized database to facilitate storage, management, transfer and exchange, and analysis of the data by researchers, planners, and other interested users should be developed and made freely available. Finally, the availability of this basic scientific information could support the development of genetic improvement programs for medicinal plants and allow a boost of biotechnological applications, based on synthetic biology tools and using bacterial, microalgal, and several other cell-/tissue-based platforms for the production of phytochemical compounds of interest, thus preventing overexploitation and species extinction of medicinal plants.

8. Conclusions

The Peruvian Amazon houses multiple medicinal plants, but the species catalog is still incomplete, because ethnopharmaceutical studies are lacking in the great majority of ethnic groups. A select number of medicinal plant species, however, have been identified as a potentially useful source of bioactive phytochemical compounds to treat various diseases such as diabetes, cancer, inflammation, and infections caused by pathogens, among other health problems. Also, for some of these bioactive phytochemical compounds, the mechanisms of action are known, which are characterized by presenting a common pattern, their pleiotropic effects, which is attributable to act on multiple targets, consequently, affecting various cellular processes. In relation to the metabolic pathways responsible for biosynthesis of these molecules, only very few are known, but for the vast majority of phytochemicals, it remains a great mystery that needs to be clarified. Therefore, we formulated a series of strategies to close these scientific knowledge gaps and achieve a sustainable exploitation of medicinal plants in the Peruvian Amazon.

Acknowledgements

This research was supported by grants from Universidad Nacional de la Amazonía Peruana (UNAP). We also thank and especially dedicate this chapter book to Janeth Braga Vela, who is a great professor and guide and an exceptional and inspiring woman.

Conflict of interest

The authors declare no conflict of interest.

Author details

Juan Carlos Castro[1*], Joseph Dylan Maddox[2,3], Marianela Cobos[4], Jae Diana Paredes[4], Anthony Jhoao Fasabi[1], Gabriel Vargas-Arana[5,6], Jorge Luis Marapara[1], Pedro Marcelino Adrianzen[1], María Zadith Casuso[4] and Segundo Levi Estela[4]

1 Specialized Unit of Biotechnology, Research Center of Natural Resources of the Amazon (CIRNA), National University of the Peruvian Amazon (UNAP), Iquitos, Peru

2 Pritzker Laboratory for Molecular Systematics and Evolution, The Field Museum of Natural History, Chicago, IL, USA

3 Environmental Sciences, American Public University System, Charles Town, WV, USA

4 Laboratory of Biotechnology and Bioenergetics, Scientific University of Peru (UCP), Iquitos, Peru

5 Laboratory of Natural Products Chemistry, Research Institute of the Peruvian Amazon (IIAP), Iquitos, Peru

6 Peruvian University of the East (UPO), Iquitos, Peru

*Address all correspondence to: juan.castro@unapiquitos.edu.pe

References

[1] Cardoso D, Särkinen T, Alexander S, Amorim AM, Bittrich V, Celis M, et al. Amazon plant diversity revealed by a taxonomically verified species list. Proceedings of the National Academy of Sciences of the United States of America. 2017;**114**:10695-10700. DOI: 10.1073/pnas.1706756114

[2] Gentry AH. Tree species richness of upper Amazonian forests. Proceedings of the National Academy of Sciences of the United States of America. 1988;**85**:156-159. DOI: 10.1073/pnas.85.1.156

[3] Holdridge LR. Life Zone Ecology. Costa Rica. Tropical Science Center; 1967. 206 p

[4] Hoorn C, Wesselingh FP, ter Steege H, Bermudez MA, Mora A, Sevink J, et al. Amazonia through time: Andean uplift, climate change, landscape evolution, and biodiversity. Science. 2010;**330**:927-931. DOI: 10.1126/science.1194585

[5] Rodríguez LO, Young KR. Biological diversity of Peru: Determining priority areas for conservation. Ambio: A Journal of the Human Environment. 2000;**29**:329-337. DOI: 10.1579/0044-7447-29.6.329

[6] van der Werff H, Consiglio T. Distribution and conservation significance of endemic species of flowering plants in Peru. Biodiversity and Conservation. 2004;**13**:1699-1713. DOI: 10.1023/B:BIOC.0000029334.69717.f0

[7] Brack A. Perú: Biodiversidad, pobreza y bionegocios. Lima, Perú: Programa de las Naciones Unidas para el Desarrollo; 2004

[8] Joppa LN, Roberts DL, Myers N, Pimm SL. Biodiversity hotspots house most undiscovered plant species. Proceedings of the National Academy of Sciences of the United States of America. 2011;**108**:13171-13176. DOI: 10.1073/pnas.1109389108

[9] Céline V, Adriana P, Eric D, Joaquina A, Yannick E, Augusto LF, et al. Medicinal plants from the Yanesha (Peru): Evaluation of the leishmanicidal and antimalarial activity of selected extracts. Journal of Ethnopharmacology. 2009;**123**:413-422. DOI: 10.1016/j.jep.2009.03.041

[10] Ruiz L, Ruiz L, Maco M, Cobos M, Gutierrez-Choquevilca A-L, Roumy V. Plants used by native Amazonian groups from the Nanay River (Peru) for the treatment of malaria. Journal of Ethnopharmacology. 2011;**133**:917-921. DOI: 10.1016/j.jep.2010.10.039

[11] Vásquez-Ocmín P, Cojean S, Rengifo E, Suyyagh-Albouz S, Amasifuen Guerra CA, Pomel S, et al. Antiprotozoal activity of medicinal plants used by Iquitos-Nauta road communities in Loreto (Peru). Journal of Ethnopharmacology. 2018;**210**:372-385. DOI: 10.1016/j.jep.2017.08.039

[12] Estevez Y, Castillo D, Pisango MT, Arevalo J, Rojas R, Alban J, et al. Evaluation of the leishmanicidal activity of plants used by Peruvian Chayahuita ethnic group. Journal of Ethnopharmacology. 2007;**114**:254-259. DOI: 10.1016/j.jep.2007.08.007

[13] Brako L, Zarucchi JL. Catalogue of the Flowering Plants and Gymnosperms of Peru. 6th ed. St. Louis, Mo: Missouri Botanical Garden; 1993. 1286 p

[14] Mittermeier RA, Mittermeier CG. Megadiversity: Earth's Biologically Wealthiest Nations. CEMEX; 1997. 501 p

[15] Bennett BC. Plants and people of the Amazonian rainforests. Bioscience. 1992;**42**:599-607. DOI: 10.2307/1311925

[16] Schultes RE. The Amazonia as a source of new economic plants. Economic Botany. 1979;**33**:259-266. DOI: 10.1007/BF02858251

[17] Peters CM, Gentry AH, Mendelsohn RO. Valuation of an Amazonian rainforest. Nature. 1989;**339**:655-656. DOI: 10.1038/339655a0

[18] Brack A. Diccionario enciclopédico de plantas útiles del Perú. Lima, Perú: Programa de las Naciones Unidas para el Desarrollo; 1999

[19] Mejía K, Rengifo E, Vila C. Plantas Medicinales de uso popular en la Amazonía Peruana. Iquitos, Perú: Agencia Española de Cooperación Internacional (AECI), Instituto de Investigaciones de la Amazonía Peruana; 2000

[20] Sanz-Biset J, Campos-de-la-Cruz J, Epiquién-Rivera MA, Cañigueral S. A first survey on the medicinal plants of the Chazuta valley (Peruvian Amazon). Journal of Ethnopharmacology. 2009;**122**:333-362. DOI: 10.1016/j.jep.2008.12.009

[21] Odonne G, Valadeau C, Alban-Castillo J, Stien D, Sauvain M, Bourdy G. Medical ethnobotany of the Chayahuita of the Paranapura basin (Peruvian Amazon). Journal of Ethnopharmacology. 2013;**146**:127-153. DOI: 10.1016/j.jep.2012.12.014

[22] Odonne G, Bourdy G, Castillo D, Estevez Y, Lancha-Tangoa A, Alban-Castillo J, et al. Ta'ta', Huayani: Perception of leishmaniasis and evaluation of medicinal plants used by the Chayahuita in Peru. Part II. Journal of Ethnopharmacology. 2009;**126**:149-158. DOI: 10.1016/j.jep.2009.07.015

[23] Valadeau C, Castillo JA, Sauvain M, Lores AF, Bourdy G. The rainbow hurts my skin: Medicinal concepts and plants uses among the Yanesha (Amuesha), an Amazonian Peruvian ethnic group. Journal of Ethnopharmacology. 2010;**127**:175-192. DOI: 10.1016/j.jep.2009.09.024

[24] Sanz-Biset J, Cañigueral S. Plants as medicinal stressors, the case of depurative practices in Chazuta valley (Peruvian Amazonia). Journal of Ethnopharmacology. 2013;**145**:67-76. DOI: 10.1016/j.jep.2012.09.053

[25] Rainer WB, Douglas S. Medicinal Plants of the Andes and the Amazon: The Magic and Medicinal Flora of Northern Peru. Trujillo, Perú: William L. Brown Center; 2015. 292 p

[26] ¿Qué es la BDPI? Base de Datos de Pueblos Indígenas u Originarios. Available from: http://bdpi.cultura.gob.pe/ [Accessed: October 23, 2018]

[27] Perú Instituto Nacional de Estadística e Informática. Available from: https://www.inei.gob.pe/ [Accessed: October 23, 2018]

[28] Wang S-C, Lu M-C, Chen H-L, Tseng H-I, Ke Y-Y, Wu Y-C, et al. Cytotoxicity of calotropin is through caspase activation and downregulation of anti-apoptotic proteins in K562 cells. Cell Biology International. 2009;**33**:1230-1236. DOI: 10.1016/j.cellbi.2009.08.013

[29] Junyuan Z, Hui X, Chunlan H, Junjie F, Qixiang M, Yingying L, et al. Quercetin protects against intestinal barrier disruption and inflammation in acute necrotizing pancreatitis through TLR4/MyD88/p38 MAPK and ERS inhibition. Pancreatology. 2018;**18**:742-752. DOI: 10.1016/j.pan.2018.08.001

[30] Van Sebille YZA, Gibson RJ, Wardill HR, Ball IA, Keefe DMK, Bowen JM. Dacomitinib-induced diarrhea: Targeting chloride secretion

with crofelemer. International Journal of Cancer. 2018;**142**:369-380. DOI: 10.1002/ijc.31048

[31] Sá MS, de Menezes MN, Krettli AU, Ribeiro IM, Tomassini TCB, Ribeiro dos Santos R, et al. Antimalarial activity of physalins B, D, F, and G. Journal of Natural Products. 2011;**74**:2269-2272. DOI: 10.1021/np200260f

[32] Wang H-Y, Kan W-C, Cheng T-J, Yu S-H, Chang L-H, Chuu J-J. Differential anti-diabetic effects and mechanism of action of charantin-rich extract of Taiwanese *Momordica charantia* between type 1 and type 2 diabetic mice. Food and Chemical Toxicology. 2014;**69**:347-356. DOI: 10.1016/j.fct.2014.04.008

[33] Kaneshima T, Myoda T, Toeda K, Fujimori T, Nishizawa M. Antimicrobial constituents of peel and seeds of camu-camu (*Myrciaria dubia*). Bioscience, Biotechnology, and Biochemistry. 2017;**81**:1461-1465. DOI: 10.1080/09168451.2017.1320517

[34] Zechmeister L. Cis-trans isomerization and stereochemistry of carotenoids and diphenyl-polyenes. Chemical Reviews. 1944;**34**:267-344. DOI: 10.1021/cr60108a004

[35] Karrer P, Helfenstein A, Widmer R, van Itallie TB. Über Bixin. (XIII. Mitteilung über Pflanzenfarbstoffe.). Helvetica Chimica Acta. 1929;**12**:741-756. DOI: 10.1002/hlca.19290120174

[36] Barber MS, Hardisson A, Jackman LM, Weedon BCL. Studies in nuclear magnetic resonance. Part IV. Stereochemistry of the bixins. Journal of the Chemical Society. 1961;**0**:1625-1630. DOI: 10.1039/JR9610001625

[37] Kumar Y, Phaniendra A, Periyasamy L. Bixin triggers apoptosis of human Hep3B hepatocellular carcinoma cells: An insight to molecular and in silico approach. Nutrition and Cancer. 2018;**70**:1-13. DOI: 10.1080/01635581.2018.1490445

[38] Rojo de la Vega M, Zhang DD, Wondrak GT. Topical bixin confers NRF2-dependent protection against photodamage and hair graying in mouse skin. Frontiers in Pharmacology. 2018;**9**:287. DOI: 10.3389/fphar.2018.00287

[39] Tao S, Park SL, Rojo de la Vega M, Zhang DD, Wondrak GT. Systemic administration of the apocarotenoid bixin protects skin against solar UV-induced damage through activation of NRF2. Free Radical Biology and Medicine. 2015;**89**:690-700. DOI: 10.1016/j.freeradbiomed.2015.08.028

[40] Rojo de la Vega M, Krajisnik A, Zhang D, Wondrak G, Rojo de la Vega M, Krajisnik A, et al. Targeting NRF2 for improved skin barrier function and photoprotection: Focus on the achiote-derived apocarotenoid bixin. Nutrients. 2017;**9**:1371. DOI: 10.3390/nu9121371

[41] Ubillas R, Jolad SD, Bruening RC, Kernan MR, King SR, Sesin DF, et al. SP-303, an antiviral oligomeric proanthocyanidin from the latex of *Croton lechleri* (Sangre de Drago). Phytomedicine. 1994;**1**:77-106. DOI: 10.1016/S0944-7113(11)80026-7

[42] Gabriel SE, Davenport SE, Steagall RJ, Vimal V, Carlson T, Rozhon EJ. A novel plant-derived inhibitor of cAMP-mediated fluid and chloride secretion. American Journal of Physiology. 1999;**276**:G58-G63

[43] Cottreau J, Tucker A, Crutchley R, Garey KW. Crofelemer for the treatment of secretory diarrhea. Expert Review of Gastroenterology & Hepatology. 2012;**6**:17-23. DOI: 10.1586/egh.11.87

[44] Yeo QM, Crutchley R, Cottreau J, Tucker A, Garey KW. Crofelemer, a novel antisecretory agent approved for the treatment of HIV-associated diarrhea. Drugs Today. 2013;**49**:239-252. DOI: 10.1358/dot.2013.49.4.1947253

[45] Tradtrantip L, Namkung W, Verkman AS. Crofelemer, an antisecretory antidiarrheal proanthocyanidin oligomer extracted from *Croton lechleri*, targets two distinct intestinal chloride channels. Molecular Pharmacology. 2010;**77**:69-78. DOI: 10.1124/mol.109.061051

[46] Simić A, Soković MD, Ristić M, Grujić-Jovanović S, Vukojević J, Marin PD. The chemical composition of some *Lauraceae* essential oils and their antifungal activities. Phytotherapy Research. 2004;**18**:713-717. DOI: 10.1002/ptr.1516

[47] dos Santos ÉRQ, Maia CSF, Fontes Junior EA, Melo AS, Pinheiro BG, Maia JGS. Linalool-rich essential oils from the Amazon display antidepressant-type effect in rodents. Journal of Ethnopharmacology. 2018;**212**:43-49. DOI: 10.1016/j.jep.2017.10.013

[48] Branch LC, da Silva MF. Folk medicine of Alter do Chao, Pará. Acta Amazonica. 1983;**13**:737-797. DOI: 10.1590/1809-4392135737

[49] Huo M, Cui X, Xue J, Chi G, Gao R, Deng X, et al. Anti-inflammatory effects of linalool in RAW 264.7 macrophages and lipopolysaccharide-induced lung injury model. Journal of Surgical Research. 2013;**180**: e47-e54. DOI: 10.1016/j.jss.2012.10.050

[50] Rodenak-Kladniew B, Castro A, Stärkel P, De Saeger C, García de Bravo M, Crespo R. Linalool induces cell cycle arrest and apoptosis in HepG2 cells through oxidative stress generation and modulation of Ras/MAPK and Akt/mTOR pathways. Life Sciences. 2018;**199**:48-59. DOI: 10.1016/j.lfs.2018.03.006

[51] Gu Y, Ting Z, Qiu X, Zhang X, Gan X, Fang Y, et al. Linalool preferentially induces robust apoptosis of a variety of leukemia cells via upregulating p53 and cyclin-dependent kinase inhibitors. Toxicology. 2010;**268**:19-24. DOI: 10.1016/j.tox.2009.11.013

[52] Shen Y-L, Wang T-Y, Chen T-Y, Chang M-Y. The proliferative inhibitor and apoptosis mechanism of linalool in breast cancer cells. Biomarkers and Genomic Medicine. 2013;**5**:131. DOI: 10.1016/j.bgm.2013.08.016

[53] Pereira I, Severino P, Santos AC, Silva AM, Souto EB. Linalool bioactive properties and potential applicability in drug delivery systems. Colloids and Surfaces B: Biointerfaces. 2018;**171**:566-578. DOI: 10.1016/j.colsurfb.2018.08.001

[54] Kohn LK, Queiroga CL, Martini MC, Barata LE, Porto PSS, Souza L, et al. In vitro antiviral activity of Brazilian plants (*Maytenus ilicifolia* and *Aniba rosaeodora*) against bovine herpesvirus type 5 and avian metapneumovirus. Pharmaceutical Biology. 2012;**50**:1269-1275. DOI: 10.3109/13880209.2012.673627

[55] Jabir MS, Taha AA, Sahib UI. Linalool loaded on glutathione modified gold nanoparticles: A drug delivery system for a successful antimicrobial therapy. Artificial Cells, Nanomedicine, and Biotechnology. 2018;**46**:1-11. DOI:10.1080/21691401.2018.1457535

[56] Ferreira GLS, Bezerra LMD, Ribeiro ILA, Morais Júnior RCD, Castro RD. Susceptibility of cariogenic microorganisms to phytoconstituents. Brazilian Journal of Biology. 2018;**78**:691-696. DOI: 10.1590/1519-6984.174147

[57] Sarrazin SLF, Oliveira RB, Maia JGS, Mourão RHV. Antibacterial activity of the rosewood (*Aniba rosaeodora* and *A. parviflora*) linalool-rich oils from the Amazon. European Journal of Medicinal Plants. 2015;**12**:1-9

[58] Pimentel RBQ, Souza DP, Albuquerque PM, Fernandes AV, Santos AS, Duvoisin S, et al. Variability and antifungal activity of volatile compounds from *Aniba rosaeodora* Ducke, harvested from Central Amazonia in two different seasons. Industrial Crops and Products. 2018;**123**:1-9. DOI: 10.1016/j.indcrop.2018.06.055

[59] de Oliveira Lima MI, Araújo de Medeiros AC, Souza Silva KV, Cardoso GN, de Oliveira Lima E, de Oliveira Pereira F. Investigation of the antifungal potential of linalool against clinical isolates of fluconazole resistant *Trichophyton rubrum*. Journal de Mycologie Médicale. 2017;**27**:195-202. DOI: 10.1016/j.mycmed.2017.01.011

[60] VM V, Dubey VK, Ponnuraj K. Identification of two natural compound inhibitors of *Leishmania donovani* spermidine synthase (SpdS) through molecular docking and dynamic studies. Journal of Biomolecular Structure and Dynamics. 2018;**36**:2678-2693. DOI: 10.1080/07391102.2017.1366947

[61] Dutra FL, Oliveira MM, Santos RS, Silva WS, Alviano DS, Vieira DP, et al. Effects of linalool and eugenol on the survival of *Leishmania* (L.) infantum chagasi within macrophages. Acta Tropica. 2016;**164**:69-76. DOI: 10.1016/j.actatropica.2016.08.026

[62] García Prado E, García Gimenez MD, De la Puerta Vázquez R, Espartero Sánchez JL, Sáenz Rodríguez MT. Antiproliferative effects of mitraphylline, a pentacyclic oxindole alkaloid of *Uncaria tomentosa* on human glioma and neuroblastoma cell lines. Phytomedicine. 2007;**14**:280-284. DOI: 10.1016/j.phymed.2006.12.023

[63] Reis SRIN, Valente LMM, Sampaio AL, Siani AC, Gandini M, Azeredo EL, et al. Immunomodulating and antiviral activities of *Uncaria tomentosa* on human monocytes infected with dengue virus-2. International Immunopharmacology. 2008;**8**:468-476. DOI: 10.1016/j.intimp.2007.11.010

[64] Sandoval-Chacón M, Thompson JH, Zhang XJ, Liu X, Mannick EE, Sadowska-Krowicka H, et al. Antiinflammatory actions of cat's claw: The role of NF-kappaB. Alimentary Pharmacology & Therapeutics. 1998;**12**:1279-1289

[65] Allen-Hall L, Arnason JT, Cano P, Lafrenie RM. Uncaria tomentosa acts as a potent TNF-alpha inhibitor through NF-kappaB. Journal of Ethnopharmacology. 2010;**127**:685-693. DOI: 10.1016/j.jep.2009.12.004

[66] Rojas-Duran R, González-Aspajo G, Ruiz-Martel C, Bourdy G, Doroteo-Ortega VH, Alban-Castillo J, et al. Anti-inflammatory activity of mitraphylline isolated from *Uncaria* tomentosa bark. Journal of Ethnopharmacology. 2012;**143**:801-804. DOI: 10.1016/j.jep.2012.07.015

[67] Montserrat-de la Paz S, de la Puerta R, Fernandez-Arche A, Quilez AM, Muriana FJG, Garcia-Gimenez MD, et al. Pharmacological effects of mitraphylline from *Uncaria tomentosa* in primary human monocytes: Skew toward M2 macrophages. Journal of Ethnopharmacology. 2015;**170**:128-135. DOI: 10.1016/j.jep.2015.05.002

[68] Fujita A, Sarkar D, Wu S, Kennelly E, Shetty K, Genovese MI. Evaluation of phenolic-linked bioactives of camu-camu (*Myrciaria dubia* mc. Vaugh) for antihyperglycemia, antihypertension,

antimicrobial properties and cellular rejuvenation. Food Research International. 2015;**77**:194-203. DOI: 10.1016/j.foodres.2015.07.009

[69] Tauchen J, Bortl L, Huml L, Miksatkova P, Doskocil I, Marsik P, et al. Phenolic composition, antioxidant and anti-proliferative activities of edible and medicinal plants from the Peruvian Amazon. Revista Brasileira de Farmacognosia. 2016;**26**:728-737. DOI: 10.1016/j.bjp.2016.03.016

[70] dos Santos AE, Kuster RM, Yamamoto KA, Salles TS, Campos R, de Meneses MD, et al. Quercetin and quercetin 3-O-glycosides from *Bauhinia longifolia* (bong.) Steud. show anti-Mayaro virus activity. Parasites & Vectors. 2014;**7**:130. DOI: 10.1186/1756-3305-7-130

[71] D'Andrea G. Quercetin: A flavonol with multifaceted therapeutic applications? Fitoterapia. 2015;**106**: 256-271. DOI: 10.1016/j.fitote.2015.09.018

[72] Wang W, Sun C, Mao L, Ma P, Liu F, Yang J, et al. The biological activities, chemical stability, metabolism and delivery systems of quercetin: A review. Trends in Food Science & Technology. 2016;**56**:21-38. DOI: 10.1016/j.tifs.2016.07.004

[73] Dajas F. Life or death: Neuroprotective and anticancer effects of quercetin. Journal of Ethnopharmacology. 2012;**143**:383-396. DOI: 10.1016/j.jep.2012.07.005

[74] Lesjak M, Beara I, Simin N, Pintać D, Majkić T, Bekvalac K, et al. Antioxidant and anti-inflammatory activities of quercetin and its derivatives. Journal of Functional Foods. 2018;**40**:68-75. DOI: 10.1016/j.jff.2017.10.047

[75] Suganthy N, Devi KP, Nabavi SF, Braidy N, Nabavi SM. Bioactive effects of quercetin in the central nervous system: Focusing on the mechanisms of actions. Biomedicine & Pharmacotherapy. 2016;**84**:892-908. DOI: 10.1016/j.biopha.2016.10.011

[76] Patel RV, Mistry BM, Shinde SK, Syed R, Singh V, Shin H-S. Therapeutic potential of quercetin as a cardiovascular agent. European Journal of Medicinal Chemistry. 2018;**155**:889-904. DOI: 10.1016/j.ejmech.2018.06.053

[77] Davies SP, Reddy H, Caivano M, Cohen P. Specificity and mechanism of action of some commonly used protein kinase inhibitors. Biochemical Journal. 2000;**351**:95-105. DOI: 10.1042/bj3510095

[78] Cao H, Pauff JM, Hille R. X-ray crystal structure of a xanthine oxidase complex with the flavonoid inhibitor quercetin. Journal of Natural Products. 2014;**77**:1693-1699. DOI: 10.1021/np500320g

[79] Zhang C, Wang R, Zhang G, Gong D. Mechanistic insights into the inhibition of quercetin on xanthine oxidase. International Journal of Biological Macromolecules. 2018;**112**:405-412. DOI: 10.1016/j.ijbiomac.2018.01.190

[80] Hamilton KE, Rekman JF, Gunnink LK, Busscher BM, Scott JL, Tidball AM, et al. Quercetin inhibits glucose transport by binding to an exofacial site on GLUT1. Biochimie. 2018;**151**:107-114. DOI: 10.1016/j.biochi.2018.05.012

[81] Sicheri F, Moarefi I, Kuriyan J. Crystal structure of the Src family tyrosine kinase Hck. Nature. 1997;**385**:602-609. DOI: 10.1038/385602a0

[82] Ugochukwu E, Soundararajan M, Rellos P, Fedorov O, Phillips C, Wang J, et al. Crystal Structure of Human Serine/Threonine Kinase 17B (STK17B) in Complex with Quercetin. RCSB PDB Protein Data Bank. 2010. DOI: 10.2210/pdb3lm5/pdb

[83] Walker EH, Pacold ME, Perisic O, Stephens L, Hawkins PT, Wymann MP, et al. Structural determinants of phosphoinositide 3-kinase inhibition by wortmannin, LY294002, quercetin, myricetin, and staurosporine. Molecular Cell. 2000;**6**:909-919

[84] Vaisberg AJ, Milla M, Planas MC, Cordova JL, de Agusti ER, Ferreyra R, et al. Taspine is the cicatrizant principle in Sangre de Grado extracted from *Croton lechleri*. Planta Medica. 1989;**55**:140-143. DOI: 10.1055/s-2006-961907

[85] Porras-Reyes BH, Lewis WH, Roman J, Simchowitz L, Mustoe TA. Enhancement of wound healing by the alkaloid taspine defining mechanism of action. Proceedings of the Society for Experimental Biology and Medicine. 1993;**203**:18-25

[86] Fayad W, Fryknäs M, Brnjic S, Olofsson MH, Larsson R, Linder S. Identification of a novel topoisomerase inhibitor effective in cells overexpressing drug efflux transporters. PLoS One. 2009;**4**:e7238. DOI: 10.1371/journal.pone.0007238

[87] Zhan Y, Zhang Y, Chen Y, Wang N, Zheng L, He L. Activity of taspine isolated from radix et *Rhizoma Leonticis* against estrogen-receptor-positive breast cancer. Fitoterapia. 2011;**82**:896-902. DOI: 10.1016/j.fitote.2011.05.004

[88] Castelli S, Katkar P, Vassallo O, Falconi M, Linder S, Desideri A. A natural anticancer agent thaspine targets human topoisomerase IB. Anti-Cancer Agents in Medicinal Chemistry. 2013;**13**:356-363

[89] Jako C, Coutu C, Roewer I, Reed DW, Pelcher LE, Covello PS. Probing carotenoid biosynthesis in developing seed coats of *Bixa orellana* (Bixaceae) through expressed sequence tag analysis. Plant Science. 2002;**163**:141-145. DOI: 10.1016/S0168-9452(02)00083-3

[90] Cárdenas-Conejo Y, Carballo-Uicab V, Lieberman M, Aguilar-Espinosa M, Comai L, Rivera-Madrid R. De novo transcriptome sequencing in *Bixa orellana* to identify genes involved in methylerythritol phosphate, carotenoid and bixin biosynthesis. BMC Genomics. 2015;**16**:877. DOI: 10.1186/s12864-015-2065-4

[91] Bouvier F, Dogbo O, Camara B. Biosynthesis of the food and cosmetic plant pigment bixin (annatto). Science. 2003;**300**:2089-2091. DOI: 10.1126/science.1085162

[92] Dubey VS, Bhalla R, Luthra R. An overview of the non-mevalonate pathway for terpenoid biosynthesis in plants. Journal of Biosciences. 2003;**28**:637. DOI: 10.1007/BF02703339

[93] Rohmer M. The discovery of a mevalonate-independent pathway for isoprenoid biosynthesis in bacteria, algae and higher plants. Natural Product Reports. 1999;**16**:565-574

[94] Zhu B-Q, Cai J, Wang Z-Q, Xu X-Q, Duan C-Q, Pan Q-H, et al. Identification of a plastid-localized bifunctional nerolidol/linalool synthase in relation to linalool biosynthesis in young grape berries. International Journal of Molecular Sciences. 2014;**15**:21992-22010. DOI: 10.3390/ijms151221992

[95] Lichtenthaler HK, Schwender J, Disch A, Rohmer M. Biosynthesis of isoprenoids in higher plant chloroplasts proceeds via a mevalonate-independent pathway. FEBS Letters. 1997;**400**:271-274. DOI: 10.1016/S0014-5793(96)01404-4

[96] Suga T, Shishibori T, Bukeo M. Biosynthesis of linalool in higher plants. Phytochemistry. 1971;**10**:2725-2726. DOI: 10.1016/S0031-9422(00)97272-8

[97] Chen C, Zheng Y, Zhong Y, Wu Y, Li Z, Xu L-A, et al. Transcriptome analysis and identification of genes related to terpenoid biosynthesis in *Cinnamomum camphora*. BMC Genomics. 2018;**19**:550. DOI: 10.1186/s12864-018-4941-1

[98] Okada K, Kasahara H, Yamaguchi S, Kawaide H, Kamiya Y, Nojiri H, et al. Genetic evidence for the role of isopentenyl diphosphate isomerases in the mevalonate pathway and plant development in *Arabidopsis*. Plant and Cell Physiology. 2008;**49**:604-616. DOI: 10.1093/pcp/pcn032

[99] Neti SS, Pan J-J, Poulter CD. Mechanistic studies of the protonation-deprotonation reactions for type 1 and type 2 isopentenyl diphosphate:dimethylallyl diphosphate isomerase. Journal of the American Chemical Society. 2018;**140**:12900-12908. DOI: 10.1021/jacs.8b07274

[100] Falcone Ferreyra ML, Rius SP, Casati P. Flavonoids: Biosynthesis, biological functions, and biotechnological applications. Frontiers in Plant Science. 2012;**3**:222. DOI: 10.3389/fpls.2012.00222

[101] Cheynier V, Comte G, Davies KM, Lattanzio V, Martens S. Plant phenolics: Recent advances on their biosynthesis, genetics, and ecophysiology. Plant Physiology and Biochemistry. 2013;**72**: 1-20. DOI: 10.1016/j.plaphy.2013.05.009

Chapter 4

Medicinal Plants Used as Galactagogues

Emelia Oppong Bekoe, Cindy Kitcher, Nana Ama Mireku Gyima, Gladys Schwinger and Mark Frempong

Abstract

The recommended diet for human infants within the first 6 months of life is breast milk. No other natural or artificial formulation has been able to match up to this gold standard. Mothers who have attempted to pursue exclusive breastfeeding can, however, attest to numerous nutritional and non-nutritional challenges mainly resulting in insufficient milk production (hypogalactia) or the absence of milk production (agalactia). There are very few and officially recommended orthodox drugs to increase lactation. The most widely used galactagogues being chlorpromazine, sulpiride, metoclopramide and domperidone are associated with very high incidences of unpleasant side effects including their extra-pyramidal effects in both mother and infant. There is therefore a need to keep searching for more acceptable galactagogues. This section reviews current literature on medicinal plants used within the local Ghanaian community to enhance lactation. Various electronic databases such as PubMed, Science Direct, SciFinder and Google Scholar as well as published books on Ghanaian medicinal plants were searched. A total of 22 plants belonging to 13 families were reviewed with regards to their medicinal values, information on lactation and toxicity.

Keywords: galactagogues, lactation, breastfeeding, medicinal plants

1. Introduction

Exclusive breast feeding involves feeding only breast milk without any added fluids or solids. It is highly recommended by the World Health Organization (WHO) for the first 6 months of life with supplemental breast feeding continuing for at least 2 years [1]. This is because optimal breastfeeding of infants has a direct impact on growth, development, and health in the neonatal period [2, 3]. Breastfeeding is known to have invaluable benefits both for the child and mother. For the mother, breast feeding causes weight reduction, provides stronger interaction with the infant as well as pleasure and pleasant emotion. It also provides a more practical approach to feeding in comparison to the use of a bottle prevents breast cancer and pregnancy and provides relief in breast pain while also being economical. For the infant, it promotes affectional bond with the mother while adequately supplying the nutritional and emotional needs [3]. In the developing world, low immunization rates, contaminated drinking water, and reduced immunity as a result of malnutrition make breast feeding crucial to reducing life threatening infections. A review of interventions in 42 developing countries estimated that exclusive breast feeding for 6 months, with partial breastfeeding continuing to 12 months, can prevent 1.3 million (13%) deaths each year in children under 5 years [3]. However exclusive breastfeeding is not without challenges.

2. Challenges with breastfeeding

The WHO's recommendation for breastfeeding has been adopted by several countries all over the World and also in West Africa, but this has presented with several challenges, hence reducing the number of children who could potentially be breastfed. In the United States, for example, less than half of infants receive any breast milk at 6 months (49.4%), and approximately one-quarter are breast-fed up to 1 year (26.7%) [4]. Breast discomfort or pain, sore nipples, mastatitis, inverted nipples, presence of breast implants, difficulty getting baby to suck, poor weight gain and hypernatremia dehydration due to insufficient milk intake are rampant challenges encountered during breast feeding [3]. Lactation failure is also common among postpartum women, resulting in insufficient milk supply which is a major reason for early weaning. It has been claimed that at least 5% of women experience lactation failure (agalactias) whiles approximately 15% of women experience inadequate supply of their breast milk (hypogalactias) [5] at 3 weeks postpartum. The number of lactating women who have produce insufficient breast milk is on the rise [2]. There are a number of well-known causes of low breast milk supply that is primarily related to breast feeding management. These factors are difficult to control and require a good knowledge of breastfeeding practices. These factors include; schedule breastfeeding, skipping breastfeeding, supplementing the diet of the baby with infant formulas and poor latching of the baby on the breast. However, there are more complicated causes of low breast milk supply such as; insufficient mammary tissue (hypoplasia), medications (hormonal contraceptive pills), retained placenta, diseases (diabetes, jaundice), metabolic conditions (obesity), previous breast surgeries, cesarean section, thyroid and other hormonal disorders. Another cause is even environmental toxins such as pesticides. A study found that daughters of women who grew up in a pesticide contaminated environment had much higher incidence of insufficient mammary tissue than those living on the hill top of the same an area [6].

3. Solutions to breastfeeding challenges

To respond to the challenge of insufficient milk production (hypogalactia) or the absence of milk production (agalactia) milk banks are being created and the use of medication that induces, maintains or increases milk production are being used [2, 7].

Throughout history, donor breast milk banks have been the choice of some parents, and it is currently recommended as second choice if the mother's own milk is not available. However, the risk of possible transmission of diseases including HIV, cytomegalovirus, and Creutzfeldt-Jakob disease has induced the need for pasteurization. There are major concerns however as to what extent pasteurized donor breast milk retains the biological properties of mother's milk. Evidence on donor milk quality is limited [3] and operational human milk banks are not able to meet demands for especially the most vulnerable neonates [8].

3.1 Synthetic galactagogues

Orthodox drugs that are widely used as galactagogues are chlorpromazine, sulpiride, metoclopramide and domperidone [2] but there are reservations as to their efficacy and their association with very high incidences of unpleasant side effects including extra-pyramidal effects in both mother and infant. There is therefore a need to keep searching for more acceptable, safe and efficacious galactagogues [2, 9]. In the United States, Canada and Europe, metoclopramide and domperidone are widely prescribed [10].

Metoclopramide though prescribed off-label as a lactation aid has one troublesome side-effect of inducing depression. Extrapyramidal symptoms also occur in about 1 in 500 patients at even usual adult doses resulting in involuntary movements of limbs, facial grimacing, torticollis, oculogyric crisis, and rhythmic protrusion of tongue, bulbar type of speech, trismus, or dystonic reactions resembling tetanus. Metoclopramide is secreted in human milk and its safety in infants has not been established. Neonates are less able to clear the drug from their systems hence dystonias and other extrapyramidal reactions are more common in this pediatric population than in adults [10]. Severe depression, seizures and intestinal discomfort have also been reported in infants that consume milk from mothers treated with metoclopramide [2, 11]. Other adverse effects additionally reported in mothers include anxiety, several gastrointestinal disorders and insomnia [2].

Domperidone use in human clinical trials has also been associated with varying findings. In some recent human data no maternal or neonatal adverse effects were reported [2]. Other studies have however reported adverse effects in mothers such as xerostomia, gastrointestinal disorders, cardiac arrhythmia, and sudden death but none in infants [2]. Domperidone is reported to also increase the risk of sudden cardiac death or could be linked with increased risk of prolonged QT syndrome (arrhythmia) [4].

Sulpiride and chlorpromazine are also typical antipsychotics that have been documented to be effective as galactagogues but are also associated with extra-pyramidal reactions and weight gain. Human growth hormone and thyrotropin-releasing hormone are other agents have also been utilized to increase breastmilk production, but these agents have very limited clinical experience behind them [2, 7]. Oxytocin, although widely used in the past, has limited scientific data as a galactagogue also [7].

3.2 Botanical galactagogues

There are numerous references in literature for herbal medicines that are used to aid breastfeeding. However these are mainly based on empirical traditions with few human studies that show evidence that milk synthesis can be increased and that these are safe [2]. Most herbal galactagogues are believed to exert their pharmacologic effects through interactions with dopamine receptors, resulting in increased prolactin levels and there by augmenting milk supply [7]. Galactagogues are useful for women who are unable to produce breast milk on their own due to infant prematurity, illness of the mother or child, adoption, or surrogate motherhood [7].

The use of medicinal plants to stimulate breastmilk production has a long history of use [10] in almost all cultures over the world but has not been extensively studied nor fully exploited for use in lactating mothers [2]. The use of herbal medicines and phytonutrients or nutraceuticals to treat various conditions is expanding rapidly worldwide [12]. Botanical galactagogues may have the advantages of various claims of efficacy, preference of consumers for natural therapies, erroneous belief that herbal products are superior to manufactured products as well as dissatisfaction with the results, cost and side effects from the orthodox galactagogues [12].

A literature search on botanical galactagogues used within Ghanaian communities revealed a number of plants that are used for such purposes but with very little information and scientific studies to back their efficacy and safety.

4. Medicinal plants used as galactagogues

4.1 Amaryllidaceae

4.1.1 *Allium sativum* L.

A. sativum (garlic) is a perennial herb cultivated in various parts of the world and widely used as a food ingredient [13, 14]. Garlic has been used as a spice, food, and medicine for over 5000 years, and is one of the earliest documented herbs utilized for the maintenance of health and treatment of disease [15]. Garlic has many medicinal properties including, anti-microbial, anti-fungal, anti-viral, anti-protozoal, anti-inflammatory, anticancer and antioxidants [13, 14]. Garlic has traditionally been used to strengthen the immune system and gastrointestinal health. Today, this intriguing herb is probably the most widely researched medicinal plant [15]. Garlic is given for nutritional purposes to enhance gestation and lactation [16]. In a study conducted to evaluate the effectiveness of naturally prepared galactagogue mixtures containing garlic on breast milk production and prolactin levels in postnatal mothers, it was observed that the galactagogue mix increased prolactin production, confirming the folkloric use of garlic as a galactagogue [17]. Garlic is also known to impart odor and flavor to breast milk when consumed and infants tend to breast-feed longer on such milk [18].

Chemical constituents isolated from *A. sativum* were diallyl trisulfide (50.43%), diallyl disulfide (25.30%), diallyl sulfide (6.25%), diallyl tetrasulfide (4.03%), 1,2-dithiolane (3.12%), allyl methyl disulfide (3.07%), 1,3-dithiane (2.12%), and allyl methyl trisulfide (2.08%) [19]. The essential oil of *A. sativum* possessed contact toxicity against overwintering *C. chinensis* [19].

4.2 Annonaceae

4.2.1 *Xylopia aethiopica A. rich*

X. aethiopica is an evergreen tree with many-branched and narrow crown; it can grow from 15 to 30 m high. It is planted for medicinal purposes, as a shade tree and as an ornamental. The fruits are used as a tonic to improve women fertility and to aid delivery. Various parts of this plant are used across Ghana and Nigeria for various medicinal purposes. Powdered samples are taken or applied directly for use. The fruits also serve as a condiment, an emmenagogue, anthelmintic, antitussive, carminative and rubefacient. Xylopia is used generally for pain and in the treatment of bronchitis, asthma, arthritis, rheumatism, headache, neuralgia and colic pain [20, 21]. The seeds are ground and used as a galactagogue, emetic, rubefacient, stimulant and vermifuge [22]. The seeds are crushed and applied on the forehead for treating headache and neuralgia and its extract for round worm infestation and as a treatment for biliousness. Decoction of leaves serves as an emetic and is used against rheumatism. The powdered leaves are rubbed on the chest for treating bronchio-pneumonia and taken as snuff for treating headaches. Roots are powdered and applied to sores and also to treat cancer. Lactating mothers take the ground seed to increase milk flow. Fruits are particularly high in zinc content, perhaps the reason behind its consumption during lactation. The fruit contains xylopic acid, volatile oils, fixed oils, rutin and zinc. Compounds isolated from *X. aethiopica* include Lupeol, 16α-hydroxy-ent-kauran-19-oic acid, 3, 4′, 5-trihydroxy-6,6″-dimethylpyrano[2,3-g]flavone, 3-O-β-sitosterol β-D-glucopyranoside, isotetrandrine and trans-tiliroside [22–24].

4.3 Asclepiadaceae

4.3.1 Secamone afzelii (Roem. & Schult.) K. Schum

S. afzelii, is a familiar creeping woody climber found on fences, unkempt farm lands, on trees and grows to a very long length of about 2–3 cm. It is often seen as a nuisance to other plants because of its domineering spread wherever it grows. It is used in traditional medicine for stomach problems, diabetes, colic, dysentery and also for kidney problems. The whole plant boiled with rice is used as purgative for children. The decoction of the entire plant is prescribed for cough and catarrhal. For the treatment of gonorrhea, the whole plant is crushed with fresh palm nuts and oil [25]. A decoction of the whole plant is used as a galactagogue [26]. Studies have shown that *S. afzelli* has antimicrobial effects and also protect cells against damage by reactive oxygen species [27–30]. The anti-inflammatory property of the leaf extract has also been demonstrated [30] in a murine model. Kaempferol-3-O-β-D-apiofuranosyl-(1 → 2)-α-L-rhamnopyranoside, rutin, myricetin 3-O-α-L-rhamnopyranosyl-(1 → 6)-β-D-glucopyranoside, kaempferol-3-O-α-L-rhamnopyranosyl-(1 → 6)-β-D-galactapyranoside, mauritianin, and vicenin-2 have been isolated from *S. afzelii* [26]. The methanol extracts of *S. afzelii* is reported to be toxic in *Artemia salina* [31].

4.4 Costaceae

4.4.1 Costus afer Ker-Gawl

C. afer, natively called the bush sugar cane is classified as an endangered medicinal plant in Nigeria. It is a perennial, rhizomatous herb that can grow to a height up to 4 m. Leaves are arranged spirally, simple and entire [32]. It can be found in the forest belt of Senegal, South Africa, Guinea, Niger, Sierra Leone, Ghana, Cameroon and Nigeria [33]. *C. afer* is a useful medicinal plant that is highly valued for its antidiabetic, anti-inflammatory and anti-arthritic properties in South-East and South-West Nigeria, the plant extract is used as fodder to treat goats with retained placenta. The decoction of the stem or powdered fruits is used as a cough remedy. Its boiled root is applied to cuts and sores. A soothing formulation for rheumatic pains is prepared with the boiled leaves [33]. The leaves and stem are cut and crushed into smaller bits and boiled together with other plants such as *Alchornea cordifolia*, pawpaw, citrus species and the bark of *Mangifera indica* for the treatment of hunch back and malaria. Also the juice of *C. afer* is used as eye drop for inflammation and other eye defects. The young and tender leaves when chewed are believed to give strength to the weak and dehydrating patient. An infusion of the inflorescence is taken to treat stomach complaints. The stem or fruit decoction mixed together with sugarcane juice are taken to treat cough, respiratory problem and sore throat [32]. Alkaloids, saponins, flavonoids, anthraquinones, cardiac glycosides, terpenoids, phenolic compounds and tannins have been found to be present in the plant [33]. This plant contains diosgenin which is used as a precursor in the synthesis of a number of steroid drugs including corticosteroids, sex hormones, oral contraceptive and anabolic agents. The rhizome also contains saponins aferosides A–C, as well as diosein and parphyllin c and flavonoid glycoside kaempterol

3-0-rhamnopyranoside [34]. Extracts from the leaves exhibits antioxidant, hypolipidemic, hepatoprotective, anti-inflammatory, and analgesic, anticancer, antimicrobial, insecticidal and nematcidal activity and also contains verbascoside, which possesses antimicrobial activities [35]. Acute and chronic toxicity studies on *C. afer* showed no inherent toxic effects in animal models [35]. Liver function experiments of this plant in rats showed significant differences in the test groups when compared with the control while there was no significant effect on kidney function [33].

4.5 Euphorbiaceae

4.5.1 *Euphorbia hirta* L.

E. hirta is a slender-stemmed, annual hairy plant with many branches from the base to the top, spreading up to 40 cm in height. *E. hirta* is often used traditionally for female disorders, respiratory ailments (cough, coryza, bronchitis, and asthma), worm infestations in children, dysentery, jaundice, pimples, gonorrhea, digestive problems, diabetes and tumors. It is reported to contain alkanes, triterpenes, phytosterols, tannins, polyphenols, and flavanoids. The root exudate exhibits nematicidal activity [3]. The decoction of the dry herb is used for skin diseases while that for the fresh herbs is used as gargle for the treatment of thrush. Roots are also used for snake bites. This herb shows antibacterial, anti-inflammatory, antimalarial, galactogenic, anti-asthmatic, anti-diarrheal, anti-cancer, anti-oxidant, anti-infertility, anti-amoebic, and anti-fungal activities [36]. The root decoction is also beneficial for nursing mothers deficient in milk [36]. *E. hirta* has shown a galactogenic activity in guinea pigs before puberty by increasing the development of the mammary glands and induction of milk secretion [36].

4.5.2 *Euphorbia thymifolia wall*

E. thymifolia is a softly hispid prostrate herb that is slender, cylindrical, pale green but often pink in color when fresh, becoming grayish green or dark purplish on drying. Stems are with white latex, spreading on the ground, 10–20 cm in length with a diameter from 1 to 3 mm [37]. *E. thymifolia* is traditionally used as a blood purifier, sedative, hemostatic, aromatic, stimulant, astringent in diarrhea and dysentery, anthelminthic, demulcent, laxative; and also in cases of flatulence, constipation; chronic cough; as an antiviral in bronchial asthma and paronychia. The dried leaves and seeds are given along with butter-milk to children in bowel complaints. Root is given in amenorrhea and gonorrhea. The oil is used as an insect repellant and in medicinal soaps for the treatment of erysipelas. It is also used as a vermifuge for dogs and farm foxes. Plant juice is employed in southern India as a cure for ring worms. The plant powder is given with wine as a remedy for bites of venomous reptiles. It is applied on the scalp with ammonium chloride to cure of dandruff. The fresh plant is considered vulnerary and used in ophthalmia and other eye troubles, ardor, sores, atrophy, dysentery and breast pain [24]. This plant is reported to be used as a galactagogue both in West-Africa and in India [24, 38].

4.5.3 *Hymenocardia acida Tul*

H. acida is a small tree of about 6 m high, gnarled and twisted with characteristic rough, rusty-red bark. It is widespread in tropical Africa [39]. The leaves of *Hymenocardia acida* are commonly used in Northern Nigeria alone or in combination with other plant parts to manage sickle cell disease. The plant contains carbohydrates, tannins, flavonoids, saponins, alkaloids, cardiac glycosides, resins, steroids and terpenes [38]. The root of this plant is reported to be used within West-Tropical Africa to stimulate lactation but [24] there are however anecdotal reports that this plant it is also given to diminish breastmilk supply. Ethnopharmacological studies of *H. acida* revealed an extensive array of medicinal uses, particularly from tropical African countries. In Senegal and Ivory Coast, an infusion or decoction of its leaves is used for the treatment of chest complaints, small pox, in baths and draughts as a febrifuge, and is taken as snuff for headaches or applied topically for rheumatic pains and toothaches. The bark and leaves are prescribed together with other plants in various ways in Nigeria for abdominal and menstrual pains and as poultices to treat abscesses and tumors. The powdered leaves of this tree are also used for the treatment of arthritis. Pharmacological activities reported on the plant include anti-ulcer, anti-plasmodial and cytotoxic activities [39].

4.5.4 Plagiostyles africana Prain exDe wild

P. africana trees grow in the lowland rainforest of south Nigeria and West Cameroons extending to Zaïre (the Democratic Republic of Congo). It reaches 16 m tall by 1.30 m in girth. The wood is light yellowish white and it is cut in Gabon to make spoons, combs and hair-pins. A wood-decoction is taken in the belief that it promotes milk-production [24]. The bark contains a white to yellowish viscid latex. The bark is used for chest-affections, and for fever [40].

4.5.5 Ricinus communis L.

R. communis (castor oil plant) is a perennial shrub whose leaves have long petiole and palm like lobed blades. Fruit is three chambered, globose capsule with soft spines. When capsules mature, they split up into three cavities and the seeds are expelled out [41]. This plant is grown worldwide for the production of castor oil. *R. communis* exhibits various biological and pharmacological activities such as abortifacient effect, acid phosphatase inhibition, acid phosphatase stimulation, agglutin activity, alkaline phosphatase inhibition, anti-conceptive activity, anti-diabetic activity, anti-infertility effects anti-inflammatory activity, antimicrobial activity, antioxidant activity, free radical scavenging activity, hepatoprotective activity, insecticidal activity and repellent properties [5, 41]. Castor oil is massaged over the breast after child-birth to increase the flow of milk as it stimulates the mammary glands. The leaves of castor can also be used to foment the breast for the same purpose [5, 24].

4.6 Leguminosae

4.6.1 Tamarindus indica L.

The tamarind (*T. indica*) is a common tree, especially in West Africa [42] and India. It is a moderate to large sized, evergreen tree that grows up to 24 m in height and 7 m in girth. *T. indica* has antimicrobial, antioxidant, anti-venom properties and it is also used as a galactagogue [43]. It is indigenous to tropical Africa and is also cultivated in subtropical China, India and Spain. Initially, the fruit shows a reddish-brown color that turns black brown, becoming more aromatic and sour on ripening. The fruit pulp is used for seasoning, as a food component and in juices. *T. indica* has antimicrobial, antioxidant, anti-venom properties and also used as a galactagogue [43]. Tamarind is most commonly used as a laxative and in the treatment of wounds and abdominal pains, followed by diarrhea, helminth infections, fever, malaria, aphrodisiac, respiratory problems and dysentery [42]. Its fruit is regarded as a digestive, carminative, laxative, expectorant and blood tonic [44]. Other parts of the plant have anti-oxidant [45], anti-hepatotoxic [46], anti-inflammatory, anti-mutagenic, anti-cancer, anti-ulcer and anti-diabetic [47] activities. The flower and leaf are eaten as vegetables, while the germ obtained from the seed is used for manufacturing tamarind gum which is well-known as a component of jelly [5, 48]. Toxicity study in rat modules showed that tamarind pulp extract was generally safe and well tolerated at 5, 200, 1000 mg/kg body weight per day for 6 months [49].

4.6.2 Acacia nicolita var. adansonaii (Guill. & Perr.) Brenan

A. nicolita also known as gum Arabic occurs as a tree which can grow up to about 50 feet high. It has a dark brown bole with deeply fissured bark. The leaves are compound and alternately arranged with about 10 to 30 elliptical pubescent leaflets on each leaf. The flowers occur as round, yellow heads situated at the end of branches. Fruits are thick, gray and are well constricted hairy pods [50]. Various parts of *A. nicolita* have been used for the treatment of various cancers in Western Africa. These include cancers of the ear, eye and testicles. Roots of the plant are used to treat tuberculosis, its wood for the treatment of smallpox, and the leaves for the treatment of ulcers [51]. In the Katsina state of Nigeria, decoction of the pod is used for postpartum wound healing [52] and here also the young shoots and pods are used to stimulate lactation [53]. When the effect of the aqueous extract of *A. nicolita* was investigated on milk production in rats, it was observed that, the extract was able to significantly stimulate the release of prolactin. Also, it was observed that the mammary glands of estrogen-primed rats treated with the extract showed clear lobuloalveolar development with milk secretion [54]. Present in *A. nicolita* are tannins, flavonoids, alkaloids, fatty acids and terpenes have been isolated from various parts of the plant. This plant is also known to have anti-inflammatory, anti-oxidant, anti-diarrheal, anti-hypertensive and anti-spasmodic, anti-bacterial, anti-helminthic, anti-platelet aggregatory, and anti-cancer activities [50]. Toxicological studies on *A. nicolita* showed that it has a low toxicity potential [55]. However it is also reported that repeated administration of doses higher than 250 mg/kg body weight for 28 days caused hepatotoxicity in rats [56].

4.6.3 Desmodium adscendens (Sw.) DC

D. adscendens is a herbaceous non-climbing perennial shrub that commonly occurs in tropical areas of Africa, South America, Asia, Australia and Oceania [57]. The plant thrives in varying habitats ranging from forests to grasslands and in secondary/disturbed vegetation. A decoction of the leave and stem is used for asthma and other diseases associated with smooth muscle contraction and epilepsy in Ghana [57]. It is used for the treatment of fever, pain and epilepsy in the Congo. In Brazil the plant is used in the treatment of ovary inflammation. It is used in Ghana to enhance lactation [22]. *D. adsendens* contains indole alkaloids, unsaturated fatty acids, tyramine, hordenine and saponins [58, 59]. Triterpenoid saponins, tetrahydroiso-quinolones, phenylethylamines and indole-3-alkyl amines have been isolated from the leaves [60]. *D. adscendens* causes dilation, relaxation of smooth muscles, anti-histamine effects and normalizes elevated liver enzyme levels [58].

4.7 Malvaceae

4.7.1 Hibiscus sabdariffa Linn

H. sabdarriffa commonly known as Roselle (English), Sobolo (Akan Ghanaian language) is widely cultivated among the tropical and subtropical regions of the world. These include some parts of Asia and West Africa. This plant was domesticated by natives of Western Sudan before 4000 BC [61]. The plant is an erect herbaceous annual and a shrub that can grow up to about 2 m in height. It consists of smooth cylindrical and typically red stems. The leaves are simple, deeply lobed, petiolate and alternately arranged with reddish reticulate veins. The flowers occur singly in the axils of the leaves. The calyces are typically red and made up of five sepals fused at the base which become fleshy and juicy upon maturity [62, 63].

The main class of phytochemicals present in *H. sabdariffa* is anthocyanins and flavonoid, as well as organic acids and polysaccharides. Citric acid, malic acid, tartaric acid and ascorbic acid are also present [64]. Some flavonoids that have been described in *H. sabdariffa* extracts include hibiscitrin, sabdaritrin, gossytrin and gossypitrin [65, 66]. Different parts of *H. sabdariffa* are used for various medicinal purposes. The calyces of the flower are commonly incorporated in hot and cold drinks due to its pleasing taste. In many parts of Africa, it has been used for its spasmolytic, antioxidant [67–69], antibacterial [70, 71], antipyretic [72], diuretic and anthelmintic properties [73]. It is also used for the treatment of high blood pressure and liver diseases. Additionally to their medicinal uses, various parts of the plants are incorporated in meals and used for other culinary purposes. In some cultures, *H. sadariffa* is included in some herbal mixtures and consumed by nursing mothers to increase milk supply [74]. In Nigeria also, the decoctions of the seeds have been reported to be used to increase lactation in cases of poor milk supply [75]. In 66 healthy mothers who took extracts of hibiscus, fennel, fennel oil, verbena, raspberry leaves, fenugreek and vitamin C, there was an increase in breastmilk production by the third day [76]. Toxicity studies have shown that the prolonged usage of the aqueous-methanolic extract of *H. sabdariffa* calyces at the dose of 250 mg/kg could cause liver injury in rats [77]. Also, the 12-week subchronic effect of *H. sabdariffa* calyx aqueous extract at the doses of 1.15, 2.30, and 4.60 g/kg induced testicular toxicity [78].

4.7.2 Gossypium herbaceum L. (Malvaceae)

G. herbaceum is an erect, shrubby, hairy plant that grows up to 2–8 m high [79]. The decoction of this plant is used traditionally across West Africa as an aphrodiasiac, galactagogue, spermatogenic, expectorant, laxative, demulcent, emenagogue, dysmenorrhea, and for the expulsion of retained placenta [80, 81]. In human studies *G. herbaceum* was shown to be efficacious, safe and cost effective in augmenting lactation in perceived insufficient milk supply [9]. This plant is known to contain carbohydrates, tannins, saponins, steroids, glycosides, phenolics, sitosterol, ergosterol, lipids, gossypol, oleic, palmitic and linoleic acid [79]. Extracts from this plant and it active constituents gossypol have shown anti-cancer, anti-infertility, anti-malarial, anti-oxidant, anti-trypanosomal, anti-viral, anti-microbial, anti-viral, hepatoprotective and anti-depressant activities in animal models [16, 82, 83].

4.8 Moraceae

4.8.1 Milicia excelsa (Welw.) C.C. Berg

M. excelsa is commonly known as odum or iroko in Ghana. It is a large, dioecious tree that grows up to 50 m high [84]. This plant is widely used in African folk medicine as a decoction to treat several ailments. A root decoction is taken to treat female sterility. A decoction of the root and stem bark is taken as an aphrodisiac. The extracts from the bark are taken to treat cough, asthma, heart trouble, lumbago, spleen pain, stomach pain, abdominal pain, edema, ascites, dysmenorrhea, gonorrhea, general fatigue, rheumatism, sprains, and as a galactagogue, aphrodisiac, tonic and purgative. Also the stem bark preparations are topically applied to treat scabies, wounds, and loss of hair, fever, venereal diseases and sprains. They are applied as an enema to cure piles, diarrhea and dysentery. The latex is applied on burns, wounds, sores, eczema and on other skin problems as well as taken to treat type 2 diabetes [85, 86]. Additionally, it is taken against stomach problems, hypertension, tumors, and obstruction of the throat and as a galactagogue [87]. Leaves are eaten to treat insanity; a leaf maceration is drunk as a galactagogue. A decoction of the leaves is taken for the treatment of gallstones. Leaf preparations are externally applied to treat snakebites and fever and as eye drops to treat filariasis. Alkaloids, flavonoids and saponins are present as well as triterpenes and glycosides [79, 88]. The leaf extract of *M. excelsa* is reported to be safe in rodents [79, 89, 90].

4.8.2 Ficus sp. L.

Ficus species comprises one of the largest genera of angiosperms with more than 800 species of trees, shrubs, hemiepiphytes, climbers, and creepers in the tropics and subtropics worldwide [91]. The bark, root, leaves, fruit and latex of this plant are frequently used for the treatment of various illnesses including gastrointestinal, liver, venereal, respiratory, metabolic and cardiovascular disorders. It is used in traditional medicine as a galactagogue [92]. The fresh juice (50–100 ml) of leaves of *F. racemosa* L. is given with water for about 10 days to treat gastrointestinal problems. Bark of *F. arnottiana* and *F. hispida* shows hypoglycaemic activity. Roots of *F. bengalensis* show anthelmintic activity. This extract is also reported to inhibit insulinase activity from liver and kidney. Fruit extracts exhibits antitumor activity. Various pharmacological actions such as anti-ulcer, anti-diabetic, lipid lowering and antifungal activities have been described for *F. exasperata*. Ethanolic leaf extract of *F. exasperata* shows anti-bacterial activity. Leaves exhibit hypotensive activity. Ethanolic and aqueous wood extracts of *F. glomerata* shows Anti-HIV-1 integrase activity. *F. religiosa* is reported to be used for the treatment of asthma, cough, sexual disorders, diarrhea, hematuria, ear-ache and toothache, migraine, eye troubles, gastric problems and scabies; leaf decoction has been used as an analgesic for toothache; fruits for the treatment of asthma, other respiratory disorders and scabies; stem bark is used in gonorrhea, bleeding, paralysis, diabetes, diarrhea, bone fracture, antiseptic, astringent and antidote. Fruit of *F. carica* shows spasmolytic activity, mediated through the activation of K^+-ATP channels along with anti-platelet activity. Hence, it can be used in gut motility and inflammatory disorders [93]. Most species of Ficus contain phenolic compounds, organic acids, and volatile compounds [91]. Some species have been reported not to be toxic in rodents [93].

4.9 Musaceae

4.9.1 Musa paradisiaca L.

M. paradisiaca is an herbaceous plant that grows up to about 9 m with a robust treelike false-stem. The unripe fruits and juice of *M. paradisiaca* is used in folk medicine to treat and manage diarrhea, dysentery, cholera, intestinal lesions, ulcerative colitis, diabetes, sprue, uremia, nephritis, gout, hypertension, cardiac disease, otalgia and hemoptysis [94, 95]. The flowers are also employed in treating dysentery, diabetes and menorrhagia [94]. The root is also used traditionally as an anthelmintic [95], for treating blood disorders and venereal diseases [94]. It is also used as an anti-inflammatory, analgesic and anti-dote for snakebites [96].

The green fruits of *M. paradisiaca* has been reported to possess anti-hypertensive [97] as well as hypoglycemic effect due to effects on insulin production and glucose utilization [98]. *M. paradisiaca* inhibits cholesterol crystallization in vitro [99]. *M. paradisiaca* has also been shown to induce atherosclerosis [100]. There have been reports of the potential of *M. paradisiaca* flower to enhance milk production of nursing rats [101, 102]. Serotonin, nor-epinephrine, tryptophan, indole compounds, tannin, starch, iron, crystallisable and non-crystallisable sugars, vitamins, albuminoids, fats, mineral salts have been found in the fruit pulp of *M. paradisiaca* [94] with several other compounds that have been isolated and identified from various parts of the plant [103].

4.10 Ranunculaceae

4.10.1 Nigella sativa L.

N. sativa is a small herb of about 45 cm long with linear-lanceolate leaves and a pale blue flower. It is used as a food and medicine frequently to treat a variety of health conditions pertaining to the respiratory system, digestive tract, kidney and liver functions, cardiovascular system, and immune system support, as well as for general well-being [104] and as a galactagogue [105].

Phytochemical analysis has revealed the presence of nigelline, nigellicine, nigelimine, nigellimine-*N*-oxide, avenasterol-5-ene, avanasterol-7-ene, campesterol, cholesterol, citrostadienol, cycloeucalenol, sitosterol, stigmasterol, stigmastanol, 24-ethyl-lophenol, obstafoliol [105]. This plant is reported to have anti-cancer, antimicrobial, analgesic, antipyretic, contraceptive and anti-fertility, anti-oxytocic, anti-tussive, anti-inflammatory, and anti-oxidant potentials. Anti-cancer activity has been demonstrated for blood, breast, colon, pancreatic, liver, lung, fibrosarcoma, prostate, and cervix cancer cell lines and in animal models as well [106–109]. Toxicological studies showed no toxic effect in rodents [105].

4.11 Solanaceae

4.11.1 Solanum torvum Swartz

S. torvum is an evergreen, widely branched, prickly shrub that grows up to 5 m tall [110]. The fruits of *S. torvum* are edible and commonly available in the markets for incorporation into stews and soups across West-Africa. A decoction of the fruits is given for cough ailments and is considered useful in cases of liver and spleen enlargement. The plant is used as a sedative and diuretic and the leaves are used as a hemostatic. The ripened fruits are used in the preparation of tonic and hemopoietin agents and also for the treatment for pain. It has antioxidant properties. It is intensively used worldwide in traditional medicine as a poison anti-dote and for the treatment of fever, wounds, tooth decay, reproductive problems and arterial hypertension [17, 111–113]. *S. torvum* fruits are reported to contain alkaloids, flavonoids, saponins, tannins, glycosides, fixed oil, vitamin B group, vitamin C and iron salts. It also has number of chemical constituents like neochlorogenin 6-O-β-D-quinovo-pyranoside, neochlorogenin 6-O-β-D-xylopyranosyl-(1 → 3)-β-D-quinovopyranoside, neochlorogenin 6-O-α-L-rhamnopyranosyl-(1 → 3)-β-Dquinovopyranoside, sola-genin 6-O-β-D-quinovopyranoside, solagenin 6-O-α-Lrhamnopyranosyl-(1 → 3)-β-D-quinovopyranoside, isoquercetin, rutin, kaempferol and quercetin [16, 113, 114]. *S. torvum* also possesses antimicrobial, antiviral, immuno-secretory, antioxidant, analgesic, anti-inflammatory, anti-ulcerogenic activities, cardiovascular, nephroprotective, antidiabetic, angiotensin and erotonin receptor blocking activities [110]. It is reported to be used in a concoction to nourish pregnant and lactating mothers with vitamins and proteins and to enhance lactation [115].

4.12 Verbanaceae

4.12.1 Lippia multiflora Moldenke

L. multiflora is an aromatic, perennial plant with woody stems growing up to 3 m high [53]. The plant is locally harvested in Ghana and Benin and the leaves are steeped in hot water for tea. It is used in the treatment of stomach aches, nausea and fever. The leaves and immature flowering stems have anti-biotic, laxative and vermifuge activities [116]. The leaves contain limonene, a-caryophyllene, trans-farnesene, caryophyllene oxide and farnesol [117]. Tea infusion of plant is used for the treatment of arterial hypertension in Ghana [118]. A herbal extract of the plant exhibits anti-malarial, anti-microbial, anti-inflammatory, diuretic, laxative, muscle relaxant and is also used in lactation failure [22]. Lippia oil is effective topically gram-negative bacteria [117] and body lice, head lice, scabies' mites [119]. This plant possesses a tranquilizer and analgesic activities as diazepam [118].

4.13 Zingiberaceae

4.13.1 Aframomum melegueta (Roscoe) K. Schum

A. melegueta is commonly known as grains of paradise or alligator pepper. It is a spicy edible perennial fruit which grows to about 1 m high. *A. melegueta* produces reddish-brown seeds, which have a strong aromatic flavor and a pungent taste. These seeds are widely employed as spices and it is also an ingredient in numerous West African ethno medical practices. *A. melegueta* is a remedy for a number of diseases such as constipation, rheumatic pains and fever [120, 121]. The medicinal uses of *A. melegueta* also include its use as an aphrodisiac, measles and leprosy. It is also taken to treat excessive lactation, post partem hemorrhage, purgation and used as a galactagogue, anthelmintic and hemostatic [122]. *A. melegueta* exhibits anti-inflammatory, anti-oxidant and anti-tumor effects [123, 124] as well as anti-protozoal activity against schistosomes [22]. The phytochemical constituents are essential oils—such as gingerol, shagaol, paradol. Alkaloids, flavonoids, saponins, tannins, cardiac glycosides, terpenoids, steroids [125] as well as essential oils and resins have also been identified in this plant [126]. The LD_{50} of 273.86 mg/kg body weight and lower than normal hemoglobin and red blood cells in animal studies seems to confirm the possibility of toxicity from this plant [125].

5. Conclusion

There are numerous references in literature for herbal medicines use to aid breastfeeding. However, the use of herbal galactagogues is mainly based on empirical traditions with little scientific data. With increase in the complexity of breastfeeding, it is imperative that these herbal galactagogues be studied. There is a need to standardize the herbal galactagogues, investigate their nutritional and phytochemical composition as well as conduct clinical trials to generate scientific evidence of their efficacy and safety, as a basis for commercial production and usage. Conducting pharmacodynamics and pharmacokinetic studies will also play a vital role in determining their metabolism in the mother and neonate. Their mechanism of action will also need to be investigated. These herbs will have the advantages of being easily available, cheaper and more tolerable to both mother and neonate.

Acknowledgements

The authors are grateful to the staff of the Ghana Herbarium for making available published literature on some of the medicinal plants.

Conflict of interest

The authors declare no conflict of interest.

Author details

Emelia Oppong Bekoe[1*], Cindy Kitcher[1], Nana Ama Mireku Gyima[1], Gladys Schwinger[2] and Mark Frempong[3]

1 Department of Pharmacognosy and Herbal Medicine, School of Pharmacy, University of Ghana, Legon, Ghana

2 Department of Plant and Environmental Science, University of Ghana, Legon, Ghana

3 Department of Obstetrics and Gynecology, University Hospital, Legon, Ghana

*Address all correspondence to: emekisseih@yahoo.com

References

[1] Hoddinott P, Tappin D, Wright C. Breast feeding. British Medical Journal. 2008;**336**(7649):881-887. DOI: 10.1136/bmj.39521.566296.BE

[2] Penagos Tabares F, Bedoya Jaramillo JV, Ruiz-Cortes ZT. Pharmacological overview of galactogogues. Veterinary Medicine International. 2014;**2014**:602894. DOI: 10.1155/2014/602894

[3] Dadalto ECV, Rosa EM. Knowledge about the benefits of breastfeeding and disadvantages of the pacifier related to the Mother's practice with preterm infants. Revista Paulista de Pediatria. 2017;**35**(4):399-406. DOI: 10.1590/1984-0462/;2017;35;4;00005

[4] Bazzano AN, Hofer R, Thibeau S, Gillispie V, Jacobs M, Theall KP. A review of herbal and pharmaceutical galactagogues for breast-feeding. The Ochsner Journal. 2016;**16**(4):511-524

[5] Padma LL, Rupalu BK. *Ricinus communis* (Castor): An overview. International Journal of Research in Pharmacology & Pharmacotherapeutics. 2014;**3**(2):136-144

[6] Elemo O, Oreagba I, Akinwunmi A, Elemo G, Nicholas-Okpara V. Lactation failure and potential traditional herbs as galactagogues. International Journal of Healthcare Sciences. 2016;**4**(1):427-434. DOI: 10.5586/asbp.3580

[7] Gabay MP. Galactogogues: Medications that induce lactation. Journal of Human Lactation. 2002;**18**(3):274-279. DOI: 10.1177/089033440201800311

[8] Kim J, Unger S. Human milk banking. Paediatrics & Child Health. 2010;**15**(9):595-602

[9] Manjula S, Sultana A, Rahman K. Clinical Efficacy of *Gossypium herbaceum* L. seeds In Perceived Insufficient Milk (PIM) supply: A randomized single-blind placebo-controlled study. Orient Pharm Exp Med. 2013;**1**(1):1-10. DOI: 10.1007/s13596-013-0121-7

[10] Abascal K, Yarnell E. Botanical galactagogues. Alternative and Complementary Therapies. 2008;**14**(6):288-294. DOI: 10.1089/act.2008.14602

[11] Zuppa AA, Sindico P, Orchi C. Safety and efficacy of Galactogogues: Substances that induce, maintain and increase Breastmilkproduction. Journal of Pharmacy and Pharmaceutical Sciences. 2010;**13**(2):162-174. DOI: 10.18433/J3DS3R

[12] Ekor M. The growing use of herbal medicines: Issues relating to adverse reactions and challenges in monitoring safety. Frontiers in Pharmacology. 2014;**4**:177. DOI: 10.3389/fphar.2013.00177

[13] Sharma R, Jaitawat A, Kantwa SM, Jain N, Rani D. Role of garlic and fenugreek during gestation and lactation. A Review Universal Journal of Environmental Research and Technology. 2014;**4**(4):265-279

[14] Bayan L, Koulivand PH, Garlic GA. A review of potential therapeutic effects. Avicenna Journal of Phytomedicine. 2014;**4**:1-14

[15] Ried K, Fakler P. Potential of garlic (*Allium sativum*) in lowering high blood pressure: Mechanisms of action and clinical relevance. Integr Blood Press Control. 2014;**7**:71-82. DOI: 10.2147/IBPC.S51434

[16] Agarwal BB, Prasad S, Reuter SR, Yadev VR, Park B, Kim JH, et al. Identification of novel anti-inflammatory agents from Ayurvedic medicine for prevention of chronic diseases: "Reverse pharmacology" and

"bedside to bench" approach. Current Drug Targets. 2011;**12**(11):1595-1653

[17] Srinivas R, Eagappan K, Sasikumar S. The effect of naturally formulated galactogogue mix on breast milk production, prolactin level and short-term catch-up of birth weight in the first week of life. International Journal of Health Sciences & Research. 2014;**4**:242-253

[18] Mennella JA, Beauchamp GK. The effects of repeated exposure to garlic-flavored milk on the nursing's behavior. Pediatric Research. 1993;**34**(6):805-808

[19] Zhao NN, Zhang H, Zhang XC, Luan XB, Zhou C, Liu QZ, et al. Evaluation of acute toxicity of essential oil of garlic (*Allium sativum*) and its selected major constituent compounds against overwintering Cacopsylla chinensis (Hemiptera: Psyllidae). Journal of Economic Entomology. 2013;**106**(3):1349-1354

[20] Obiri DD, Osafo N, Ayande PG, Antwi AO. Xylopia aethiopica (Annonaceae) fruit extract suppresses Freund's adjuvant-induced arthritis in Sprague-Dawley rats. Journal of Ethnopharmacology. 2014;**152**(3): 522-531. DOI: 10.1016/j.jep.2014.01.035

[21] Woode E, Ameyaw EO, Boakye-Gyasi E, Abotsi WK. Analgesic effects of an ethanol extract of the fruits of Xylopia Aethiopica (Dunal) A. rich (Annonaceae) and the major constituent, Xylopic acid In murine models. Journal of Pharmacy & Bioallied Sciences. 2012;**4**(4):291

[22] Science and Technology Research Institute (STEPRI). In: Bussia K, editor. Ghana Herbal Pharmacopoeia. Accra, Ghana: QualiType Limited; 2007

[23] Kuete V, Sandjo LP, Mbaveng AT, Zeino M, Efferth T. Cytotoxicity of compounds from Xylopia Aethiopica towards multi-factorial drug-resistant Cancer cells. Phytomedicine. 2015;**22**(14):1247-1254. DOI: 10.1016/j.phymed.2015.10.008

[24] Burkill HM. The Useful Plants of West Tropical Africa, Families E–I. Vol. 2. Kew: Royal Botanic Gardens; 1994

[25] Gill LS. Ethnomedical Uses of Plants in Nigeria. Benin City, Nigeria: University of Benin Press; 1992. p. 103

[26] Magid A, Yao-Kouassi PA, Gossan DPA, Mairot C, Voutquenne-Nazabadioko L. New antioxidant flavonoids from the aerial parts of Secamone afzelii. Journal of Antioxidant Activity. 2016;**2**(1):8

[27] Houghton PJ, Hylands PJ, Mensah AY, Hensel A, Deters AM. In vitro tests and ethnopharmacological investigations: Wound healing as an example. Journal of Ethnopharmacology. 2005;**100**:100-107. DOI: 10.1016/j.jep.2005.07.001

[28] Mensah AY, Houghton PJ, Agyare C, Komlaga G, Mensah MLK, Fleisher TC, et al. Investigation of activities related to wound healing of *Secamone afzelii*. Journal of Science and Technology (Ghana). 2007;**26**:83-89. DOI: 10.4314/just.v26i3.33008

[29] Mensah AY, Houghton PJ, Akyirem GNA, Fleischer TC, Mensah MLK, Sarpong K, et al. Evaluation of the antioxidant and free radical scavenging properties of *Secamone afzelii* Rhoem. Phytotherapy Research. 2004;**18**: 1031-1032. DOI: 10.1002/ptr.1614

[30] Mohanty I, Senapati MR, Jena D, Behera PC. Ethnoveterinary importance of herbal Galactogogues—A review. Veterinary World. 2014;**7**(5):325-330. DOI: 10.14202/vetworld.2014.325-330

[31] Lagnika L, Anago E, Sanni A. Screening for antibacterial, antioxidant activity and toxicity of some medicinal plants used in Benin folkloric medicine.

Journal of Medicinal Plant Research. 2011;**5**(5):773-777. DOI: 10.5897/JMPR

[32] Omokhua GE. Medicinal and socio-cultural importance of *Costus afer* (Ker Grawl) in Nigeria. International Multidisciplinary Journal, Ethiopia. 2011;**5**(5):282-287. DOI: 10.4314/afrrev.v5i5.22

[33] Ezejiofor AN, Orish CN, Orisakwe OE. Effect of aqueous leaves extract of *Costus afer* Ker Gawl (Zingiberaceae) on the liver and kidney of male albino Wistar rat. Ancient Science of Life. 2013;**33**(1):4-9. DOI: 10.4103/0257-7941.134554

[34] Aweke G. Plant Resources of Tropical Africa (PROTA). The Netherlands: Wageningen; 2007

[35] Tcheghebe OT, Sipowo Tala VR, Fouodjouo M. Ethnobotanical uses, phytochemical and pharmacological profiles, and toxicity of *Costus afer* Ker Gawl.: An overview. Journal of Scientific Research in Allied Science. 2018;**1**(4):01-11

[36] Kumar S, Malhotra R, Kumar D. Euphorbia hirta: Its chemistry, traditional and medicinal uses, and pharmacological activities. Pharmacognosy Reviews. 2010;**4**(7):58-61. DOI: 10.4103/0973-7847.65327

[37] Mali PY, Panchal SS. A review on Phyto-pharmacological potentials of *Euphorbia thymifolia* L. Ancient Science of Life. 2013;**32**(3):165-172. DOI: 10.4103/0257-7941.123001

[38] Ibrahim H, Sani FS, Danladi BH, Ahmadu AA. Phytochemical and antisickling studies of the leaves of *Hymenocardia acida* Tul (Euphorbiaceae). Pakistan Journal of Biological Sciences. 2007;**10**(5):788-791. DOI: 10.3923/pjbs.2007.788.79122

[39] Sofidiya MO, Odukoya OA, Afolayan AJ, Familoni OB. Phenolic contents, antioxidant and antibacterial activities of *Hymenocardia acida*. Natural Product Research. 2009;**23**(2):168-177. DOI: 10.1080/14786410801915838

[40] List the plant. *Plagiostyles africana* (Müll.-Arg.) Prain [family Euphorbiaceae]. 2018. Available from: http://plants.jstor.org/stable/10.5555/al.ap.upwta.2_249

[41] Marwat SL, ur-Rehman F, Khan EA, Baloch MS, Sadiq M, Ullah I, et al. *Ricinus communis*: Ethnomedicinal uses and pharmacological activities Pak. Journal of Pharmaceutical Sciences. 2017;**30**(5):1815-1827

[42] Havinga RM, Hartl A, Putscher J, Prehsler S, Buchmann C, Vogl CR. *Tamarindus indica* L. (Fabaceae): Patterns of use in traditional African medicine. Journal of Ethnopharmacology. 2010;**127**(3):573-588. DOI: 10.1016/j.jep.2009.11.028

[43] Sahu SP. Study on biochemical correlation of galactogogue effect of *Tamarindus indica* seed in cross bred dairy cows Veterinary Biochemistry College of Veterinary Science and Animal Husbandary 2015: Theis: Orissa University of Agriculture and Technology, BHUBANESWAR-751003

[44] Komutarin T, Azadi S, Butterworth L, Keil D, Chitsomboon B, Suttajit M, et al. Extract of the seed coat oof *Tamarindus indica* inhibits nitric oxide production by murine macrophages in vitro and in vivo. Food and Chemical Toxicology. 2004;**42**(4):649-658. DOI: 10.1016/j.fct.2003.12.001

[45] Tsuda T, Watanabe M, Ohshima K, Yamamoto A, Kawakishi S, Osawa T. Antioxidative components isolated from the seed of tamarind (*Tamarindus indica* L.). Journal of Agricultural and Food Chemistry. 1994;**42**:2671-2674. DOI: 10.1021/jf00048a004

[46] Joyeux M, Mortier F, Fleurentin J. Screening of antiradical, antilipoperoxidant and hepatoprotective effects of nine plant extracts used in

caribbean folk medicine. Phytotherapy Research. 1995;**9**:228-230. DOI: 10.1002/ptr.2650090316

[47] Maiti R, Jana D, Das UK, Ghosh D. Antidiabetic effect of aqueous extract of seed of *Tamarindus indica* in streptozotocin-induced diabetic rats. Journal of Ethnopharmacology. 2004;**92**:85-91. DOI: 10.1016/j.jep.2004.02.002

[48] Phakruschaphan T. Comparison of peeling and extraction methods in the production of tamarind seed gum. The Kasetsart Journal of Natural Sciences. 1982;**16**(2):74-81

[49] Iskandar I, Setiawan F, Sasongko LD, Adnyana IK. Six-month chronic toxicity study of tamarind pulp (*Tamarindus indica* L.) water extract. Scientia Pharmaceutica. 2017;**85**(1). DOI: 10.3390/scipharm85010010

[50] Luqman JR, Shahid-ul-Islam MF. *Acacia nilotica* (L.): A review of its traditional uses, phytochemistry, and pharmacology. Sustainable Chemistry and Pharmacy. 2015;**2**:12-30

[51] Kalaivani T, Matthew L. Free radical scavenging activity from leaves of *Acacia nilotica* (L.) Wild. Ex Delile, an Indian medicinal tree. Food Chem Toxicol. 2010;**48**(1):298-305. DOI: 10.1016/j.fct.2009.10.013. Epub 2009 Oct 29

[52] Kankara SS, Mohd IH, Muskhazli M, Rusea G. Ethnobotanical survey of medicinal plants used for traditional maternal healthcare in Katsina state, Nigeria. South African Journal of Botany. 2015;**97**:165-175. DOI: 10.1016/j.sajb.2015.01.007

[53] Burkill HM. The Useful Plants of West Tropical Africa. 2nd ed. Vol. 3. Kew: Royal Botanic gardens; 1995

[54] Lompo-Ouedraogo Z, van er Heide D, van der Beek EM, Swarts HJ, Mattheij JA, Sawadogo L. Effect of aqueous extract of *Acacia nilotica* ssp adansonii on milk production and prolactin release in the rat. The Journal of Endocrinology. 2004;**182**(2):257-266

[55] Al-Mustafa ZH, Dafallah AA. A study on the toxicology of Acacia nilotica. The American Journal of Chinese Medicine. 2000;**28**(1):123-129

[56] Lukman AA, Abdulfatai AA, Oluwakanyinsola AS, Musbau AA. Toxicological studies of aqueous extract of *Acacia nilotica*. Interdisciplinary Toxicology. 2015;**8**(1):48-54

[57] Francois C, Fares M, Baiocchi C, Maixent JM. Safety of *Desmodium adscendens* extract on hepatocytes and renal cells. Protective effect against oxidative stress. Journal of Intercultural Ethnopharmacology. 2015;**4**(1):1-5. DOI: 10.5455/jice.20141013041312

[58] McManus OB, Harris GH, Giangiacomo KM, Feigenbaum P, Reuben JP, Addy ME, et al. An activator of calcium-dependent potassium channels isolated from a medicinal herb. Biochemistry. 1993;**32**(24):6128-6133. DOI: 10.1021/bi00075a002

[59] Addy ME, Schwartzman ML. An extract of *Desmodium adscendens* inhibits NADPH-dependent oxygenation of arachidonic acid by kidney cortical Microsomes. Phytotherapy Research. 1992;**6**(5):245-250. DOI: 10.1002/ptr.2650060505

[60] Addy ME. Several chromatographically distinct fractions of *Desmodium Adscendens* inhibit smooth muscle contractions. International Journal of Crude Drug Research. 1989;**27**(2):81-91. DOI: 10.3109/13880208909053942

[61] Murdock GP. Africa, its Peoples and their Culture History. New York: McGraw-Hills; 1959

[62] Ross IA. Medicinal Plants of the World: Chemical Constituents, Traditional and Modern Medicinal Uses. Vol. 1. Totowa, NJ: Humana Press Inc; 2003

[63] Morton JF. Fruits of Warm Climates. Miami: Florida Flair Books; 1987

[64] Da-Costa-Roch I, Bonnlaender B, Sievers H, Pischel I, Heinrich M. *Hibiscus sabdariffa* L.—A phytochemical and pharmacological review. Food and Chemical Toxicology. 2014;**165**:424-443. DOI: 10.1016/j.foodchem.2014.05.002

[65] McKay DL, Chen CY, Saltzman E, Blumberg JB. Can Hibiscus tea lower blood pressure? AfroFood Industry Hi-Tech. 2009;**20**(6):40-42

[66] Williamson EM, Driver SB, Baxter K. Stockley's Herbal Medicines Interactions: A Guide to the Interactions of Herbal Medicines, Dietary Supplements and Nutraceuticals with Conventional Medicines. London: Pharmaceutical Press; 2013

[67] Duh P, Yen G. Antioxidative activity of three herbal water extracts. Food Chemistry. 1997;**60**(4):639-645

[68] Odebunmi EO, Oluwaniyi OO, Awolola GV, Adediji OD. Proximate and nutritional composition of Kola nut (*Cola nitida*), bitter cola (*Garcinia cola*) and Alligator pepper (*Afromomum melegueta*). African Journal of Biotechnology. 2009;**8**(2):308-310

[69] Olalye MT, Rocha JB. Commonly used tropical medicinal plants exhibit distinct in vitro antioxidant activities against hepatotoxins in rat liver. Experimental and Toxicologic Pathology. 2007;**56**(6):433-438

[70] Liu KS, Tsao SM, Yin MC. In vitro antibacterial activity of Roselle Calyx and Procatechuic acid. Phytotherapy Research. 2005;**19**(11):942-945. DOI: 10.1002/ptr.1760

[71] Afolabi OC, Ogunsola FT, Coker AO. Susceptibility of cariogenic *Streptococcus mutans* to extracts of *Garcinia kola*, *Hibiscus sabdariffa* and *Solanum americanu*. The West African Journal of Medicine. 2008;**27**(4):230-233

[72] Reanmongkol W, Itharat A. Antipyretic activity of the extracts of *Hibiscus sabdariffa* calyces L. in experimental animals. Songklanakarin Journal of Science and Technology. 2007;**29**(1):29-38

[73] Leung A, Foster S. Encyclopedia of Common Natural Ingredients Used in Food, Drugs, and Cosmetics. New York: John Wiley and Sons; 1996

[74] Scott CR, Jacobson H. A selection of international nutritional and herbal remedies for breastfeeding concerns. Midwifery Today with International Midwife. 2005;**75**:38-39

[75] Gaya IB, Mohammad OMA, Suleiman AM, Maje MI, Adekunle AB. Toxicological and lactogenic studies on the seeds of *Hibiscus sabdariffa* Linn (Malvaceae) extract on serum prolactin levels of albino Wistar rats. The Internet Journal of Endocrinology. 2009;**5**(2):1-6

[76] Turkyilmaz C, Onal E, Hirfanoglu IM, et al. The effect of galactagogue herbal tea on breast milk production and short-term catch-up of birth weight in the first week of life. Journal of Alternative and Complementary Medicine. 2011;**17**(1):39-42. DOI: 10.1089/acm.2010.0090

[77] Akindahunsi AA, Olaleye MT. Toxicological investigation of aqueous-methanolic extract of the calyces of *Hibiscus sabdariffa* L. Journal of Ethnopharmacology. 2003;**89**: 161-164. DOI: 10.1016/S0378-8741(03)00276-9

[78] Orisakwe OE, Husaini DC, Afonne OJ. Testicular effects of sub-chronic administration of *Hibiscus sabdariffa* calyx aqueous extract

in rats. Reproductive Toxicology. 2004;**18**:295-298. DOI: 10.1016/j.reprotox.2003.11.001

[79] Khaleequr R, Arshiya S, Shafeequr R. *Gossypium herbaceum* Linn: An ethnopharmacological review. Journal of Pharmaceutical and Scientific Innovation. 2016;**1**(5):1-5

[80] Ghani N. KhazianulAdvia. New Delhi: Idarae Kitabus Shifa; 2002. p. 339

[81] Kabiruddin M. Makhzul Mufredat. New Delhi: Idarae Kitabus Shifa; 2007. pp. 136-137

[82] Wang X, Howell CP, Chen F, Yin J, Jiang Y. Gossypol-A polyphenolic compound from cotton plant. Advances in Food and Nutrition Research. 2009;**58**:215-263. DOI: 10.1016/S1043-4526(09)58006-0

[83] Khalid MS, Hasan SK, Suresh DK, Hasan R, MAF S, Farooqui Z. Antiulcer activity of Ethanolic extract of *Gossypium herbaceum* flowers. Journal of Pharmaceutical Sciences. 2011;**1**(1):79-84

[84] Ofori DA. Genetic Diversity and its Implications for the Management and Conservation of Milicia Species [PhD thesis]. United Kingdom: University of Aberdeen; 2001. p. 158

[85] Udegbunam SO, Nnaji TO, Udegbunam RI, Okafor JC, Agbo I. Evaluation of herbal ointment formulation of *Milicia excelsa* (Welw) C.C berg for wound healing. African Journal of Biotechnology. 2013;**12**:3351-3359. DOI: 10.5897/AJB12.1201

[86] Dzeufiet PDD, Tchamadeu M, Bilanda DC, Ngadena YS, Poumeni MK, Nana D, et al. Preventive effect of *Milicia excelsa* (Moraceae) aqueous extract on dexamethasone induced insulin resistance in rat. Journal of Pharmacy & Pharmaceutical Sciences. 2014;**5**:1232-1241

[87] Betti JL. An ethnobotanical study of medicinal plants among the Baka pygmies in the DJA Biospher reserve, Cameroon. African Study Monographs. 2004;**25**(1):1-27

[88] Ouete JL, Sandjo LP, Kapche DW, Yeboah SO, Mapitse R, Abegaz BM. Excelsoside: A new benzylic diglycoside from the leaves of *Milicia excelsa*. Zeitschrift für Naturforschung. Section C. 2014;**69**(7-8): 271-275

[89] Akinpelu LA, Akanmu MA, Obuotor EM. Antipsychotic effects of ethanol leaf extract and fractions of *Milicia excelsa* (Moraceae) in mice. Journal of Pharmaceutical Research International. 2018;**22**(6):1-10

[90] Akpalo E, Tete-Benissan A, Awaga K, Akpagana K. Review of twelve west African medicinal plants: Active phytochemical combinations in direct biochemically wound healing process. Journal of Medicinal Plant Research. 2015;**9**(34):908-917

[91] Mawa S, Husain K, Jantan I. *Ficus carica* L. (Moraceae): Phytochemistry, traditional uses and biological activities. Evidence-based Complementary and Alternative Medicine. 2013;**2013**:974256. DOI: 10.1155/2013/974256

[92] Khare CP. Encyclopedia of Indian Medicinal Plants. New York: Springer publication; 2004

[93] Pattar J, Shridhar NB, Vijaykumar M, Krishna S, Satyanarayana, ML. Toxicological studies of ficus virens in wistar albino rats. International research journal of pharmacy. 2012;**3**(12): 84-87. DOI: 10.1186/s12944-015-0013-6

[94] Ghani A. Medicinal Plants of Bangladesh: Chemical Constituents and Uses. (Revised and Enlarged). Old Nimtali, Dhaka: Asiatic Society of Bangladesh; 2003. pp. 196-197

[95] Khare CP. Indian Medicinal Plants. Vol. 426. New York, USA: Springer Science+BusinessMedia; 2007

[96] Coe FG, Anderson GJ. Ethnobotany of the Sumu (Ulwa) of southeastern Nicaragua and comparisons with Miskitu plant loreLa EtnobotÁNica de los Sumu (Ulwa) del Sudeste de Nicaragua y Comparaciones con El saber BotÁNico De los Miskitus. Economic Botany. 1999;**54**(3):363-386

[97] Osim EE, Ibu JO. The effect of plantains (*Musa paradisiaca*) on DOCA-induced hypertension in rats. Pharmaceutical Biology. 1991;**29**(1):9-13

[98] Ojewole JAO, Adewunmi CO. Hypoglycemic effect of methanolic extract of *Musa paradisiaca* (Musaceae) green fruits in normal and diabetic mice. Methods and Findings in Experimental and Clinical Pharmacology. 2003;**25**(6):453-456

[99] Saraswathi NT, Gnanam FD. Effect of medicinal plants on the crystallization of cholesterol. Journal of Crystal Growth. 1997;**179**:611-617. DOI: 10.1016/S0022-0248(97)00172-3

[100] Parmar HS, Kar A. Protective role of *Citrus sinensis*, *Musa paradisiaca*, and *Punica granatum* peels against diet-induced atherosclerosis and thyroid dysfunctions in rats. Nutrition Research. 2007;**27**(11):710-718

[101] Mahmood A, Omar MN, Ngah N, Yahaya A. Galactagogue effects of *Musa paradisiaca* flower extract on lactating rats. Advances in Bioresearch. 2012;**3**(4):46-52

[102] Mahmood A, Omar MN, Ngarh N. Galactagogue effects of *Musa x paradisiaca* flower extract on lactating rats. Asian Pacific Journal of Tropical Medicine. 2012;**3**(4):882-886

[103] Dutta PK, Das AK, Banerji N. A tetracyclic triterpenoid from *Musa paradisiaca*. Phytochemistry. 1983;**22**(11):2563-2564

[104] Ahmad A, Husain A, Mujeeb M, Khan SA, Najmi AK, Siddique NA. A review on therapeutic potential of *Nigella sativa*: A miracle herb. Asian Pacific Journal of Tropical Biomedicine. 2013;**3**(5):337-352. DOI: 10.1016/S2221-1691(13)60075-1

[105] Paarakh PM. *Nigella sativa* Linn—A comprehensive review. Indian Journal of Natural Product and Resources. 2009;**1**(4):409-429

[106] Shafiq H, Ahmad A, Masud T, Kaleem M. Cardio-protective and anti-cancer therapeutic potential of *Nigella sativa*. Iranian Journal of Basic Medical Sciences. 2014;**17**(12):967-979

[107] Forouzanfar F, Bazzaz BSF, Hosseinzadeh H. Black cumin (*Nigella sativa*) and its constituent (Thymoquinone): A review on antimicrobial effects. Iranian Journal of Basic Medical Sciences. 2014;**17**(12):929-938

[108] Amin B, Hosseinzadeh H. Black cumin (*Nigella sativa*) and its active constituent, thymoquinone: An overview on the analgesic and anti-inflammatory effects. Planta Medica. 2015;**82**(1-2):8-16. DOI: 10.1055/s-0035-1557838

[109] Hosseinzadeh H, Eskandari M, Ziaee T. Antitussive effect of thymoquinone, a constituent of *Nigella sativa* seeds, in Guinea pigs. Pharmacology. 2008;**2**:480-484

[110] Jaiswal BS. *Solanum torvum*: A review of its traditional uses, phytochemistry and pharmacology. International Journal of Pharma and Bio Sciences. 2012;**3**(3):104-111

[111] Siemonsma J, Piluek K. Plant Resources of South-East Asia (PROSEA). Vol. 8. Indonesia: Bogor; 1994. p. 412

[112] Kala CP. Ethnomedicinal botany of the Apatani in the Eastern Himalayan region of Indian. Journal

of Ethnobiology and Ethnomedicine. 2005;**1**:1-8. DOI: 10.1186/1746-4269-1-11

[113] Sivapriya M, Srinivas L. Isolation and purification of a novel antioxidant protein from the water extract of Sundakai (*Solanum torvum*) seeds. Food Chemistry. 2007;**104**:510-517. DOI: 10.1016/j.foodchem.2006.11.060

[114] Mahmood U, Agrawal PK, Thakur RS, Torvonin AA. Spirostane Saponin from *Solanum torvum* Leaves. Phytochemistry. 1985;**24**(10):2456-2457. DOI: 10.1016/S0031-9422(00)83069-1

[115] Dickson RA, Amponsah IK, Annan K, Fleischer TC. Nutritive Potential of a Polyherbal Preparation from some Selected Ghanaian Herbs. 2014

[116] Achigan-Dako EG, Pasquini MW, Assogba Komlan F, N'danikou S, Yédomonhan H, Dansi A, et al. Traditional Vegetables in Benin. Cotonou: Institut National des Recherches Agricoles du Bénin, Imprimeries du CENAP; 2010

[117] Bassole IHN, Ouattara AS, Nebie R, Ouattara CAT, Kabore ZI, Traore SA. Chemical composition and antibacterial activities of the essential oils of *Lippia chevalieri* and *Lippia multiflora* from Burkina Faso. Phytochemistry. 2003;**62**(2): 209-212. DOI: 10.1016/S0031-9422(02)00477-6

[118] Brankov K, Hadzovic S, Erdeljan D. Efficiency of reactivators and spasmolytics after Amitone poisoning in vitro. Arhiv za Higijenu Rada i Toksikologiju. 1976;**27**(2):123-130

[119] Oladimeji FA, Orafidiya OO, Ogunniyi TAB, Adewunmi TA. Pediculocidal and scabicidal properties of *Lippia multiflora* essential oil. Journal of Ethnopharmacology. 2000;**72**(1-2):305-311. DOI: 10.1016/S0378-8741(00)00229-4

[120] Fernandez X, Pintaric C, Lizzani-Cuvelier L, Loiseau AM, Morello A, Pellerin P. Chemical composition of absolute and supercritical carbon dioxide extract of Afra*momum melegueta*. Flavour and Fragrance Journal. 2006;**21**(1):162-165

[121] Ajaiyeoba EO, Ekundayo O. Essential oil constituents of *Aframomum melegueta* (roscoe) K. Schum. Seeds (alligator pepper) from Nigeria. Flavour and Fragrance Journal. 1999;**14**(2):109-111

[122] Iwu MW, Duncan AR, Okunji CO. New antimicrobials of plant origin. In: Perspectives on New Crops and New Uses. Alexandria, VA: ASHS Press; 1999. pp. 457-462

[123] Ilic NM, Dey M, Poulev AA, Logendra S, Kuhn PE, Raskin I. Anti-inflammatory activity of grains of paradise (*Aframomum melegueta* Schum) extract. Journal of Agricultural and Food Chemistry. 2014;**62**(43):10452-10457

[124] Chung WY, Jung YJ, Surh YJ, Lee SS, Park KK. Antioxidative and antitumor promoting effects of [6]-Paradol and its homologs. Mutation Research/Genetic Toxicology and Environmental Mutagenesis. 2001;**496**(1):199-206

[125] Akpanabiatu MI, Ekpo ND, Ufot UF, Udoh NM, Akpan EJ, Etuk EU. Acute toxicity, biochemical and haematological study of *Aframomum melegueta* seed oil in male Wistar albino rats. Journal of Ethnopharmacology. 2013;**150**(2):590-594. DOI: 10.1016/j.jep.2013.09.006

[126] Okwu DE. Phytochemicals vitamins and mineral contents of two Nigerian medicinal plant. International Journal of Molecular Medicine and Advance Sciences. 2005;**1**(4):375-381

Chapter 5

Medicinal Plants Used by Indigenous Communities of Oaxaca, Mexico, to Treat Gastrointestinal Disorders

Mónica Lilian Pérez-Ochoa, José Luis Chávez-Servia, Araceli Minerva Vera-Guzmán, Elia Nora Aquino-Bolaños and José Cruz Carrillo-Rodríguez

Abstract

The use of medicinal plants for the treatment of gastrointestinal disorders and ethnodiseases such as diarrhea, stomachache, dysentery, "empacho" (blockage), and bile is a common strategy among indigenous communities. It is estimated that approximately 34% of medicinal plants are used to treat diseases of the digestive tract. In Mexico, gastrointestinal infections caused by bacteria, parasites, or viruses represent one of the main causes of death in children in rural populations. Our objective was to document the use of medicinal plants used by the indigenous groups of Oaxaca, Mexico, for the treatment of gastrointestinal disorders, based on previous studies, experiences, and field observations in indigenous communities and supplemented with bibliographic references. In Oaxaca, there are 16 indigenous groups, the largest being the speakers of the Zapoteco, Mixteco, Mazateco, Mixe, Chinanteco, Amuzgo, Tacuate, Chatino, and Cuicateco languages. In this review of the medicinal plants used for gastrointestinal disorders, 186 species were grouped into 147 genera and 71 botanical families, among which the largest number of species belonged to Asteraceae (29), Fabaceae (15), Euphorbiaceae (9), Solanaceae (9), and Lamiaceae (9). Different pharmacological studies showed potential for preventing microbial and fungal pathogens that cause gastrointestinal disease.

Keywords: ethnodiseases, bioculture, indigenous knowledge, plant diversity

1. Introduction

Medicinal plants are key elements of traditional medicine because they are part of the collection of knowledge and cultural heritage of sociocultural communities. Communities are often repositories and users of medicinal plants, and both rural and urban social groups with rural or indigenous origins have knowledge of these plants. Based on ethnobotanical, ethnomedicinal, and ethnopharmacological studies, the plants that are used by different healers and families of the Tarahumara, Yaqui, Chontal, Nahuatl, Mazahua, Otomi, Mixteco, Zapoteco, Mixe, Maya and Tzotzil groups, and all Mexican indigenous groups are symbolic [1].

In Mexico, gastrointestinal diseases are common in communities that are highly marginalized and poverty-stricken and are often transmitted through the fecal-oral route and the consumption of contaminated water and food. The infant population is the most vulnerable, both in terms of incidence and vulnerability [2]. In 2012, approximately 20% of the population of Chiapas, Guerrero, and Oaxaca did not have access to an adequate quality of water. This problem was exacerbated because only between 65 and 75% of houses have adequate waste management systems. Gastrointestinal diseases in children under 5 years of age directly affect mortality rates (19.2–19.4%) and mainly occur in marginalized communities [3]. These observations suggest that minimizing gastrointestinal diseases is dependent on the social environment of the community, access to clean water and food safety. As such, the symptoms and syndromes of diarrhea, stomachache, gastric atrophy, and enteric fever are associated with bacterial, fungal, parasitic, and rotavirus agents [2], and the frequency of these symptoms among children varies from community to community.

Medicinal plants are commonly used by communities for the treatment of gastrointestinal disorders through plant infusions, maceration, chewing, poultices, and different types of extracts (alcoholic or aqueous) [1]. Some studies have documented the traditional uses of medicinal plants by healers, their conservation, and their cultural importance in different indigenous groups [4–9]. Other studies have contributed ethnobotanical knowledge of medicinal plants [10–12]. The evaluation of phytochemical compounds with medicinal activity is also a subject of interest [13–16]. One aspect in which different authors have devoted a great amount of attention to is the antiparasitic and antimicrobial effects of medicinal plants for the treatment of diarrhea and other gastrointestinal disorders [17–25].

Research in natural products is often based on ethnobotanical information. One goal of ethnopharmacology is to improve the understanding of the pharmacological effects of plants on health, especially for indigenous communities that are highly marginalized and poverty-stricken. In this study, we examined plants used for the treatment of gastrointestinal disorders such as diarrhea, dysentery, and abdominal pain. The objective of this work was to document the use of medicinal plants used by the indigenous groups of Oaxaca, Mexico for the treatment of gastrointestinal disorders, based on previous unreported studies, experiences, and field observations in indigenous communities. Our results are supplemented with bibliographic reviews.

2. Sociocultural and ethnographic context of Oaxaca, Mexico

Mexico has an indigenous population of 12.25 million (10.1% of the total), of which 7.38 million speak an indigenous language [26]. It is estimated that there are 1.2 million speakers in Oaxaca over 3 years of age that speak an indigenous language. Oaxaca is the state with the largest indigenous population (32.2% of its total population) and has 245 municipalities where more than 40% of the population speaks indigenous languages [26–28]. However, in Mexico, 24.4 million people consider themselves indigenous [26, 29], a figure that is higher than the total number of inhabitants of several European countries and is of great importance in the preservation of culture, biodiversity, and biocultural heritage. Indigenous peoples are also associated with the use of medicinal plants.

Based on the vegetation, ecosystem, biome, and indigenous settlement maps, Toledo et al. [30] identified 26 indigenous regions in Mexico. These regions coincide with the zones of greatest biodiversity and pluriculturality or indigenous settlements and are also where protected natural areas are located. In Oaxaca, eight indigenous regions were identified: Mixteca, Cañada, Papaloapan, Sierra Norte, Istmo, Costa, Sierra Sur, and Valles Centrales Different indigenous communities can be found in each of these regions. The Mixteca region is dominated by the Mixteco, Triqui, Chocho and Nahuatl groups, the Cañada by the Cuicateco and Mazateco groups, and so on. The topography of the mountainous areas and valleys of Oaxaca is rugged, with contrasting climates ranging from humid temperate at 2000–3000 masl, to temperate to subtemperate in intermediate zones from 1000 to 2000 masl, to tropical and subtropical regions (<1000 masl) [31]. Thus, indigenous communities are located in various climates, altitudes and vegetation, and consequently have access to and knowledge of different medicinal plants. We should note that among Oaxaca indigenous regions, the differences are not extreme in terms of climatic conditions, flora, fauna, topography, crops, handicrafts, and the use of traditional medicinal plants (**Table 1**); however, there are sociocultural differences in the knowledge associated with the use of plants for treating ethnodiseases and diseases with clinical diagnoses.

Among indigenous communities from distant ethnic regions and origins, and occupying different geographical territories, the use of plants for the treatment of gastrointestinal disorders is different, even though the symbolic or cosmological meanings may be the same. Thus, there is similar understanding of how plants are

Indigenous region (n[1])	Main indigenous groups	Climate and precipitations	Altitude (m)
Mixteca (155)	Mixtecos, Triquis, Nahuas	Tropical subhumid, semitropical subhumid to temperate subhumid, annual precipitation from 550 to 2177 mm. Includes a semi-dry region	1200–2800
Cañada (45)	Mazatecos, Cuicatecos, Ixcatecos, Nahuas	Semidesert with variations of very warm, semiwarm and temperate in high areas, annual precipitation from 372.8 to 643.7 mm	1180–2700
Papaloapan (20)	Chinantecos, Zapotecos, Mazatecos, Mixes	Tropical humid, semitropical humid to humid temperate, and precipitation from 2000 to 4500 mm. The rainiest region of Oaxaca	0–2000
Sierra Norte (68)	Zapotecos de la Sierra, Mixes, Chinantecos, Mazatecos, Cuicatecos	Tropical subhumid, semitropical subhumid to temperate subhumid, annual precipitation from 1000 to 3000 mm	1000–3200
Valles Centrales (121)	Zapotecos de Valles, Mixtecos, Mixes	Subtropical to semidry, annual precipitation from 600 to 800 mm	1000–2000
Istmo (41)	Zapotecos, Huaves, Zoques, Chontales	Tropical subhumid to semitropical subhumid, annual precipitation from 800 to 2500 mm.	0–1600
Sierra Sur (70)	Zapotecos de la Sierra Sur, Amuzgos, Mixtecos, Chatinos, Triquis	Tropical subhumid, semitropical subhumid to humid temperate, annual precipitation from 800 to 2000 mm	1000–2600
Costa (50)	Zapotecos de la Costa, Mixtecos, Amuzgos, Chatinos, Chontales	Tropical subhumid, semitropical subhumid to temperate, delimited region by Sierra Madre del Sur, annual precipitation from 731.9 to 2050 mm	0–2000

[1]*Number of municipalities; sources: Arellanes et al. [31].*

Table 1.
Ecogeographic descriptions of eight indigenous regions of Oaxaca, Mexico.

used to treat stomach, intestinal, diarrhea, or psychosomatic diseases (e.g., "susto" (fright), stomachaches, "mal aire" (bad air) with vomiting, and "empacho" (blockage), but the species of plant used, form of use, and application differ significantly between ethnic groups. In severe cases of illness, indigenous peoples resort to the community healers or alternate among medical professionals, pharmaceutical medicine, and the use of medicinal plants recommended by the family or healers [32, 33].

3. Relationship between indigenous groups and endemic medicinal plants used for gastrointestinal disorders

Among rural and indigenous communities, the concept of health and disease is holistic. As such, the human body develops its organic and metabolic functions without physical deterioration and includes mental, mystical-spiritual, and psychological aspects (symbolic reality). Social, cultural, and ethnic concepts are implicit in the perceptions of health and disease, and based on these concepts, the healing-therapeutic benefits of medicinal plants are sought. From the indigenous perspective, the causal explanations of illness are complex. The body suffers symptomatic imbalances resulting from physical, emotional, or mental deterioration, which are consequences of "susto" (fright), anger, interpersonal conflicts, cold currents, harmful foods (cold, hot, types of meat, cravings, etc.), sexual relations, witchcraft, etc. [34–38]. Consequently, the factors that produce imbalances in the body, in this case stomach problems, are to be avoided.

The knowledge and use of medicinal plants in indigenous communities is changing due to the introduction of pharmaceutical products recommended by health professionals. Giovannini et al. [39] note two trends in support of this fact: the complete displacement of medicinal plants by pharmaceutical products and the coexistence between clinical medicine and the use of medicinal plants. Thus far, local indigenous knowledge for the treatment of cardiovascular diseases, cancers, diabetes, and other prevalent diseases has been disseminated, which is why patent medicine is used. However, there are some examples of healing via the use of medicinal plants. In cases of chronic diarrhea caused by pathogens, the use of plants has been beneficial, such as plants used to treat diarrhea caused by *Salmonella* spp. [24]. In Oaxaca, acute diarrhea and acute respiratory infections are the main causes of mortality in children under 5 years of age [40].

The prevalence among Oaxacan children of microbial or parasitic gastrointestinal diseases, which cause acute diarrhea and other problems, has forced communities to resort to medicinal plants. Consequently, under these circumstances, there is a set of common species among indigenous communities that are used similarly, provided that their ecological conditions are also similar. It should also be noted that knowledge may be treated differently between different ethnic communities, especially when faced with common health problems. For example, the Mixe, Mixteco, and Zapoteco groups of the Sierras, located in temperate regions, commonly use *Chenopodium graveolens*, *Lantana achyranthifolia*, *Baccharis salicifolia*, and *Miconia mexicana*, although the local names used by each region are different. Additionally, the Chinanteco groups and Zapoteco of the Istmo use similar plant species (**Table 2**).

3.1 Healers and medicinal plants

Within Oaxacan indigenous groups, the healers play essential roles as therapists or ethnopractitioners and are not referred to as shamans, witch doctors, or herbalists. Here, we only refer to the cures or treatments using plants recommended by healers for the treatment of gastrointestinal disorders. The indigenous healers have

Indigenous group (climate at the communities)	Species	Spanish name	References
Mixtecos, Mixe, Zapotecos de las Sierras (temperate)	*Chenopodium graveolens* Willd.	Epazote de zorrillo	[14, 17]
Mixtecos, Mixe, Zapotecos de las Sierras (temperate)	*Lantana achyranthifolia* Desf.	Cinco negritos, Hierba mariposa	[8, 16]
Mixtecos, Mixe, Zapotecos de las Sierras (temperate)	*Baccharis salicifolia* (Ruiz & Pavón) Pers.	Jara, cacho de venado	[1, 4, 5, 13]
Mixtecos, Mixe, Zapotecos de las Sierras (temperate)	*Miconia mexicana* (Bonpl.) Naudin	Itswa	[21]
Mixe, Mixtecos (temperate)	*Loeselia mexicana* (Lam.) Brand.	Espinosilla	[21, 41]
Chinantecos, Zapotecos del Istmo (tropical and subtropical)	*Gomphrena serrata* L.	Cabezona, amor seco, amor de soltero	[1, 42, 43]
Chinantecos, Zapotecos del Istmo (tropical and subtropical)	*Byrsonima crassifolia* (L.) Kunth	Nanche amarillo (corteza)	[6, 14, 24, 41]
Chinantecos, Zapotecos del Istmo (tropical and subtropical)	*Cuphea pinetorum* Benth.	Cenicilla, Hierba de gallina	[18, 25]
Chinantecos, Mixe, Zapotecos del Istmo (tropical and subtropical)	*Gouania lupuloides* (L.) Urb.	Bejuco de reuma	[17, 44, 45]

Table 2.
Common plants used by indigenous groups for the treatment of gastrointestinal disorders in Oaxaca, Mexico.

social recognition in the communities as persons of knowledge, skills, and healing practices. These healers have the facilities to explain the physical and nonphysical causes of diseases through a symbolic, verbal and corporal language, and resort to deities to exercise healing techniques. The body of knowledge is a legacy inherited or acquired from their ethnic medical culture and becomes a depository with the capacity to incorporate medical experiences regarding the descriptions of diseases, anatomy, and physiology of the human body [1, 34, 38, 46, 47].

The healer's diagnosis is based on the spirit, soul, and body, which are closely interconnected, to define health and disease. In Oaxacan communities, Mixe and Mazateco healers use psychotropic or hallucinogenic plants and mushrooms for successful diagnoses and healing. These hallucinogens are used as a mechanism to access supernatural forces and as interlocutors to ward off malignant agents [34, 46, 47]. The remedies or treatments recommended by healers for gastrointestinal problems vary from diets, teas, maceration or poultices of medicinal plants, changes in eating habits such as avoiding foods considered "hot" or "cold," avoiding animals or people, sun exposure, or environmental changes in temperature, such as avoiding cold water, etc.

María Sabina was a well-known healer among the Mazateco Indians of the Sierra de Huautla de Jiménez in Oaxaca and throughout Mexico. After her death, she was recognized as a symbolic character of the Mexican healers. She used mushrooms (e.g., *Psilocybe zapotecorum and Psilocybe mexicana*) and hallucinogenic plants (e.g., *Salvia divinorum*) to obtain divine powers both to diagnose and to restore the health of the patient. In the case of gastrointestinal diseases, all recommendations are preventive/curative and are accompanied by psychospiritual rituals of protection, reintegration, and cleanliness of the soul. She is known to have said, "The health services provided by healers and Western medicine should not be lucrative," [48, 49].

3.2 Plants used in indigenous communities for the treatment of gastrointestinal disorders

Medicinal plants are essential natural resources in the indigenous communities of Oaxaca, Mexico; they are easily accessible and there is a high diversity of species and forms of use for the treatment of diseases of the digestive tract. The region has the greatest level of diversity and endemism of species of phytotherapeutic use [50]. Based on a bibliographical compilation and field notes of visits to the indigenous communities of Oaxaca, a short list of medicinal plants used for gastrointestinal disorders was obtained (**Table 1A**). The compilation consists of 71 botanical families, among which the greatest number of species is in the families Asteraceae (29), Fabaceae (15), Euphorbiaceae (9), Solanaceae (9), Lamiaceae (9), Verbenaceae (6), Myrtaceae (5), Malvaceae (5), and Fagaceae (5). These families included 147 genera and 186 endemic species [50]. The genera used most frequently were *Croton* (5), *Quercus* (4), *Piper* (4), *Psidium* (3), *Ocimum* (3), and *Tagetes* (3). The medicinal species introduced to Mexico were excluded from this list, despite being widely used by Oaxacan indigenous groups.

Among indigenous communities, plants are grouped according to gastrointestinal physiological alterations, among which the most common refer to diarrhea (112 plants), stomach pain (90 plants), and dysentery (79 plants). Acute diarrhea is a symptom of gastrointestinal tract infection, which is commonly caused by pathogenic bacteria (e.g., *Escherichia coli*, *Salmonella* spp., *Vibrio cholerae*, *Clostridium perfringens*, *Bacillus cereus*, *Staphylococcus aureus*, *Vibrio parahaemolyticus*, *Campylobacter jejuni, Campylobacter coli, Shigella* spp., *and Aeromonas* spp.*)*, viruses (rotavirus, adenovirus, enterovirus, and norovirus), or parasites (*Giardia lamblia* and *Entamoeba histolytica)* and is frequently accompanied by abdominal pain, stomach pain, fever, and vomiting [51]. For the treatment of vomiting, constipation and parasites, between 28 and 31 plant species are used. For the condition known locally as "empacho" (gastrointestinal disease) as well as for indigestion, ulcers and gastritis, between 17 and 39 species are utilized (**Table 1A**). It is important to note that we refer to the local descriptions of symptoms and the disease names that are used by Oaxacan indigenous communities.

The indigenous knowledge of medicinal plants includes the different phases of use, correct identification of the species (although they do not have systematic botanical studies), wild or cultivated origin, collection time (morning, noon, afternoon, or night), plant part to be used, and processing required for use. Each of these elements affects the effectiveness of the plant [8, 17, 51]. The leaves, stems and flowers are the most used parts, and the bark, roots and seeds are used less often (**Table 1A**). The form of use or extraction preparation ranges from infusion and cooking in water, maceration in ethyl alcohol (*Dorstenia drakena* L. and *Barkleyanthus salicifolius* (Kunth) H. Rob. & Brettell) or cane alcohol (*Saccharum officinarum* L.) and consumed as tea (oral), or as a topical application between the stomach and intestines. Additionally, the fresh crushed leaves or leaves macerated in ethyl alcohol can be ingested or applied topically (rubbed onto the affected part). Plants for treating dysentery are used as purgatives or for treating constipation as rectal washes and include *Eryngium foetidum* L., *Capraria biflora* L., *Prosopis laevigata*, and *Solanum rostratum* Dunal (**Table 1A**).

Bark is often cooked or used as an infusion in hot or cold water; it is a common treatment for diarrhea, dysentery and related symptoms. The bark of *Semialarium mexicanum* (Miers) Mennega, *Hymenaea courbaril* L., *Quercus oleoides, Hintonia latiflora*, and *Guaiacum coulteri* is used to treat ulcers or gastritis, and the bark of *Amphipterygium adstringens* is used to treat stomach cancer. The roots of some plants have shown to be beneficial to treat diarrhea, stomach pain, and intestinal infection. In addition, the use of fruits and seeds to treat diarrhea, dysentery, constipation, and "empacho" is mentioned. For example, the fruits and seeds of the chili pepper (*Capsicum annuum* L.) are used for the treatment of dyspepsia (inflammation of the digestive tract), diarrhea, and dysentery. An infusion of guava leaves and roots (*Psidium* spp.) is used to treat diarrhea, dysentery, stomach pain, flatulence, and vomiting. The peel of the fruits of *Curatella americana* L. and *Persea americana* Mill. and the stigmas of the corn flower (*Zea mays* L.) are made into an infusion to treat stomachaches. The seeds of *Carica papaya* L. are used to treat diarrhea, vomiting, fever, intestinal inflammation, and parasites (**Table 1A**).

"Empacho" is a digestive ethnodisease recognized by traditional Mexican people. This disorder primarily occurs in children and does not correspond to a specific clinical diagnosis, but is culturally recognized in all Mexican rural communities. Empacho is characterized by discomfort caused by the intake of food that is difficult to unfold, and the healer or mother of the child indicates that food is "stuck" to the stomach or intestine. Symptoms include abdominal pain, lack of appetite, diarrhea, flatulence, and vomiting. The treatment includes the use of ash- or salt-containing oral plant infusions, purgatives, and massages [52]. Some traditional treatments recommend infusions made from the bark and/or leaves of *Guazuma ulmifolia* Lam. complemented with spoonful of castor oil and massages (sobadas) that "release the empacho" [53].

Another ethnodisease associated with gastrointestinal disorders is "bile or bile leakage." The healer and adults report "pounding" (vibrations) from an area near the stomach, which is accompanied by pain in the esophagus. Symptoms include loss of appetite, headache, feeling of "bitterness" in the mouth upon waking up, and fatigue. *Pseudognaphalium attenuatum* DC., *Agastache mexicana* spp. Xolocotziana, *Hintonia latiflora*, *Loeselia mexicana*, *Tecoma stans*, *Zornia thymifolia*, *Anoda cristata*, *Oenothera rosea*, *Verbena litoralis*, and *Calea ternifolia* var. *Ternifolia* are used to treat bile (**Table 1A**). For gastrointestinal intestinal disorders in children, *Psidium guajava*, *Byrsonima crassifolia*, and *Quercus* spp. are used [53]. Mixe communities use fruit and bark infusions of *G. ulmifolia* to treat diarrhea and hemorrhages [14], whereas *Cestrum nocturnum* is used among the Zapotecas from the southern highlands and the Chinantecos of Oaxaca [53, 54].

Several studies have shown the importance of flavonoids, tannins, terpenoids, and alkaloids present in medicinal plants used for the treatment of gastrointestinal diseases. Other mechanisms of action include antispasmodic activity, delaying of intestinal transit, suppression of intestinal motility, stimulation of the adsorption of water, and a reduction in the secretion of electrolytes [20]. The compounds most frequently reported are terpenoids (monoterpenes, sesquiterpenes, di-, and triterpenes), flavonoids (flavones, flavonols), tannins (condensed and hydrolysable), and volatile compounds, which are derived from the essential oils in aromatic plants.

Root extracts of *Tagetes erecta* have shown to have high efficacy against Gram-positive bacteria (*Staphylococcus aureus*, *Bacillus subtilis*, and *Micrococcus luteus*), Gram-negative bacteria (*Escherichia coli* and *Pseudomonas aeruginosa*), and fungi (*Candida albicans* and *Aspergillus niger*). Flowers of *T. erecta* have been shown to contain thiophene derivatives, terpenoids, alkaloids, flavonoids, and carotenoids [55]. Similarly, methanol extracts of *Tagetes lucida* yielded coumarins with high antimicrobial activity against Gram-positive and Gram-negative bacterial strains, with greater inhibition of *V. cholerae* as well as antifungal activity. The antifungal activity of *T. lucida* results from the presence of dimethoxy: 6,7-dimethoxy-4-methylcoumarin and scoparone (6,7-dimethoxycoumarin) [56] and is effective against *Helicobacter pylori* [57]. In traditional Oaxacan medicine, the anthelminthic effects of *Chenopodium ambrosioides* (epazote) along with the epimastigotes of *Trypanosoma cruzi* have demonstrated efficacy against *Entamoeba histolytica* infections due to the effect of limonene [58].

4. Antipathogenic efficacy of medicinal plants

A natural question about the use of medicinal plants for treating gastrointestinal disorders is: how effective are the uses of plants in controlling or preventing infections by pathogenic agents? Several in vitro studies have been conducted that aimed to evaluate the biological activity of plant extracts against enteropathogenic bacteria (*Escherichia coli, Shigella sonnei, Shigella flexneri, Salmonella, and Campylobacter*) and parasites (*Giardia lamblia and Entamoeba histolytica*) responsible for diarrhea, dysentery and/or gastric disorders [59–61]. Several chemical compounds (alkaloids, tannins, flavonoids, and terpenes) responsible for the pharmacological effects of these plants have been identified and isolated [62, 63]. Examples of biological activity of native plants of Oaxaca, Mexico, used for the prevention and control of gastrointestinal disorders are listed in **Table 3**.

The experiences in the communities of Oaxaca indicate that the roots and aerial parts of *Geranium mexicanum* Kunth and the flowers of *Chiranthodendron pentadactylon* are effective to treat diarrhea, dysentery, and stomach pain (**Table 3**). The methanolic or aqueous extracts of these plants showed high antibacterial activity against *Shigella flexneri* and *Shigella sonnei* at minimum inhibitory concentrations of 8 mg/mL. Both extracts can be considered an alternative strategy to treat enteric pathogens resistant to common drugs [60]. In biological experiments using mice, it was demonstrated that the molecule (−)-epicatechin, which is isolated from *Geranium mexicanum*, has high antiprotozoal activity (*Giardia lamblia*) in concentrations of 0.072 μmol/kg, which is the dose required to kill 50% of microorganisms [59].

Calzada et al. [69], found that (−)-epicatechin and tiliroside, isolated from extracts of *C. pentadactylon* flowers, were effective against *E. histolytica, G. lamblia, E. coli, S. sonnei, S. flexneri, Salmonella* sp., and *Vibrio cholerae*. In another work, Calzada et al. [11] determined that root extracts of *G. mexicanum* had a greater hyperperistaltic effect than the extracts of *Lygodium venustum*, *Chenopodium ambrosoides*, and *C. pentadactylon*, which was similar to the effect of the drug loperamide, which is used to control acute and constant diarrhea associated with intestinal inflammation. In experiments with mice, the methanolic extracts of *G. mexicanum*, *Bocconia frutescens*, and *C. pentadactylon* in a concentration of 300 mg/kg of body weight had high inhibitory or intestinal antisecretory activity against *V. cholerae*. The activity of these extracts exceeds the effect of the drug loperamide [72]. A similar effect was determined with extracts of *C. pentadactylon* flowers [73]. *B. frutescens* also showed inhibitory activity against *S. aureus* and *E. coli* [60]. These results show that *G. mexicanum, C. pentadactylon*, and *B. frutescens* have medicinal properties and are effective for the treatment of diarrhea, among other gastrointestinal problems (**Table 3**).

The methanolic extracts *Ocimum basilicum* and *Artemisia ludoviciana* have inhibitory effects against *V. cholerae*, and the minimum bactericidal concentration varies from 0.5 to 3.0 mg/mL. The extracts have a degradative effect on the cellular membranes of *V. cholerae*, which increases membrane permeability, decreases cytoplasmic pH, hyperpolarizes the membrane, decreases the cellular ATP concentration, and consequently causes cell death [65]. This result indicates a chemical modification of the growth medium and induction of the death of the pathogen. For example, Hussain et al. [62] reported that basil contains essential oils (linalool, epi-α-cadinol, α-bergamotene, and γ-cadinene) that exert antimicrobial activity against *S. aureus* and *B. subtilis*. Similarly, the essential oil of *A. ludoviciana* contains camphor, 1,8-cineole, and camphene, which were effective against *Acanthamoeba castellanii*, *Leishmania infantum,* and *Trichomonas vaginalis* [66].

Plant species	Gastro-intestinal disorders (parts[1])	Chemical compounds	Antimicrobial activity	References
Ambrosia artemisiifolia L.	Stomachache and intestinal parasites (All)	Isabelin (germacranolide sesquiterpene dilactone)	*S. aureus* *C. albicans*	[64]
Artemisia ludoviciana Nutt	Chronic active gastritis and peptic ulcer (St, L)	Camphor, 1,8-cineole and camphene, sesquiterpene lactones, and flavonoids	*V. cholerae* *H. pylori* *A. castellanii,* *L. infantum* *T. vaginalis*	[57, 65–67]
Geranium mexicanum Kunth	Diarrhea, dysentery, and stomachache (R, St, L)	(−)-Epicatechin	*S. flexneri* *S. sonnei,* *E. histolytica* *G. lamblia*	[59–61]
Ocimum basilicum	Diarrhea, dysentery, stomachache and vomit (St, L)	Linalool, epi-α-cadinol, α-bergamotene, and γ-cadinene	*V. cholerae* *S. aureus* and *B. subtilis*	[62, 65]
Lantana achyranthifolia Desf.	Gastro-intestinal disease (AP)	Carvacrol, isocaryophyllene, α-bisabolol, bisabolene, and 1,8-cineole	*V. cholerae,* *S. boydii,* *Y. enterocolitica* *F. moniliforme*	[8, 68]
Chiranthodendron pentadactylon	Antimicrobial and antidiarrheal activities (F)	Epicatechin and tiliroside	*S. flexneri* *S. sonnei* *E. histolytica* *G. lamblia* *E. coli* *Salmonella* spp. *V. cholerae.*	[60, 69]
Anoda cristata	Stomachache (L)	Acacetin and diosmetin	*H. pylori*	[63, 70]
Bocconia frutescens	Diarrhea, dysentery stomachache ulcers (L)		*E. coli* and *S. aureus.*	[63]
Lippia graveolens H.B.K.	Diarrhea, dysentery, indigestion (AP)	Carvacrol, α-terpinyl acetate, m-cymene, and thymol	*R. solani* *E. coli* *P. aeruginosa* *S. aureus*	[68, 71]
Guaiacum coulteri A. Gray	Chronic active gastritis and peptic ulcer (OB)	Alkaloids	*Helicobacter pylori*	[57]

[1]All, all parts; AP, aerial parts; L, leaf; St, stem; and OB, outer bark.

Table 3.
Antimicrobial activity of native medicinal plants of Oaxaca, Mexico.

Aqueous extracts of *A. ludoviciana ssp. Mexicana* and methanolic extracts of *Guaiacum coulteri* showed high growth inhibitory activity against *Helicobacter pylori* at minimum inhibitory concentrations of 125 and < 15.6 μg/mL, respectively [57].

H. pylori is the etiological agent of chronic active gastritis and peptic ulcer and is related to gastric carcinoma. It was also shown that *A. ludoviciana* has activity against *Campylobacter jejuni* and *C. coli* at minimum bactericidal concentrations of 0.5 mg/mL [74]. Ruiz-Cancino et al. [67] determined that the sesquiterpene lactones (douglanin, ludovicin A, 1α, 3α-dihydroxyarbusculin B, santamarin, arglanin, artemorin, chrysartemin B, armefolin, ridentin, eudesmanolide 3α-hydroxyreynosin, etc.) and flavonoids (eupatilin and jaceosidin) of *A. ludoviciana* spp. *mexicana* are the molecules responsible for the inhibitory properties against the nuclear transcription factor kappa B, NF-κB [14]. NF-κB is involved in critical mechanisms related to the development of cancer. The signaling cascades of NF-κB may be the main malignant gastrointestinal mediators that favor esophageal, gastric, and colon cancer [75].

The essential oils of *Lantana achyranthifolia* consist of monoterpenes and sesquiterpenes (carvacrol, isocaryophyllene, α-bisabolol, α-bisabolene, and 1,8-cineole), have antibacterial activities against Gram-positive and Gram-negative bacteria, *V. cholerae, Shigella boydii*, and *Yersinia enterocolitica* [76]. The antibacterial activity results from the compounds carvacrol, 1,8-cineole and linalool [77]. The essential oils of *L. achyranthifolia* and *Lippia graveolens* have antifungal activity [68] and contain carvacrol, α-terpinyl acetate, β-caryophyllene, geranyl acetate, terpinyl acetate, bornyl acetate, and limonene [77, 78]. More research is required on other medicinal species with similar potential.

The extracts of *Cnidoscolus aconitifolius*, *Crotalaria pumila*, and *Anoda cristata* (**Table 3**) inhibit bacterial growth. The flavonoids acacetin and diosmetin from *A. cristata* have been shown to inhibit up to 90% of *H. pylori* growth. These data suggest that, through the use of nutraceutical food plants, *H. pylori* infections can be prevented [70]. *Ambrosia artemisiifolia* L. is used to treat stomach pain and contains isabelin, a germacranolide sesquiterpene dilactone with antimicrobial activity against *S. aureus* and *Candida albicans* [64].

5. Remarks

Medicinal plants continue to play an indispensable role in the daily life of rural and urban communities. However, their use is controversial, and they are often only used in teas or hot drinks; they are not associated with healing properties. Through interactions with the indigenous communities of Oaxaca, Mexico, it was found that all households use the inherited knowledge of medicinal plants. In the regions furthest from the urban centers where the hospitals are located, medicinal plants are part of the survival strategy.

In the communities of Oaxaca and other regions of Mexico, healers (the generic name for traditional practitioners) are called "yerberos" (herbalists) because they only use plants. The consultation or intervention of the healers occurs when the symptoms of the disease or ethnodisease continue after the patient takes the "remedies" (teas, crushed, chewed, potions, etc.), which are prepared by the adults of the family. We define ethnodisease as a disorder that has no somatic symptoms, description of organic or metabolic dysfunction, or association with clinical symptomatology. Thus, "empacho" is often associated with indigestion, but has a broader sociocultural description than a gastroenterological disorder.

Based on our field notes and previous documentation of the indigenous communities in Oaxaca, Mexico, as well as our bibliography, a brief list of medicinal plants used for gastrointestinal disorders was compiled. This list comprises 71 botanical families, among which the most speciose were Asteraceae (29), Fabaceae (15), Euphorbiaceae (9), Solanaceae (9), Lamiaceae (9), Verbenaceae (6), Myrtaceae (5),

Malvaceae (5), and Fagaceae (5). The families included 147 genera and 186 endemic species. The most frequently used genera were *Croton* (5), *Quercus* (4), *Piper* (4), *Psidium* (3), *Ocimum* (3), and *Tagetes* (3) (**Table 1A**). The medicinal species introduced to Mexico were excluded from this list, despite being widely used by Oaxacan indigenous groups.

The use of antibiotics for infectious gastrointestinal diseases is unconscionable among the users of pharmacological medicine and has generated collateral damage, including antibiotic resistance of pathogenic microorganisms. Cases of antibiotic resistance are increasingly frequent, and thus, medicinal plants will fill an important niche once their antibacterial, antiprotozoal, antisecretory, spasmolytic, and anti-inflammatory protective effects are demonstrated. In addition to these benefits, antiradical and antioxidant activity effective against gastroenterological disorders have been shown after the frequent consumption of teas. Advances have been made in the knowledge of antipathogenic effects of medicinal plants and their association with specific compounds. However, not all plants used by the indigenous groups of Mexico and Latin America are being studied and documented.

Acknowledgements

The authors are grateful for the financial support provided by the Instituto Politecnico Nacional (project nos. 1922 and 20181030).

A. Appendix

Family/ species[1]	Gastrointestinal disorders (used parts[2])	Bioactive compounds	References
Acanthaceae			
Justicia spicigera Schltdl.	Stomachache, diarrhea, dysentery, nausea, cramps (L, St, F)	Phenolics, flavonoids, lignans	[14, 17, 51, 53, 79–81]
Amaranthaceae			
Dysphania ambrosioides (L.)	Diarrhea, vomiting, stomach pain and inflammation, parasites (AP, L)	Terpenoids, flavonoids	[4, 11, 53, 54, 60, 82–85]
Dysphania graveolens (Willd.) Mosyakin & Clemants	Stomach pain, diarrhea, parasites, dysentery, indigestion, *empacho*, vomiting (AP)	Terpenoids, flavonoids	[17, 53, 57, 86]
Anacardiaceae			
Amphipterygium adstringens (Schltdl.) Standl.	Ulcers, stomach cancer, gastritis, stomach pain, intestinal infection, and inflammation (Se, St, Bark)	Triterpenes, phenolic, lipids	[41, 53, 57, 87, 88]
Spondias mombin L.	Diarrhea, stomach pain, dysentery, *empacho* (OB)	Phenols, flavonoids, saponins	[53, 89–91]
Spondias purpurea L.	Diarrhea in children (OB, R)	Phenols, flavonoids, tannins, phenolic acid derivatives, terpenoids	[14, 17, 41, 92, 93]

Family/ species[1]	Gastrointestinal disorders (used parts[2])	Bioactive compounds	References
Annonaceae			
Annona glabra L.	Dysentery, diarrhea (R, L, Sh)	Flavonoids, diterpenoids	[53, 94, 95]
A. reticulata L.	Diarrhea, stomach pain, intestinal pain (bark, L, Sh)	Acetogenins, terpenoids, alkaloids, phenols	[14, 53, 92, 96–100]
Apiaceae			
Donnellsmithia juncea (Spreng.) Mathias & Constance	Diarrhea, vomiting (All)		[53]
Eryngium foetidum L.	Diarrhea, dysentery, stomach pain (L)	Tannins, saponins, terpenoids, flavonoids, phenols, eryngial	[53, 54, 92, 101–103]
Apocynaceae			
Plumeria rubra L.	Intestinal parasites, diarrhea, purgative (Steam latex)	Terpenoids, iridoids, phenols, flavonoids	[53, 104, 105]
Thevetia ahouai (L.) A. DC.	Ulcers, purgative (All)	Cardenolide glycosides	[53, 106]
Araceae			
Anthurium schlechtendalii Kunth ssp. Jimenezii	Diarrhea (All)		[92]
A. schlechtendalii Kunth ssp. Schlechtendalii	Diarrhea (All)		[92]
Aristolochiaceae			
Aristolochia leuconeura Linden	Diarrhea, colics (All)		[84]
Asclepiadaceae			
Asclepias curassavica L.	Intestinal parasites, purgative (AP)	Cardenolides, glycosides, protease	[14, 92, 107]
Asteraceae			
Ageratum conyzoides L.	Stomach pain (All)	Terpenoids, flavonoids, benzofuranes, and coumarins	[92, 108, 109]
Ambrosia artemisiifolia L.	Stomach pain, intestinal parasites (L)	Terpenoids, sterols	[53]
Artemisia ludoviciana ssp. mexicana Nutt.	Stomach pain, vomiting, dysentery, colic, parasites, indigestion, diarrhea, flatulence (L, St)	Sesquiterpene lactones, flavonoids	[4–6, 10, 11, 14, 53, 57, 60, 67, 72, 84]
Baccharis conferta Kunth	Diarrhea, vomiting, indigestion, colic, and stomach pain (All)	Flavonoids, terpenoids	[10, 41, 43, 53, 110]
B. salicifolia (Ruiz & Pav.) Pers.	Stomach infection, stomach pain; diarrhea, dysentery (All)	Flavonoids, terpenoids	[5, 9, 13, 53]
Barkleyanthus salicifolius (Kunth) H. Rob. & Brettell	Vomiting, diarrhea, fever (St, L)	Terpenoids, alkaloids, flavonoids	[9, 53, 111]

Family/ species[1]	Gastrointestinal disorders (used parts[2])	Bioactive compounds	References
Bidens pilosa L.	Diarrhea, vomiting, stomach pain, and inflammation, ulcers (F, L, B)	Terpenoids	[53, 112]
Calea ternifolia Kunth var. *ternifolia*	Stomach pain, diarrhea, indigestion, malaria, *bilis* (L)	Terpenoids	[10, 53, 113]
C. urticifolia (Miller) DC.	Dysentery, diarrhea, malaria, stomach pain, heartburn (All)	Terpenoids	[14, 17, 53, 92, 113]
Chaptalia nutans L. Pollak	Dysentery, intestinal parasites (R, L, St)	7-O-beta-D-glucopyranosyl-nutanocoumarin	[17, 41, 53, 114]
Chrysactinia mexicana A. Gray	Diarrhea, dysentery, colic (AP)	Terpenoids	[11, 53, 60, 115–117]
Dyssodia papposa (Vent.) Hitchc.	Diarrhea, stomach pain, vomiting (All)		[53]
Heterotheca inuloides Cass	Gastritis, ulcers (AP)	Terpenoids, flavonoids, phenolics, steroids	[53, 57, 118–120]
Koanophyllon albicaule (Sch. Bip. ex Klatt) R.M. King & H. Rob.	Diarrhea (L)	Sterols, flavonoids, tannins	[53]
Melampodium divaricatum (Rich.) DC	Dysentery, vomiting, nausea (All)	Terpenoids, coumarins, glycoside derivatives	[53, 121]
Mikania houstoniana (L.) B.L. Rob.	Stomach pain (St)		[53]
Parthenium hysterophorus L.	Stomach pain, fever, *empacho*, malaria, parasites (All)	Resin, alkaloids	[53]
Pinaropappus roseus (Less.) Less.	Constipation (L, R, F)		[53]
Piqueria trinervia Cav.	Intestinal infections, diarrhea, typhoid, *empacho*, stomach pain, purgative, parasites, malaria (F, L, R)	Terpenoids	[53, 122]
Pluchea odorata (L.) Cass.	Vomiting, stomach pain (L)	Flavonoids, terpenoids	[41, 53, 123]
Porophyllum macrocephalum DC.	Laxative (R, L)	Terpenoids, sulfur compounds	[10, 53]
Pseudognaphalium attenuatum DC.	Stomach pain, gastritis, *bilis* (AP)		[53, 92]
Sanvitalia procumbens Lam.	Diarrhea, dysentery, indigestion, vomiting, stomach pain (All)	Terpenoids	[53]
Tagetes erecta L.	Stomach pain, *empacho*, diarrhea, colic, vomiting, indigestion, parasites (L, F)	Thiophene derivative, terpenoids, flavonoids, carotenoids	[53, 54, 124–126]
T. filifolia Lag.	Stomach pain, flatulence (All)	Terpenoids	[41, 53, 127]

Family/ species[1]	Gastrointestinal disorders (used parts[2])	Bioactive compounds	References
T. lucida Cav.	Stomach pain, colic, diarrhea, dysentery, *empacho*, typhoid, vomiting (L, F)	Coumarins, terpenoids, flavonoids	[53, 56, 57, 92, 124]
Tithonia diversifolia (Hemsl.) A. Gray	Vomiting, stomach pain, diarrhea, malaria (L)	Terpenoids, flavonoids, phenols	[5, 10, 57, 84, 128]
Vernonanthura patens (Kunth) H. Rob.	Dysentery (L, Sh, B)	Terpenoids	[53, 129, 130]
Zinnia peruviana L.	Diarrhea, stomach pain (All)		[53, 131]
Bignoniaceae			
Dolichandra uncata (Andrews) L.G. Lohmann	Intestinal inflammation, fever (L, B9		[53]
Parmentiera aculeata (Kunth) Seem.	Dysentery, *empacho* (Bark, Fr)	Flavonoids, sterols, tannins	[7, 41, 53, 132]
Tabebuia rosea (Bertol.) A. DC.	Dysentery, fever, stomach inflammation (Bark)		[41, 43, 53]
Tecoma stans (L.) Juss ex Kunth	Stomach pain, dysentery, *bilis*, gastritis, poor digestion, *empacho*, intestinal atony (L, St, B, OB)	Alkaloids, terpenoids, flavonoids, phenolic acids	[6, 22, 41, 53, 133, 134]
Brassicaceae			
Nasturtium officinale R. Br.	Indigestion (All)		[53]
Burseraceae			
Bursera microphylla A. Gray	Stomach pain (B, gum)	Lignans, terpenoids, flavonoids	[53, 135]
Bursera simaruba L. Sarg.	Dysentery, stomach pain, diarrhea, intestinal infection, purgative (OB)	Tannins, flavonoids, saponins	[41, 53, 135]
Caricaceae			
Carica papaya L.	Diarrhea, dysentery, colic, intestinal parasites, constipation (Fr, L, Se, Latex)	Papain	[6, 11, 53, 72, 92]
Celastraceae			
Semialarium mexicanum (Miers) Mennega	Ulcers, stomach pain, colic, diarrhea, dysentery (R)	Terpenoids	[11, 53, 60]
Chrysobalanaceae			
Chrysobalanus icaco L.	Diarrhea, dysentery (Se, Fr)		[53]
Convolvulaceae			
Ipomoea bracteata Cav.	Diarrhea (T)		[53, 54]
Ipomoea pes-caprae (L.)	Dysentery (L)	Aromatic compounds	[41, 53]
Cruciferae			

Family/ species[1]	Gastrointestinal disorders (used parts[2])	Bioactive compounds	References
Lepidium virginicum L.	Diarrhea, dysentery, stomach pain, flatulence, colic, vomiting, indigestion, *empacho*, purgative, intestinal parasites (All)		[53]
Cucurbitaceae			
Cucurbita pepo L.	Intestinal parasites (Se)	Steroids, alkaloids, flavonoids, terpenoids, glycosides, pyrrolidine, sterols	[53]
Sechium edule (Jacq.) Sw.	Intestinal parasites, vomiting, constipation (L)		[6, 92]
Dilleniaceae			
Curatella americana L.	Stomach pain, diarrhea (Fr, L)	Flavonoids, terpenoids	[41, 53]
Eduphorbiaceae			
Phyllanthus niruri L.	Diarrhea, stomach pain (All)		[53]
Ericaceae			
Arctostaphylos pungens Kunth	Diarrhea, stomach pain, *empacho* (L, Fr)	Pyrocatechin, resin, and tannins	[53]
Euphorbiaceae			
Acalypha alopecuroidea Jacq.	Diarrhea, ulcers (All)	Flavonoids, polyphenols, saponins, tannins	[53]
Croton ciliatoglandulifer Ortega	*Empacho*, intestinal inflammation, purgative (All)	Isoquinoline derivatives	[53]
C. draco Schltdl. & Cham.	Diarrhea, vomiting, stomach pain, *empacho* (OB)		[41, 53, 96]
C. glandulosus L.	Stomach pain	Terpenoids, alkaloids	[92]
C. repens Schlecht.	Diarrhea, dysentery (R)		[53, 92]
C. soliman Cham. & Schltdl.	Intestinal inflammation, parasites (R)		[53]
Euphorbia tithymaloides L.	Intestinal parasites, purgative, gastritis (Latex)	Alkaloids, steroids, sterols, terpenoids	[53, 92]
Hura polyandra Baill.	Stomach pain, constipation, intestinal parasites, purgative (Se)		[10, 53, 92, 96]
Jatropha curcas L.	Diarrhea, vomiting, constipation (R)		[53, 136]
Fabaceae			
Chamaecrista hispidula (Vahl) H.S. Irwin & Barneby			[84]

Family/ species[1]	Gastrointestinal disorders (used parts[2])	Bioactive compounds	References
Crotalaria longirostrata Hook. & Arn.	Indigestion (L, B)		[41, 53]
Desmodium incanum DC.	Diarrhea, stomach pain (L)		[53]
Diphysa carthagenensis Jacq.	Diarrhea, dysentery (OB)		[53]
Enterolobium cyclocarpum (Jacq.) Griseb.	Diarrhea, purgative, indigestion (Fr, gum, bark)	Terpenoids	[53]
Gliricidia sepium (Jacq.) Kunth ex Walp.	*Empacho*, parasites (L, St)	Flavonoids	[41, 53, 96]
Hymenaea courbaril L.	Dysentery, diarrhea, ulcers (OB, L)	Tannins flavonoids, terpenoids	[41, 53, 92]
Leucaena diversifolia (Schltdl.) Benth.	Parasites (All)		[53]
Machaerium floribundum Benth.	Diarrhea (All)		[43, 53, 92]
Mimosa albida Humb. & Bonpl. Ex Willd.	Diarrhea, dysentery (B)		[41, 53]
Pithecellobium dulce (Roxb.) Benth.	Diarrhea, stomach pain, dysentery, constipation, indigestion (OB)	Flavonoids, glucoside derivatives, sterols, terpenoids	[53]
Prosopis juliflora (Sw.) DC.	Stomach pain, dysentery, indigestion, purgative, parasites (L)	Alkaloids, terpenoids, flavonoids	[53]
P. laevigata (Humb. & Bonpl. ex Willd.) M.C. Johnst.	Colic, intestinal inflammation, dysentery, stomach pain (OB)		[53]
Senna skinneri (Benth.) H.S. Irwin & Barneby	Dysentery, *empacho*, fever (L)		[53]
Vachellia farnesiana (L.) Wight & Arn.	*Empacho*, dysentery, dyspepsia, diarrhea, typhoid (All)	Sterols, alkaloids, flavonoids, phenols	[53]
Zornia thymifolia Kunth	Stomach pain, *bilis*, ulcer (St, L)		[53, 92, 96]
Fabaceae			
Quercus crassipes Bonpl.	Diarrhea (OB)		[53]
Q. glaucescens Bonpl.	Diarrhea (OB)	Tannins	[92]
Q. oleoides Schltdl. & Cham.	Diarrhea, gastritis, *empacho* (OB)	Tannins	[17, 53, 92]
Q. sapotifolia Liebm.	Diarrhea (OB)	Tannins	[92]
Geraniaceae			
Geranium mexicanum Kunth	Diarrhea, dysentery, stomach pain (R, AP)	Sterols, flavonoids, tyramine	[11, 53, 60, 61, 72]
Gesneriaceae			
Sinningia incarnata (Aubl.) D.L. Denham	Diarrhea, dysentery (T)		[14, 92]
Heliconiaceae			

Family/ species[1]	Gastrointestinal disorders (used parts[2])	Bioactive compounds	References
Heliotropium indicum L.			[84]
Krameriaceae			
Krameria paucifolia (Rose) Rose	Diarrhea (AP)		[137]
Lamiaceae			
Agastache mexicana Bye, E.L. Linares and Ramam.	Colic, stomach pain, *bilis* (F, L, St)	Terpenoids, oleic acid, flavonoids	[138, 139]
A. mexicana ssp. *Mexicana*	Colic, stomach pain, intestinal pain, *empacho*, indigestion (L)	Terpenoids, flavonoids	[138, 140–142]
Clinopodium macrostemum var. laevigatum (Moc. & Sessé ex Benth.) Kuntze	Stomach pain, dysentery, hangover (L, F)	Terpenoids	[14, 53, 143]
Ocimum basilicum L.	Diarrhea, dysentery, stomach pain, vomiting, *empacho* (AP)		[9, 11, 41, 43, 53, 57, 60, 72, 140, 144]
O. campechianum Mill.	Intestinal inflammation, ulcers, gastritis, fever, dysentery, *empacho*, vomiting, stomach pain vermifuge (L, B)	Terpenoids	[53, 54, 145, 146]
O. carnosum (Spreng.) Link & Otto ex Benth	Stomach pain, flatulence, diarrhea, dysentery, abdominal pain and intestinal parasites (L)	Phenols, terpenoids	[53]
Salvia hispanica L.	Diarrhea (Se)	Unsaturated fatty acids, flavonoids	[53, 147, 148]
S. microphylla Kunth	Diarrhea, dysentery, *empacho*, infection and inflammation of the stomach, vomiting (B)	Terpenoids, alkaloids, tannins	[53, 146]
Vitex mollis Kunth	Colic, intestinal inflammation, diarrhea, dysentery, stomach pain (L, Sh)		[53]
Lauraceae			
Litsea glaucescens Kunth	Stomach pain, *empacho*, children's diarrhea, indigestion (L)	Terpenoids	[53, 54, 149, 150]
Persea americana Mill.	Stomach pain, parasites, diarrhea, dysentery, constipation, flatulence, vomiting (Fr, L)	Terpenoids	[41, 57, 92, 151–153]
Liliaceae			
Milla biflora Cav.	Vomiting, stomach pain, nausea, diarrhea (F)		[53]
Loganiaceae			
Buddleja americana L.	Stomach pain, stomach infection, ulcers (L)	Lignans, flavonoids, alkaloids, tannins	[14, 53, 92]
Lygodiaceae			

Family/ species[1]	Gastrointestinal disorders (used parts[2])	Bioactive compounds	References
Lygodium venustum Sw.	Diarrhea, dysentery, nausea (AP)		[11, 53, 60, 72]
Lythraceae			
Cuphea hyssopifolia Kunth	Stomach pain (All)		[53]
Magnoliaceae			
Chiranthodendron pentadactylon Larreat	Diarrhea, dysentery, colic (F)	Flavonoids, steroids, phenols	[11, 53, 60, 72, 133, 144]
Magnolia mexicana DC.	Stomach pain, parasites (F)		[6, 53]
Magnolia schiedeana Schltdl.	Stomach pain (F)		[6]
Malpighiaceae			
Byrsonima crassifolia (L.) Kunth	Diarrhea, dysentery, *empacho*, stomach pain, indigestion, constipation (OB)	Tannins, proanthocyanidines, phenolic acids, terpenoids	[4, 6, 10, 41, 53, 84, 92]
Malpighia mexicana A. Juss.	*Empacho*, diarrhea, dysentery (OB)		[53]
Malvaceae			
Anoda cristata (L.) Schltdl.	Stomach pain, *empacho*, intestinal inflammation, *bilis* (AP, R)		[53]
Malvaviscus arboreus Cav.	Dysentery, diarrhea, stomach pain (AP)	Flavonoids, sterols, tannins	[14, 17, 53, 92, 96]
Pavonia schiedeana Steud.	*Empacho*, diarrhea (L, St)	Sterols, tannins	[53]
Sida acuta Burm. f.	Diarrhea, dysentery, *empacho* (L)		[53]
Sida rhombifolia L.	Stomach pain, gastritis, ulcers, diarrhea, dysentery (B)	Alkaloids	[41, 53, 146]
Melastomataceae			
Conostegia xalapensis (Bonpl.) D. Don	Diarrhea (L)		[41, 53]
Meliaceae			
Swietenia humilis L.	*Empacho*, stomach pain, diarrhea, fever, amoebic dysentery (Se, OB)		[41, 53]
Swietenia macrophylla G. King	Diarrhea, fever (Se)		[53]
Menispermaceae			
Cissampelos pareira L.	Dysentery, diarrhea, snake bite (L, St, R)	Alkaloids, sterols	[14, 17, 53, 54, 92]
Molluginaceae			
Mollugo verticillata L.	Intestinal inflammation, dysentery, diarrhea, *empacho*, colic, and stomach pain (B, L)		[41, 53]

Family/ species[1]	Gastrointestinal disorders (used parts[2])	Bioactive compounds	References
Moraceae			
Dorstenia drakena L.	Diarrhea, dysentery, stomach pain (R)		[6, 53, 137]
Ficus cotinifolia Kunth	Malaria, ulcers (L, latex)		[53]
Muntingiaceae			
Muntingia calabura L.	Diarrhea, stomach pain, *empacho*, vomiting, dysentery, intestinal infection (OB)	Flavonoids	[53, 96]
Myrtaceae			
Eugenia acapulcensis Steud.	Diarrhea, dysentery (L, OB)	Tannins	[14, 17, 92]
E. capuli (Schltdl. & Cham.) Hook. & Arn	Diarrhea, dysentery (B)		[53]
Psidium guajava L.	Diarrhea, stomach pain, dysentery (All)	Sterols, terpenoids, flavonoids, tannins	[4, 6, 14, 43, 53, 54, 84, 92]
P. guineense Sw.	Diarrhea, dysentery, flatulence, vomiting (L, Fr, R)		[53, 92]
P. salutare (Kunth) O. Berg	Diarrhea (Fr, L, R)		[4, 6, 84]
Nyctaginaceae			
Boerhavia coccinea Mill	Purgative (L)		[53]
Mirabilis jalapa L.	Stomach pain, purgative (All)	Terpenoids, sterols, flavonoids, alkaloids	[53, 57]
Oleaceae			
Fraxinus uhdei (Wenz.) Lingelsh.	Diarrhea, infection intestinal, purgante (All)		[53]
Onagraceae			
Oenothera rosea L'Hér. ex	Stomach pain, inflammation or infection, colic, diarrhea, *bilis*, *empacho*, constipation (AP)		[53]
Papaveraceae			
Argemone mexicana L.	Purgative (Se)	Alkaloids, flavonoids y glycosides	[53]
Bocconia frutescens L	Diarrhea, dysentery, stomach pain, ulcers (AP)		[11, 53, 60, 72]
Passifloraceae			
Passiflora exsudans Zucc.	Dysentery (R)		[53]
Phytolaccaceae			
Petiveria alliacea L.	Stomach pain, dyspepsia, *susto* (R)	Alkaloids, sterols	[53]
Pinaceae			
Pinus oocarpa Schiede ex Schltdl.	Dysentery (L)		[53]

Family/ species[1]	Gastrointestinal disorders (used parts[2])	Bioactive compounds	References
Piperaceae			
Piper aduncum L.	Diarrhea (All)		[53]
P. auritum Kunth	Stomach pain, lack of appetite and constipation (L)	Terpenoids	[53, 54, 84, 96]
P. sanctum (Miq.) Schltdl. ex C. DC.	Stomach pain, diarrhea (L)	Aromatic compounds	[53, 54, 154]
Piper schiedeanum Steudel	*Empacho* (All)		[53]
Plantaginaceae			
Scoparia dulcis L.	Diarrhea, colic, stomach pain, dysentery (AP)	Flavonoid, glucosides, terpenoids	[53, 92]
Poaceae			
Lasiacis ruscifolia (Kunth) Hitchc.	Diarrhea (All)		[53, 54]
Zea mays L.	Diarrhea, stomach pain, constipation, dysentery, vomiting (cob, tassel)	Polysaccharides	[6, 17, 41, 53, 92]
Polemoniaceae			
Loeselia mexicana (Lam.) Brand	*Bilis*, dysentery, stomach pain or inflammation, indigestion, typhoid, vomiting, laxative (AP)		[14, 21, 41, 53, 92]
Polygalaceae			
Polygala longicaulis Kunth	Stomach pain (All)		[53]
P. variabilis Kunth	Abdominal pain (All)		[92]
Portulacaceae			
Portulaca oleracea L.	Intestinal infection, constipation, parasites (All)	Tannins, alkaloids, steroids	[53, 155]
Primulaceae			
Myrsine juergensenii (Mez) Ricketson & Pipoly	Stomach pain (All)		[53]
Rhamnaceae			
Karwinskia humboldtiana (Schult.) Zucc.	Dysentery (L)		[53]
Rhizophoraceae			
Rhizophora mangle L.	Dysentery, diarrhea (R, OB)	Phenolics, tannins	[53]
Rubiaceae			
Galium mexicanum Kunth	Stomach pain, *empacho*, diarrhea (All)		[53]
Hintonia latiflora (Sessé & Moc. ex DC.) Bullock	*Bilis*, gastric ulcer, *empacho*, parasites, malaria, gastroenteritis (OB)	Phenylcoumarins, cucurbitacins, glucocucurbitacins	[53, 156]
Randia echinocarpa Sessé & Moc. ex DC.	Diarrhea, malaria (All)		[53]

Family/ species[1]	Gastrointestinal disorders (used parts[2])	Bioactive compounds	References
Sapindaceae			
Serjania triquetra Radlk.			[53, 84]
Sapotaceae			
Pouteria sapota (Jacq.) H.E. Moore & Stearn	Diarrhea, *empacho*, stomach pain (All)	Phenolics, carotenoids, δ-tocopherol	[41, 53, 96, 157]
Scrophulariaceae			
Capraria biflora L.	Dysentery, inflammation of the stomach, gastroenteritis, intestinal fever (L)	Alkaloids, terpenoids, naphthoquinone	[53, 158, 159]
Russelia sarmentosa Jacq.	Stomach pain (L)		[14, 53, 92]
Selaginellaceae			
Selaginella pallescens (Presl) Spring	Diarrhea (All)		[53, 54]
Smilacaceae			
Smilax laurifolia L.	Diarrhea (All)	Taninos ausentes, 1B	[92]
Solanaceae			
Calibrachoa parviflora (A. Juss.) D'Arcy	Flatulence (All)		[53]
Capsicum annuum L.	Dyspepsia, diarrhea, dysentery (Fr, S)	Alkaloids, capsaicinoids, carotenoids, tocopherols, sapogenins, phenolic acids	[53, 160]
Cestrum dumetorum Schltdl.	Intestinal inflammation (All)	Sterols, tannins	[53]
C. nocturnum L.	Stomach pain (L, St, F)	Sapogenins, coumarins, sitosterols, flavonoids	[41, 43, 53, 54, 161]
Physalis coztomatl Moc. & Sessé ex Dunal	Diarrhea with blood from amoebic infection or other parasites, diarrhea, stomach pain, dysentery (R, B)	Alkaloids, glycosides	[53]
P. lagascea R. & S.	Stomach pain (L)		[53]
Solanum rostratum Dunal	Purgative, stomach pain, diarrhea (L, F)		[53]
S. amictum Moric. ex Dunal.	Stomach pain (L)		[53]
S. torvum Sw.	Diarrhea, dolor de estómago (All)	Sapogenins, alkaloids	[53]
Sterculiaceae			
Guazuma ulmifolia Lam.	Diarrhea, intestinal infection, dysentery, *empacho* (All)	Procyanidins, Tannins	[6, 10, 14, 41, 53, 92]
Melochia pyramidata L.	Purgative (AP)		[53]
Waltheria indica L.	Diarrhea, dysentery, *empacho*, fever (All)	Flavonoids, esters, alkaloids	[53]
Verbenaceae			
Lantana achyranthifolia Desf.	Diarrhea, dysentery, *empacho* (All)	Terpenoids, flavonoids, and phenylpropanoids	[8, 16, 53, 68]

Family/ species[1]	Gastrointestinal disorders (used parts[2])	Bioactive compounds	References
L. camara L.	Stomach pain or inflammation, intestinal pain, parasites, vomiting (L, St)	Terpenoids, flavonoids, phenols	[53, 162–164]
Lippia alba (Mill.) N.E. Br. ex Britton & P. Wilson	Diarrhea, dysentery, stomach pain, colic, indigestion (AP)	Terpenoids	[4, 11, 53, 60, 61, 72, 92, 133, 146]
L. graveolens Kunth	Diarrhea, dysentery, *empacho*, indigestion (AP)	Terpenoids, flavonoids	[53, 165, 166]
Stachytarpheta jamaicensis (L.) Vahl	Stomach pain, intestinal inflammation (L)		[53, 92]
Verbena litoralis Kunth	Stomach pain, *bilis*, vomiting, malaria (L)		[53, 146]
Zygophyllaceae			
Guaiacum coulteri A. Gray	Ulcers (OB)	Alkaloids	[41, 53, 57]

1*Checklist of native vascular plants of Mexico [50].*
[2]*L, leaves; St, stem; F, flower; AP, aerial parts; Se, seeds; R, root; All, whole plant; Sh, shoots; B, branches; Fr, Fruit; T, tuber; OB, outer bark.*

Table 1A.
List of plants used by the indigenous groups of Oaxaca for the treatment of gastrointestinal disorders.

Author details

Mónica Lilian Pérez-Ochoa[1], José Luis Chávez-Servia[1]*, Araceli Minerva Vera-Guzmán[1] Elia Nora Aquino-Bolaños[2] and José Cruz Carrillo-Rodríguez[3]

1 CIIDIR-Oaxaca, Instituto Politécnico Nacional, Oaxaca, México

2 Instituto de Ciencia Básica, Universidad Veracruzana, Jalapa, México

3 Instituto Tecnológico del Valle de Oaxaca, México

*Address all correspondence to: jchavezs@ipn.mx

References

[1] UNAM. Biblioteca Digital de la Medicina Tradicional Mexicana [Internet]. 2009. Available from: http://www.medicinatradicionalmexicana.unam.mx/index.php [Accessed: 2018-09-27]

[2] Hernández C, Aguilera MG, Castro G. Situación de las enfermedades gastrointestinales en México. Enfermedades Infecciosas y Microbiología. 2011;**31**(4):137-151 http://www.medigraphic.com/pdfs/micro/ei-2011/ei114f.pdf

[3] Secretaria de Salud. Informe sobre la Salud de los Mexicanos 2015: Diagnóstico general de la salud poblacional. [Internet]. 2015. Available from: https://www.gob.mx/cms/uploads/attachment/file/64176/INFORME_LA_SALUD_DE_LOS_MEXICANOS_2015_S.pdf [Accessed: 2018-09-27]

[4] Heinrich M, Ankli A, Frei B, Weimann C, Sticher O. Medicinal plants in Mexico: Healers' consensus and cultural importance. Social Science & Medicine. 1998;**47**(11):1859-1871. DOI: 10.1016/S0277-9536(98)00181-6

[5] Heinrich M, Robles M, West JE, Ortiz-de-Montellano BR, Rodriguez E. Ethnopharmacology of Mexican Asteraceae (Compositae). Annual Review of Pharmacology and Toxicology. 1998;**38**:539-565. DOI: 10.1146/annurev.pharmtox.38.1.539

[6] Frei B, Sticher O, Viesca C, Heinrich M. Medicinal and food plants: Isthmus sierra Zapotec criteria for selection. Angewandte Botanik. 1998;**72**:82-86 http://discovery.ucl.ac.uk/1381118/1/Heinrich_Applied%20Botany_Frei_1998.pdf

[7] Ankli A, Heinrich M, Bork P, Wolfram L, Bauerfeind P, Brun R, et al. Yucatec Mayan medicinal plants: Evaluation based on indigenous uses. Journal of Ethnopharmacology. 2002;**79**(1):43-52. DOI: 10.1016/S0378-8741(01)00355-5

[8] Hernández T, Canalez M, Caballero J, Durán A, Lira R. Análisis cuantitativo del conocimiento tradicional sobre plantas utilizadas para el tratamiento de enfermedades gastrointestinales en Zapotitlán de Las Salinas, Puebla, México. Interciencia. 2005;**30**(9):529-535 http://www.redalyc.org/articulo.oa?id=33910803

[9] Valdés-Cobos A. Conservación y uso de plantas medicinales: El caso de la región de la Mixteca Alta Oaxaqueña, México. Ambiente y Desarrollo. 2013;**17**(33):87-97 http://revistas.javeriana.edu.co/index.php/ambienteydesarrollo/article/view/7044

[10] Heinrich M. Ethnobotany and natural products: The research for new molecules, new treatments of old diseases or a better understanding of indigenous cultures? Current Topics in Medicinal Chemistry. 2003;**3**(2):29-42. DOI: 10.2174/1568026033392570

[11] Calzada F, Arísta R, Pérez H. Effect of plants used in Mexico to treat gastrointestinal disorders on charcoal-gum acacia-induced hyperperistalsis in rats. Journal of Ethnopharmacology. 2010;**128**(1):49-51. DOI: 10.1016/j.jep.2009.12.022

[12] Juárez-Vázquez MC, Carranza-Álvarez C, Alonso-Castro AJ, González-Alcaraz VF, Bravo-Acevedo E, Chamarro-Tinajero FJ, et al. Ethnobotany of medicinal plants used in Xalpatlahuac, Guerrero, México. Journal of Ethnopharmacology. 2013;**148**(2):521-527. DOI: 10.1016/j.jep.2013.04.048

[13] Loayza I, Abujder D, Aranda R, Jakupovic J, Collin G, Deslauriers

H, et al. Essential oils of *Baccharis salicifolia*, *B. latifolia* and *B. dracunculifolia*. Phytochemistry. 1995;**38**(2):381-389. DOI: 10.1016/0031-9422(94)00628-7

[14] Bork PM, Scmitz LL, Kuhtnt M, Escher C, Heinrich M. Sesquiterpene lactone containing Mexican Indian medicinal plants and pure sesquiterpene lactones as potent inhibitors of transcription facto NF-kB. FEBS Letters. 1997;**402**(1):85-90. DOI: 10.1016/S0014-5793(96)01502-5

[15] Savithramma N, Rao ML, Ankanna S. Screening of traditional medicinal plants for secondary metabolites. International Journal of Research in Pharmaceutical Sciences. 2011;**2**(4):643-647 https://www.researchgate.net/profile/S_Ankanna/publication/267690135_Screening_of_Medicinal_Plants_for_Secondary_Metabolites/links/55ed339808aeb6516268d1e2/Screening-of-Medicinal-Plants-for-Secondary-Metabolites.pdf

[16] Sousa EO, Costa JGM. Genus lantana: Chemical aspects and biological activities. Brazilian Journal of Pharmacognosy. 2012;**22**(5):1155-1180. DOI: 10.1590/S0102-695X2012005000058

[17] Heinrich M, Kuhnt M, Wright CW, Rimpler H, Phillipson JD, Schandelmaier A, et al. Parasitological and microbiological evaluation of Mixe indian medicinal plantas (Mexico). Journal of Ethnopharmacology. 1992;**36**(1):81-85. DOI: 10.1016/0378-8741(92)90063-W

[18] Calzada F. Additional antiprotozoal constituents from *Cuphea pinetorum*, a planta used in Mayan traditional medicine to treat diarrhea. Phytotherapy Research. 2005;**19**(8): 725-727. DOI: 10.1002/ptr.1717

[19] Atta AH, Mouneir SM. Evaluation of some medicinal plant extracts for anitidiarrhoeal activity. Phytoterapy Research. 2005;**19**(6):481-485. DOI: 10.1002/ptr.1639

[20] Palombo EA. Phytochemicals from traditional medicinal plants used in the treatment of diarrhea: Modes of action and effects on intestinal function. Phytotherapy Research. 2006;**20**(9): 717-724. DOI: 10.1002/ptr.1907

[21] Navarro-García VM, Rojas G, Zepeda LG, Aviles M, Fuentes M, Herrera A, et al. Antifungal and antibacterial activity of four selected Mexican medicinal plants. Pharmaceutical Biology. 2006;**44**(4):297-300. DOI: 10.1080/13880200600715837

[22] Robles-Zepeda RE, Velázquez-Contreras CA, Garibay-Escobar A, Gálvez-Ruiz JC, Ruiz-Bustos E. Antimicrobial activity of northwestern Mexican plants against *Helicobacter pylori*. Journal of Medicinal Food. 2011;**14**(10):1280-1283. DOI: 10.1089/jmf.2010.0263

[23] Cushnie TP, Lamb AJ. Recent advances in understanding the antibacterial properties of flavonoids. International Journal of Antimicrobial Agents. 2011;**38**(2):99-107. DOI: 10.1016/j.ijantimicag.2011.02.014

[24] Arrieta-Baez D, de Esparza RR, Jiménez-Estrada M. Mexican plants used in the salmonellosis treatment. In: Kumar Y, editor. Salmonella—A Diversified Superbug. Rijeka, Croatia: Intech; 2012. pp. 169-184. DOI: 10.5772/31291

[25] Ramírez-Moreno E, Soto-Sanchez J, Rivera G, Marchat LA. Mexican medicinal plants as an alternative for the development of new compounds against protozoan parasites. In: Khater H, Govindarajan M, Benelli G, editors. Natural Remedies in the Fight against Parasites. Rijeka, Croatia: Intech; 2017. pp. 62-91. DOI: 10.5772/67259

[26] Instituto Nacional de Estadística, Geografía e Informática (INEGI). Resultados de Encuesta Intercensal 2015. Instituto Nacional de Estadística, Geografía e Informática, Aguascalientes, México. [Internet]. 2015. Available from: http://www.beta.inegi.org.mx/proyectos/enchogares/especiales/intercensal/?init=1 [Accessed: 2018-09-27]

[27] García-Vargas LA. Radiografía demográfica de la población indígena en Oaxaca. Oaxaca Población Siglo XXI. 2018;**41**:7-20 http://www.digepo.oaxaca.gob.mx/recursos/revistas/revista42.pdf

[28] Instituto Nacional de Lenguas Indígenas (INALI). Catálogo de las lenguas indígenas nacionales. Variantes lingüísticas de México con sus autodenominaciones y referencias geoestadísticas. México DF: INALI; 2010. 371 p. Available from: https://site.inali.gob.mx/pdf/catalogo_lenguas_indigenas.pdf [Accessed: 2018-09-27]

[29] Grupos H-DJ, de Oaxaca I. Situación sociodemográfica. Oaxaca, México: Universidad Autónoma Benito Juárez de Oaxaca; 2005. 139 p

[30] Toledo VM, Alarcón-Chaires P, Moguel P, Olivo M, Cabrera A, Leyequien E, et al. El atlas etnoecológico de México y Centroamérica: Fundamentos, métodos y resultados. Etnoecología. 2001;**6**(8):7-41 https://ccp.ucr.ac.cr/bvp/pdf/cambiodemografico/atlas_etnologico.pdf

[31] Arellanes A, de la Cruz V, Romero MA, Sánchez C, Ruiz FJ, Martínez VR, et al. Historia y Geografía de Oaxaca. Carteles: Oaxaca, México; 2006. 207 p

[32] Heinrich M. Herbal and symbolic medicines of the lowland Mixe (Oaxaca, Mexico). Disease concepts, healer's roles, and plant use. Anthropos. 1994;**89**:73-83 https://www.jstor.org/stable/40463843

[33] Pérez-Nicolas M, Vibrans H, Romero-Manzanares A, Saynes-Vásquez A, Luna-Cavazos M, Flores-Cruz M, et al. Patterns of knowledge and use of medicinal plants in Santiago Camotlán, Oaxaca, Mexico. Economic Botany. 2017;**71**(3):209-223. DOI: 10.1007/s12231-017-9384-0

[34] Rubel AJ, Browner CH. Antropología de la salud en Oaxaca. Alteridades. 1999;**9**(17):85-94 http://alteridades.izt.uam.mx/index.php/Alte/article/view/461/460

[35] Ugent D. Medicine, myths and magic the folk healers of a Mexican market. Economic Botany. 2000;**54**(4):427-438. DOI: 10.1007/BF02866542

[36] Berenzon-Gorn S, Hernández-Hernández J, Saavedra-Solano N. Percepciones y creencias en torno a la salud-enfermedad mental, narradas por curanderos urbanos de la ciudad de México. Gazeta de Antropologia. 2001;**17**:21 http://digibug.ugr.es/handle/10481/7481

[37] Berenzon-Gorn S, Ito-Sugiyama E, Vargas-Guadarrama LA. Enfermedades y padeceres por los que se recurre a terapeutas tradicionales de la Ciudad de México. Salud Pública de México. 2006;**48**(1):45-56 http://saludpublica.mx/index.php/spm/article/view/6670/8292

[38] Lámbarri-Rodríguez A, Flores-Palacios F, Berezon-Gorn S. Curanderos, malestar y daños: una interpretación social. Salud Mental. 2012;**35**(2):123-128 http://revistasaludmental.mx/index.php/salud_mental/article/view/1464/1462

[39] Giovannini P, Reyes-García V, Waldstein A, Heinrich M. Do pharmaceuticals displace local knowledge and use of medicinal plants? Estimates from a cross-sectional study in a rural indigenous community,

Mexico. Social Science & Medicine. 2011;**72**(6):928-936. DOI: 10.1016/j.socscimed.2011.01.007

[40] Instituto Nacional de Salud Pública (INSP). Encuesta Nacional de Salud y Nutrición 2012. Resultados Nacionales. 2nd ed. Cuernavaca, México: Instituto Nacional de Salud Pública. 2013. 190 p. Available from: https://ensanut.insp.mx/informes/ENSANUT2012ResultadosNacionales2Ed.pdf Accessed: 2018-09-27

[41] Luna-José AL, Rendón-Aguilar B. Recursos vegetales útiles en diez comunidades de la Sierra Madre del Sur, Oaxaca, Mexico. Polibotánica. 2008;**26**:193-242 http://www.scielo.org.mx/pdf/polib/n26/n26a11.pdf

[42] Salas-Morales SH, Saynes-Vásquez A, Schibli L. Flora de la costa de Oaxaca, México: Lista florística de la región de Zimatán. Boletín de la Sociedad Botánica de México. 2003;**72**:21-58 http://www.redalyc.org/pdf/577/57707202.pdf

[43] Aguilar-Stoen M, Moe SR, Camargo-Ricalde SL. Home gardens sustain crop diversity and improve farm resilience in Candelaria Loxicha, Oaxaca, Mexico. Human Ecology. 2009;**37**(1):55-77. DOI: 10.1007/s10745-008-9197-y

[44] Pool A. Taxonomic revision of Gouania (Rhamnaceae) for North America. Annals of the Missouri Botanical Garden. 2014;**99**(3):490-552. DOI: 10.3417/2013016

[45] Meave JA, Rincón-Gutiérrez A, Ibarra-Maríquez G, Gallardo-Hernández C, Romero-Romero MA. Checklist of the vascular flora of a portion of the hyper-humid region of La Chinantla, Northern Oaxaca range, Mexico. Botanical Sciences. 2017;**95**(4):722-759. DOI: 10.17129/botsci.1812

[46] Zacharias S. Mexican Curanderismo as ethnopsychotherapy: A qualitative study on treatment practices, effectiveness, and mechanisms of change. International Journal of Disability, Development and Education. 2006;**53**(4):381-400. DOI: 10.1080/10349120601008522

[47] Montiel-Tafur M, Crowe TK, Torres E. A review of curanderismo and healing practices among Mexicans and Mexican Americans. Occupational Therapy International. 2009;**16**(1):82-88. DOI: 10.1002/oti.265

[48] Ciofalo N. Indigenous women's ways of knowing and healing in Mexico. Women & Therapy. 2018;**41**(1-2):52-68. DOI: 10.1080/02703149.2017.1323478

[49] Maqueda AE. The use of *Salvia divinorum* from a Mazatec perspective. In: Labate BC, Cavnar C, editors. Plant Medicines, Healing and Psychedelic Science. Cham, Switzerland: Springer International Publishing AG; 2018. pp. 55-70. DOI: 10.1007/978-3-319-76720-8_4

[50] Villaseñor JL. Checklist of the native vascular plants of Mexico. Revista Mexicana de Biodiversidad. 2016;**87**(3):559-902. DOI: 10.1016/j.rmb.2016.06.017

[51] Sepúlveda-Jiménez G, Reyna-Aquino C, Chaires-Martinez L, Bermúdez-Torres K, Rodríguez-Monroy M. Antioxidant activity and content of phenolic compounds and flavonoids from *Justicia spicigera*. Journal of Biological Sciences. 2009;**9**(6):629-632. DOI: 10.3923/jbs.2009.629.632

[52] UNAM. Diccionario enciclopédico de la medicina tradicional mexicana. [Internet]. 2009. Biblioteca Digital de la Medicina Tradicional Mexicana. Available from: http://www.medicinatradicionalmexicana.unam.mx/alfa.php?opcion=D&p=a [Accessed: 2018-09-27]

[53] Argueta A, Gallardo VM, editors. Atlas de las plantas de la medicina

tradicional mexicana. 1st ed. México: Instituto Nacional Indigenista; 1994. 1786 p

[54] Lipp FJ. Ethnobotany of the Chinantec indians, Oaxaca, Mexico. Economic Botany. 1971;**25**:234-244. DOI: 10.1007/BF02860760

[55] Li W, Gao Y, Zhao J, Wang Q. Phenolic, flavonoid, and lutein ester content and antioxidant activity of 11 cultivars of Chinese marigold. Journal of Agricultural and Food Chemistry. 2007;**55**(21):8478-8484. DOI: 10.1021/jf071696j

[56] Céspedes CL, Avila JG, Martínez A, Serrato B, Calderón-Mugica JC, Salgado-Garciglia R. Antifungal and antibacterial activities of Mexican tarragon (*Tagetes lucida*). Journal of Agricultural and Food Chemistry. 2006;**54**(10):3521-3527. DOI: 10.1021/jf053071w

[57] Castillo-Juárez I, González V, Jaime-Aguilar H, Martínez G, Linares E, Bye R, et al. Anti-*Helicobacter pylori* activity of plants used in Mexican traditional medicine for gastrointestinal disorders. Journal of Ethnopharmacology. 2009;**122**(2):402-405. DOI: 10.1016/j.jep.2008.12.021

[58] Kiuchi F, Itano Y, Uchiyama N, Honda G, Tsubouchi A, Nakajima-Shimada J, et al. Monoterpene hydroperoxides with trypanocidal activity from *Chenopodium ambrosioides*. Journal of Natural Products. 2002;**65**(4):509-512. DOI: 10.1021/np010445g

[59] Barbosa E, Calzada F, Campos R. *In vivo* antigiardial activity of three flavonoids isolated of some medicinal plants used in Mexican traditional medicine for the treatment of diarrhea. Journal of Ethnopharmacology. 2007;**109**(3):552-554. DOI: 10.1016/j.jep.2006.09.009

[60] Alanis AD, Calzada F, Cervantes JA, Torres J, Ceballos GM. Antibacterial properties of some plants used in Mexican traditional medicine for the treatment of gastrointestinal disorders. Journal of Ethnopharmacology. 2005;**100**(1-2):153-157. DOI: 10.1016/j.jep.2005.02.022

[61] Calzada F, Cervantes-Martínez JA, Yépez-Mulia L. *In vitro* antiprotozoal activity from the roots of *Geranium mexicanum* and its constituents on *Entamoeba histolytica* and *Giardia lamblia*. Journal of Ethnopharmacology. 2005;**98**(1-2):191-193. DOI: 10.1016/j.jep.2005.01.019

[62] Hussain AI, Anwar F, Sherazi STH, Przybylski R. Chemical composition, antioxidant and antimicrobial activities of basil (*Ocimum basilicum*) essential oils depends on seasonal variations. Food Chemistry. 2008;**108**(3):986-995

[63] Sánchez-Arreola E, Hernández-Molina LR, Sánchez-Salas JL, Martínez-Espino G. Alkaloids from *Bocconia frutescens* and biological activity of their extracts. Pharmaceutical Biology. 2006;**44**(7):540-543. DOI: 10.1080/13880200600883106

[64] Molinaro F, Tyc O, Beekwilder J, Cankar K, Bertea CM, Negre M, et al. The effect of isabelin, a sesquiterpene lactone from *Ambrosia artemisiifolia* on soil microorganisms and human pathogens. FEMS Microbiology Letters. 2018;**365**(4):fny001. DOI: 10.1093/femsle/fny001

[65] Sánchez E, García S, Heredia N. Extracts of edible and medicinal plants damage membranes of *Vibrio cholerae*. Applied and Environmental Microbiology. 2010;**76**(20):6888-6894. DOI: 10.1128/AEM.03052-09

[66] Baldemir A, Karaman Ü, Ilgun S, Kacmaz G, Demirci B. Antiparasitic efficacy of *Artemisia ludoviciana* Nutt. (Asteraceae) essential oil for

Acanthamoeba castellanii, *Leishmania infantum* and *Trichomonas vaginalis*. Indian Journal of Pharmaceutical Education and Research. 2018; **52**(3):416-425. DOI: 10.5530/ijper.52.3.48

[67] Ruiz-Cancino A, Cano AE, Delgado G. Sesquiterpene lactones and flavonoids from *Artemisia ludoviciana* ssp. *mexicana*. Phytochemistry. 1993;**33**(5):1113-1115. DOI: 10.1016/0031-9422(93)85032-M

[68] Hernández T, Canales M, García AM, Duran Á, Meráz S, Dávila P, et al. Antifungal activity of the essential oils of two verbenaceae: *Lantana achyranthifolia* and *Lippia graveolens* of Zapotitlán de las Salinas, Puebla (México). Boletin Latinoamericano y del Caribe de Plantas Medicinales y Aromaticas. 2008;7(4):202-206 https://www.blacpma.usach.cl/sites/blacpma/files/007-004.pdf

[69] Calzada F, Juárez T, García-Hernández N, Valdes M, Ávila O, Mulia LY, et al. Antiprotozoal, antibacterial and antidiarrheal properties from the flowers of *Chiranthodendron pentadactylon* and isolated flavonoids. Pharmacognosy Magazine. 2017;**13**(50):240-244 http://www.phcog.com/text.asp?2017/13/50/240/204564

[70] Gomez-Chang E, Uribe-Estanislao GV, Martinez-Martinez M, Gálvez-Mariscal A, Romero I. Anti-*Helicobacter pylori* potential of three edible plants known as Quelites in Mexico. Journal of Medicinal Food. 2018. DOI: 10.1089/jmf.2017.0137

[71] Arana-Sánchez A, Estarrón-Espinosa M, Obledo-Vázquez EN, Padilla-Camberos E, Silva-Vázquez R, Lugo-Cervantes E. Antimicrobial and antioxidant activities of Mexican oregano essential oils (*Lippia graveolens* HBK) with different composition when microencapsulated in β-cyclodextrin. Letters in Applied Microbiology. 2010;**50**(6):585-590. DOI: 10.1111/j.1472-765X.2010.02837.x

[72] Velázquez C, Calzada F, Torres J, González F, Ceballos G. Antisecretory activity of plants used to treat gastrointestinal disorders in Mexico. Journal of Ethnopharmacology. 2006;**103**(1):66-70. DOI: 10.1016/j.jep.2005.06.046

[73] Velázquez C, Calzada F, Esquivel B, Barbosa E, Calzada S. Antisecretory activity from the flowers of *Chiranthodendron pentadactylon* and its flavonoids on intestinal fluid accumulation induced by Vibrio cholerae toxin in rats. Journal of Ethnopharmacology. 2009;**126**(3):455-458. DOI: 10.1016/j.jep.2009.09.016

[74] Castillo SL, Heredia N, Contreras JF, García S. Extracts of edible and medicinal plants in inhibition of growth, adherence, and cytotoxin production of *Campylobacter jejuni* and *Campylobacter coli*. Journal of Food Science. 2011;**76**(6):M421-M426. DOI: 10.1111/j.1750-3841.2011.02229.x

[75] Gambhir S, Vyas D, Hollis M, Aekka A, Vyas A. Nuclear factor kappa B role in inflammation associated gastrointestinal malignancies. World Journal of Gastroenterology. 2015;**21**(11):3174-3183. DOI: 10.3748/wjg.v21.i11.3174

[76] Hernández T, Canales M, Avila JG, García AM, Martínez A, Caballero J, et al. Composition and antibacterial activity of essential oil of *Lantana achyranthifolia* Desf. (Verbenaceae). Journal of Ethnopharmacology. 2005;**96**(3):551-554. DOI: 10.1016/j.jep.2004.09.044

[77] Cimanga K, Apers S, de Bruyne T, Van Miert S, Hermans N, Totté J, et al. Chemical composition and antifungal activity of essential oils of some aromatic medicinal plants growing in the Democratic Republic

of Congo. Journal of Essential Oil Research. 2002;**14**(5):382-387. DOI: 10.1080/10412905.2002.9699894

[78] Deena MJ, Thoppil JE. Antimicrobial activity of the essential oil of *Lantana camara*. Fitoterapia. 2000;**71**(4):453-455. DOI: 10.1016/S0367-326X(00)00140-4

[79] Euler KL, Alam M. Isolation of kaempferitrin from *Justicia spicigera*. Journal of Natural Products. 1982;**45**(2):220-221. DOI: 10.1021/np50020a020

[80] Vega-Avila E, Espejo-Serna A, Alarcón-Aguilar F, Velasco-Lezama R. Cytotoxic activity of four Mexican medicinal plants. Proceedings of the Western Pharmacology Society. 2009;**52**:78-82

[81] Corrêa GM, Alcântara AF. Chemical constituents and biological activities of species of Justicia: A review. Revista Brasileira de Farmacognosia. 2012;**22**(1):220-238. DOI: 10.1590/S0102-695X2011005000196

[82] Kliks MM. Studies on the traditional herbal anthelmintic *Chenopodium ambrosioides* L.: Ethnopharmacological evaluation and clinical field trials. Social Science & Medicine. 1985;**21**(8):879-886. DOI: 10.1016/0277-9536(85)90144-3

[83] Ávila-Blanco ME, Rodríguez MG, Moreno-Duque JL, Muñoz-Ortega M, Ventura-Juárez J. Amoebicidal activity of essential oil of *Dysphania ambrosioides* (L.) Mosyakin & Clemants in an amoebic liver abscess hamster model. Evidence-based Complementary and Alternative Medicine. 2014:1-7. DOI: 10.1155/2014/930208

[84] Geck MS, Réyes-García AJ, Casu L, Leonti M. Acculturation and ethnomedicine: A regional comparison of medicinal plant knowledge among the Zoque of southern Mexico. Journal of Ethnopharmacology. 2016;**187**:146-159. DOI: 10.1016/j.jep.2016.04.036

[85] Barros L, Pereira E, Calhelha RC, Dueñas M, Carvalho AM, Santos-Buelga C, et al. Bioactivity and chemical characterization in hydrophilic and lipophilic compounds of *Chenopodium ambrosioides* L. Journal of Functional Foods. 2013;**5**(4):1732-1740. DOI: 10.1016/j.jff.2013.07.019

[86] Álvarez-Ospina H, Rivero Cruz I, Duarte G, Bye R, Mata R. HPLC determination of the major active flavonoids and GC–MS analysis of volatile components of *Dysphania graveolens* (Amaranthaceae). Phytochemical Analysis. 2013;**24**(3):248-254. DOI: 10.1002/pca.2405

[87] Oviedo-Chávez I, Ramírez-Apan T, Soto-Hernández M, Martínez-Vázquez M. Principles of the bark of *Amphipterygium adstringens* (Julianaceae) with anti-inflammatory activity. Phytomedicine. 2004;**11**(5):436-445. DOI: 10.1016/j.phymed.2003.05.003

[88] Rivero-Cruz I, Acevedo L, Guerrero JA, Martínez S, Bye R, Pereda-Miranda R, et al. Antimycobacterial agents from selected Mexican medicinal plants. The Journal of Pharmacy and Pharmacology. 2005;**57**(9):1117-1126. DOI: 10.1211/jpp.57.9.0007

[89] Igwe CU, Onyeze GO, Onwuliri VA, Osuagwu CG, Ojiako AO. Evaluation of the chemical compositions of the leaf of *Spondias mombin* Linn from Nigeria. Australian Journal of Basic and Applied Sciences. 2010;**4**(5):706-710. http://www.ajbasweb.com/old/ajbas/2010/706-710.pdf

[90] Alves-Brito S, Ferreira de Almeida CL, Italo de Santana T, Da Silva AR, Bezerra do Nascimento JC, Torres-Souza I, et al. Antiulcer activity and potential mechanism of action of the leaves of

Spondias mombin L. Oxidative Medicine and Cellular Longevity. 2018:1-20. DOI: 10.1155/2018/1731459

[91] Cristofoli NL, Lima CA, Vieira MM, Andrade KS, Ferreira SR. Antioxidant and antimicrobial potential of cajazeira leaves (*Spondias mombin*) extracts. Separation Science and Technology. 2018;**12**:1-1. DOI: 10.1080/01496395.2018.1508233

[92] Heinrich M, Rimpler H, Barrera NA. Indigenous phytotherapy of gastrointestinal disorders in a lowland Mixe community (Oaxaca, Mexico): Ethnopharmacologic evaluation. Journal of Ethnopharmacology. 1992;**36**:63-80. DOI: 10.1016/0378-8741(92)90062-V

[93] Sameh S, Al-Sayed E, Labib RM, Singab AN. Genus Spondias: A phytochemical and pharmacological review. Evidence-based Complementary and Alternative Medicine. 2018:1-13. DOI: 10.1155/2018/5382904

[94] Galvão SDL, Monteiro AD, Siqueira EP, Bomfim MR, Dias-Souza MV, Ferreira GF, et al. *Annona glabra* flavonoids act as antimicrobials by binding to *Pseudomonas aeruginosa* cell walls. Frontiers in Microbiology. 2016;**21**(7):1-9. DOI: 10.3389/fmicb.2016.02053

[95] Nhiem NX, Hien NT, Tai BH, Anh HL, Hang DT, Quang TH, et al. New ent-kauranes from the fruits of *Annona glabra* and their inhibitory nitric oxide production in LPS-stimulated RAW264. 7 macrophages. Bioorganic & Medicinal Chemistry Letters. 2015;**25**(2):254-258. DOI: 10.1016/j.bmcl.2014.11.059

[96] Abe F, Nagafuji S, Yamauchi T, Okabe H, Maki J, Higo H, et al. Trypanocidal constituents in plants. 1. Evaluation of some Mexican plants for their trypanocidal activity and active constituents in Guaco, roots of *Aristolochia taliscana*. Biological & Pharmaceutical Bulletin. 2002;**25**(9):1188-1191. DOI: 10.1248/bpb.25.1188

[97] Chang FR, Wu YC, Duh CY, Wang SK. Studies on the acetogenins of Formosan annonaceous plants. II. Cytotoxic acetogenins from *Annona reticulata*. Journal of Natural Products. 1993;**56**:1688-1694. DOI: 10.1021/np50100a005

[98] Chavan SS, Shamkuwar PB, Damale MG, Pawar DP. A comprehensive review on *Annona reticulata*. International Journal of Pharmaceutical Sciences and Research. 2014;**5**(1):45-50. DOI: 10.13040/IJPSR.0975-8232.5(1).45-50

[99] Jamkhande PG, Wattamwar AS, Kankudte AD, Tidke PS, Kalaskar MG. Assessment of *Annona reticulata* Linn. leaves fractions for in vitro antioxidative effect and antimicrobial potential against standard human pathogenic strains. Alexandria Journal of Medicine. 2016;**52**:19-25. DOI: 10.1016/j.ajme.2014.12.007J

[100] Quílez AM, Fernández-Arche MA, García-Giménez MD, De la Puerta R. Potential therapeutic applications of the genus Annona local and traditional uses and pharmacology. Journal of Ethnopharmacology. 2018;**225**:244-270. DOI: 10.1016/j.jep.2018.06.014

[101] Paul JH, Seaforth CE, Tikasingh T. *Eryngium foetidum* L.: A review. Fitoterapia. 2011;**82**(3):302-308. DOI: 10.1016/j.fitote.2010.11.010

[102] Rojas-Silva P, Graziose R, Vesely B, Poulev A, Mbeunkui F, Grace MH, et al. Leishmanicidal activity of a daucane sesquiterpene isolated from *Eryngium foetidum*. Pharmaceutical Biology. 2014;**52**(3):398-401. DOI: 10.3109/13880209.2013.837077

[103] Forbes WM, Gallimore WA, Mansingh A, Reese PB, Robinson RD. Eryngial (trans-2-dodecenal), a bioactive compound from *Eryngium*

foetidum: Its identification, chemical isolation, characterization and comparison with ivermectin in vitro. Parasitology. 2014;**141**(2):269-278. DOI: 10.1017/S003118201300156X

[104] Hassan EM, Shahat AA, Ibrahim NA, Vlietinck AJ, Apers S, Pieters L. A new monoterpene alkaloid and other constituents of *Plumeria acutifolia*. Planta Medica. 2008;**74**(14):1749-1750. DOI: 10.1055/s-0028-1088317

[105] Srivastava A, Gupta AK, Rajendiran A. Phytochemical screening and in-vitro anthelmintic activity of methanolic extract from the stem bark of *Plumeria rubra* Linn. International Journal of Pharmaceutical Sciences and Research. 2017;**8**(12):5336-5341. DOI: 10.13040/IJPSR.0975-8232.8(12).5336-41

[106] Endo H, Warashina T, Noro T, Castro VH, Mora GA, Poveda LJ, et al. Cardenolide glycosides from *Thevetia ahouai* (LINN.) a. DC. Chemical & Pharmaceutical Bulletin. 1997;**45**(9):1536-1538. DOI: 10.1248/cpb.45.1536

[107] Li JZ, Qing C, Chen CX, Hao XJ, Liu HY. Cytotoxicity of cardenolides and cardenolide glycosides from *Asclepias curassavica*. Bioorganic & Medicinal Chemistry Letters. 2009;**19**(7): 1956-1959. DOI: 10.1016/j.bmcl.2009.02.045

[108] Shirwaikar A, Bhilegaonkar PM, Malini S, Kumar JS. The gastroprotective activity of the ethanol extract of *Ageratum conyzoides*. Journal of Ethnopharmacology. 2003;**86**(1):117-121. DOI: 10.1016/S0378-8741(03)00050-3

[109] Kouame BF, Toure D, Kablan L, Bedi G, Tea I, Robins R, et al. Chemical constituents and antibacterial activity of essential oils from flowers and stems of *Ageratum conyzoides* from Ivory Coast. Records of Natural Products. 2018;(2):160-168. DOI: 10.25135/rnp.22.17.06.040

[110] Weimann C, Göransson U, Pongprayoon-Claeson U, Claeson P, Bohlin L, Rimpler H, et al. Spasmolytic effects of *Baccharis conferta* and some of its constituents. The Journal of Pharmacy and Pharmacology. 2002;**54**(1):99-104. DOI: 10.1211/0022357021771797

[111] Romo de Vivar A, Pérez-Castorena AL, Arciniegas A, Villaseñor JL. Secondary metabolites from Mexican species of the tribe Senecioneae (Asteraceae). Journal of the Mexican Chemical Society. 2007;**51**(3):160-172 http://www.scielo.org.mx/pdf/jmcs/v51n3/v51n3a7.pdf

[112] Shen Y, Sun Z, Shi P, Wang G, Wu Y, Li S, et al. Anticancer effect of petroleum ether extract from *Bidens pilosa* L and its constituent's analysis by GC-MS. Journal of Ethnopharmacology. 2018;**217**:126-133. DOI: 10.1016/j.jep.2018.02.019

[113] Lima TC, de Jesus Souza R, da Silva FA, Biavatti MW. The genus *Calea* L.: A review on traditional uses, phytochemistry, and biological activities. Phytotherapy Research. 2018;**32**(5):769-795. DOI: 10.1002/ptr.6010

[114] Torrado-Truiti MD, Sarragiotto MH, Abreu-Filho BA, Vataru-Nakamura C, Dias-Filho BP. In vitro antibacterial activity of a 7-O-beta-D-glucopyranosyl-nutanocoumarin from *Chaptalia nutans* (Asteraceae). Memórias do Instituto Oswaldo Cruz. 2003;**98**(2):283-286. DOI: 10.1590/S0074-02762003000200020

[115] Cárdenas-Ortega NC, Zavala-Sánchez MA, Aguirre-Rivera JR, Pérez-González C, Pérez-Gutiérrez S. Chemical composition and antifungal activity of essential oil of *Chrysactinia mexicana* Gray. Journal of Agricultural

and Food Chemistry. 2005;**53**(11): 4347-4349. DOI: 10.1021/jf040372h

[116] Guerra-Boone L, Alvarez-Román R, Salazar-Aranda R, Torres-Cirio A, Rivas-Galindo VM, Waksman de Torres N, et al. Chemical compositions and antimicrobial and antioxidant activities of the essential oils from *Magnolia grandiflora*, *Chrysactinia mexicana*, and *Schinus molle* found in Northeast Mexico. Natural Product Communications. 2013;**8**(1):135-138

[117] Zavala-Mendoza D, Grasa L, Zavala-Sánchez MÁ, Pérez-Gutiérrez S, Murillo MD. Antispasmodic effects and action mechanism of essential oil of *Chrysactinia mexicana* A. Gray on rabbit ileum. Molecules. 2016;**21**(6):783. DOI: 10.3390/molecules21060783

[118] Sagrero-Nieves L, Bartley JP. Volatile components from the leaves of *Heterotheca inuloides* Cass. Flavour and Fragrance Journal. 1996;**11**(1):49-51. DOI: 10.1002/(SICI)1099-1026(199601)11:1<49::AID-FFJ538>3.0.CO;2-J

[119] Egas V, Salazar-Cervantes G, Romero I, Méndez-Cuesta CA, Rodríguez-Chávez JL, Delgado G. Anti-*Helicobacter pylori* metabolites from *Heterotheca inuloides* (Mexican arnica). Fitoterapia. 2018;**127**:314-321. DOI: 10.1016/j.fitote.2018.03.001

[120] García-Pérez JS, Cuéllar-Bermúdez SP, Arévalo-Gallegos A, Rodríguez-Rodríguez J, Iqbal H, Parra-Saldivar R. Identification of bioactivity, volatile and fatty acid profile in supercritical fluid extracts of Mexican arnica. International Journal of Molecular Sciences. 2016;**17**(9):1528. DOI: 10.3390/ijms17091528

[121] Borges-Del-Castillo J, Martinez-Martir AI, Rodriguez-Luis F, Rodriguez-Ubis JC, Vazquez-Bueno P. Isolation and synthesis of two coumarins from *Melampodium divaricatum*. Phytochemistry. 1984;**23**(4):859-861. DOI: 10.1016/S0031-9422(00)85043-8

[122] Rufino-González Y, Ponce-Macotela M, Jiménez-Estrada M, Jiménez-Fragoso CN, Palencia G, Sansón-Romero G, et al. *Piqueria trinervia* as a source of metabolites against *Giardia intestinalis*. Pharmaceutical Biology. 2017;**55**(1):1787-1791. DOI: 10.1080/13880209.2017.1325912

[123] Wollenweber E, Mann K, Arriaga FJ, Yatskievych G. Flavonoids and terpenoids from the leaf resin of *Pluchea odorata*. Zeitschrift für Naturforschung. Section C. 1985;**40**:321-324. DOI: 10.1515/znc-1985-5-607

[124] Vasudevan P, Kashyap S, Sharma S. Tagetes: A multipurpose plant. Bioresource Technology. 1997;**62**:29-35. DOI: 10.1016/S0960-8524(97)00101-6

[125] Pérez-Gutiérrez RO, Hernández-Luna HE, Hernández-Garrido SE. Antioxidant activity of *Tagetes erecta* essential oil. Journal of the Chilean Chemical Society. 2006;**51**(2):883-886. DOI: 10.4067/S0717-97072006000200010

[126] Xu LW, Juan CH, Qi HY, Sshi YP. Phytochemicals and their biological activities of plants in *Tagetes* L. Chinese Herbal Medicines. 2012;**4**(2):103-117. DOI: 10.3969/j.issn.1674-6384.2012.02.004

[127] Camarillo G, Rodríguez C. Biological activity of *Tagetes filifolia* (Asteraceae) on *Trialeurodes vaporariorum* (Hemiptera: Aleyrodidae). Revista Colombiana de Entomologia. 2009;**35**(2):177-184 http://www.scielo.org.co/pdf/rcen/v35n2/v35n2a12.pdf

[128] Tagne AM, Marino F, Cosentino M. *Tithonia diversifolia* (Hemsl.) A. Gray as a medicinal plant: A comprehensive review of its ethnopharmacology, phytochemistry, pharmacotoxicology

and clinical relevance. Journal of Ethnopharmacology. 2018;**220**:94-116. DOI: 10.1016/j.jep.2018.03.025

[129] Santana PI, Osorio MS, Sterner O, Garcìa EL. Phytochemical studies of fractions and compounds present in *Vernonanthura patens* with antifungal bioactivity and potential as antineoplastic. In: Rao V, editor. Phytochemicals—A Global Perspective of their Role in Nutrition and Health. InTech; 2012. pp. 503-518. DOI: 10.5772/28961

[130] Manzano PI, Miranda M, Abreu-Payrol J, Silva M, Sterner O, Peralta EL. Pentacyclic triterpenoids with antimicrobial activity from the leaves of *Vernonanthura patens* (Asteraceae). Emirates Journal of Food and Agriculture. 2013;**1**:539-543. DOI: 10.9755/ejfa.v25i7.15989

[131] Satorres SE, Chiaramello AI, Tonn CE, Laciar AL. Antibacterial activity of organic extracts from *Zinnia peruviana* (L.) against gram-positive and gram-negative bacteria. Emirates Journal of Food and Agriculture. 2012;**24**(4): 344-347 https://www.ejfa.me/index.php/journal/article/view/894

[132] Lim TK. *Parmentiera aculeata*. In: Edible Medicinal and Non-Medicinal Plants. Dordrecht: Springer; 2012. pp. 508-511. DOI: 10.1007/978-90-481-8661-7_67

[133] Abad MJ, Bermejo P, Villar A, Sanchez Palomino S, Carrasco L. Antiviral activity of medicinal plant extracts. Phytotherapy Research. 1997;**11**(3):198-202. DOI: 10.1002/(SICI)1099-1573(199705)11:3<198::AID-PTR78>3.0.CO;2-L

[134] Mohan SC, Anand T, Priya RM. Protective effect of *Tecoma stans* flowers on gentamicin-induced nephrotoxocity in rats. Asian Journal of Biochemistry. 2016;**11**(1):59-67. DOI: 10.3923/ajb.2016.59.67

[135] Marcotullio M, Curini M, Becerra J. An ethnopharmacological, phytochemical and pharmacological review on lignans from Mexican *Bursera* spp. Molecules. 2018;**23**:1976. DOI: 10.3390/molecules23081976

[136] Mujumdar AM, Misar AV. Anti-inflammatory activity of *Jatropha curcas* roots in mice and rats. Journal of Ethnopharmacology. 2004;**90**(1):11-15. DOI: 10.1016/j.jep.2003.09.019

[137] Frei B, Heinrich M, Bork PM, Herrmann D, Jaki B, Kato T, et al. Multiple screening of medicinal plants from Oaxaca, Mexico: Ethnobotany and bioassays as a basis for phytochemical investigation. Phytomedicine. 1998;**5**(3):177-186. DOI: 10.1016/S0944-7113(98)80025-1

[138] Estrada-Reyes R, Aguirre-Hernández E, García-Argáez A, Soto-Hernández M, Linares E, Bye R, et al. Comparative chemical composition of *Agastache mexicana* subsp. mexicana and *A. mexicana* subsp. xolocotziana. Biochemical Systematics and Ecology. 2004;**32**(7):685-694. DOI: 10.1016/j.bse.2004.01.005

[139] Juárez ZN, Hernández LR, Bach H, Sánchez-Arreola E, Bach H. Antifungal activity of essential oils extracted from *Agastache mexicana* ssp. xolocotziana and *Porophyllum linaria* against post-harvest pathogens. Industrial Crops and Products. 2015;**74**:178-182. DOI: 10.1016/j.indcrop.2015.04.058

[140] Méndez-Hernández A, Hernández-Hernández AA, López-Santiago MD, Morales-López J, editors. Herbolaria Oaxaqueña para la Salud. 1st ed. México; 2009. pp. 1-143

[141] Hernández-Abreu O, Durán-Gómez L, Best-Brown R, Villalobos-Molina R, Rivera-Leyva J, Estrada-Soto S. Validated liquid chromatographic method and analysis of content of tilianin on several extracts obtained

from *Agastache mexicana* and its correlation with vasorelaxant effect. Journal of Ethnopharmacology. 2011;**138**(2):487-491. DOI: 10.1016/j.jep.2011.09.041

[142] Zielińska S, Matkowski A. Phytochemistry and bioactivity of aromatic and medicinal plants from the genus *Agastache* (Lamiaceae). Phytochemistry Reviews. 2014;**13**(2):391-416. DOI: 10.1007/s11101-014-9349-1

[143] Villa-Ruano N, Pacheco-Hernández Y, Cruz-Durán R, Lozoya-Gloria E. Volatiles and seasonal variation of the essential oil composition from the leaves of *Clinopodium macrostemum* var. laevigatum and its biological activities. Industrial Crops and Products. 2015;77:741-747. DOI: 10.1016/j.indcrop.2015.09.050

[144] Calzada F, Yépez-Mulia L, Aguilar A. In vitro susceptibility of *Entamoeba histolytica* and *Giardia lamblia* to plants used in Mexican traditional medicine for the treatment of gastrointestinal disorders. Journal of Ethnopharmacology. 2006;**108**(3): 367-370. DOI: 10.1016/j.jep.2006.05.025

[145] Caamal-Herrera IO, Muñoz-Rodríguez D, Madera-Santana T, Azamar-Barrios JA. Identification of volatile compounds in essential oil and extracts of *Ocimum micranthum* Willd leaves using GC/MS. International Journal of Applied Research in Natural Products. 2016;**9**(1):31-40 http://www.ijarnp.org/index.php/ijarnp/article/view/331/pdf

[146] Pérez-Nicolás M, Vibrans H, Romero-Manzanares A. Can the use of medicinal plants motivate forest conservation in the humid mountains of northern Oaxaca, México? Botanical Sciences. 2018;**96**(2):267-285. DOI: 10.17129/botsci.1862

[147] Reyes-Caudillo E, Tecante A, Valdivia-López MA. Dietary fibre content and antioxidant activity of phenolic compounds present in Mexican chia (*Salvia hispanica* L.) seeds. Food Chemistry. 2008;**107**(2):656-663. DOI: 10.1016/j.foodchem.2007.08.062

[148] Porras-Loaiza P, Jiménez-Munguía MT, Sosa-Morales ME, Palou E, López-Malo A. Physical properties, chemical characterization and fatty acid composition of Mexican chia (*Salvia hispanica* L.) seeds. International Journal of Food Science and Technology. 2014;**49**(2):571-577. DOI: 10.1111/ijfs.12339

[149] Jiménez-Pérez ND, Lorea-Hernández FG, Jankowski CK, Reyes-Chilpa R. Essential oils in Mexican bays (Litsea spp., Lauraceae): Taxonomic assortment and ethnobotanical implications. Economic Botany. 2011;**65**(2):178-189. DOI: 10.1007/s12231-011-9160-5

[150] Guzmán-Gutiérrez SL, Gómez-Cansino R, García-Zebadúa JC, Jiménez-Pérez NC, Reyes-Chilpa R. Antidepressant activity of *Litsea glaucescens* essential oil: Identification of β-pinene and linalool as active principles. Journal of Ethnopharmacology. 2012;**143**(2): 673-679. DOI: 10.1016/j.jep.2012.07.026

[151] Sagrero-Nieves L, Bartley JP. Volatile components of avocado leaves (*Persea americana* mill) from the Mexican race. Journal of the Science of Food and Agriculture. 1995;**67**(1):49-51. DOI: 10.1002/jsfa.2740670109

[152] Abe F, Nagafuji S, Okawa M, Kinjo J, Akahane H, Ogura T, et al. Trypanocidal constituents in plants. 5. Evaluation of some Mexican plants for their trypanocidal activity and active constituents in the seeds of *Persea americana*. Biological & Pharmaceutical Bulletin. 2005;**28**(7):1314-1317. DOI: 10.1248/bpb.28.1314

[153] Granados-Echegoyen C, Pérez-Pacheco R, Alonso-Hernández N,

Vásquez-López A, Lagunez-Rivera L, Rojas-Olivos A. Chemical characterization and mosquito larvicidal activity of essential oil from leaves of *Persea americana* mill (Lauraceae) against Culex quinquefasciatus (say). Asian Pacific Journal of Tropical Disease. 2015;**5**(6):463-467. DOI: 10.1016/S2222-1808(15)60816-7

[154] Mata R, Morales I, Pérez O, Rivero-Cruz I, Acevedo L, Enriquez-Mendoza I, et al. Antimycobacterial compounds from *Piper sanctum*. Journal of Natural Products. 2004;**67**(12):1961-1968. DOI: 10.1021/np0401260

[155] Catap ES, Kho MJ, Jimenez MR. In vivo nonspecific immunomodulatory and antispasmodic effects of common purslane (*Portulaca oleracea* Linn.) leaf extracts in ICR mice. Journal of Ethnopharmacology. 2018;**215**:191-198. DOI: 10.1016/j.jep.2018.01.009

[156] Argotte-Ramos R, Ramírez-Avila G, Rodríguez-Gutiérrez MD, Ovilla-Muñoz M, Lanz-Mendoza H, Rodríguez MH, et al. Antimalarial 4-phenylcoumarins from the stem bark of *Hintonia latiflora*. Journal of Natural Products. 2006;**69**(10):1442-1444. DOI: 10.1021/np060233p

[157] Yahia EM, Gutiérrez-Orozco F, Arvizu-de Leon C. Phytochemical and antioxidant characterization of mamey (*Pouteria sapota* Jacq. HE Moore & Stearn) fruit. Food Research International. 2011;**44**(7):2175-2181. DOI: 10.1016/j.foodres.2010.11.029

[158] Vasconcellos MC, Montenegro RC, Militão GC, Fonseca AM, Pessoa OD, Lemos TL, et al. Bioactivity of biflorin, a typical o-naphthoquinone isolated from *Capraria biflora* L. Zeitschrift für Naturforschung. Section C. 2005;**60**(5-6):394-398. DOI: 10.1515/znc-2005-5-605

[159] Collins DO, Gallimore WA, Reynolds WF, Williams LA, Reese PB. New skeletal sesquiterpenoids, caprariolides A–D, from *Capraria biflora* and their insecticidal activity. Journal of Natural Products. 2000;**63**(11):1515-1518. DOI: 10.1021/np000280w

[160] Imran M, Butt MS, Suleria HA. *Capsicum annuum* bioactive compounds: Health promotion perspectives. In: Jean-Michel M, Ramawat KG, editors. Bioactive Molecules in Food. Cham: Springer; 2018. pp. 1-22. DOI: 10.1007/978-3-319-54528-8_47-1

[161] Khaled RN, Ćirić A, Glamočlija J, Calhelha RC, Ferreira ICFR, Soković M. Identification of the bioactive constituents and the antibacterial, antifungal and cytotoxic activities of different fractions from *Cestrum nocturnum* L. Jordan Journal of Biological Sciences. 2018;**11**(3):273-279

[162] Zoubiri S, Baaliouamer A. GC and GC/MS analyses of the Algerian *Lantana camara* leaf essential oil: Effect against *Sitophilus granarius* adults. Journal of Saudi Chemical Society. 2012;**16**(3):291-297. DOI: 10.1016/j.jscs.2011.01.013

[163] Hernández T, García-Bores AM, Serrano R, Ávila G, Dávila P, Cervantes H, et al. Fitoquímica y actividades biológicas de plantas de importancia en la medicina tradicional del Valle de Tehuacán-Cuicatlán. TIP. Revista Especializada en Ciencias Químico-Biológicas. 2015;**18**(2):116-121. DOI: 10.1016/j.recqb.2015.09.003

[164] Sousa EO, Miranda CM, Nobre CB, Boligon AA, Athayde ML, Costa JG. Phytochemical analysis and antioxidant activities of *Lantana camara* and *Lantana montevidensis* extracts. Industrial Crops and Products. 2015;**70**:7-15. DOI: 10.1016/j.indcrop.2015.03.010

[165] Lin LZ, Mukhopadhyay S, Robbins RJ, Harnly JM. Identification

and quantification of flavonoids of Mexican oregano (*Lippia graveolens*) by LC-DAD-ESI/MS analysis. Journal of Food Composition and Analysis. 2007;**20**(5):361-369. DOI: 10.1016/j.jfca.2006.09.005

[166] Hernández T, Canales M, Avila JG, García AM, Meraz S, Caballero J, et al. Composition and antibacterial activity of essential oil of *Lippia graveolens* HBK (Verbenaceae). Boletin Latinoamericano y del Caribe de Plantas Medicinales y Aromaticas. 2009;**8**(4):295-300

Chapter 6

Anticancer Activity of Uncommon Medicinal Plants from the Republic of Suriname: Traditional Claims, Preclinical Findings, and Potential Clinical Applicability against Cancer

Dennis R.A. Mans and Euridice R. Irving

Abstract

Despite much progress in our understanding of the essence of cancer, remarkable advances in methods for early diagnosis, the expanding array of antineoplastic drugs and treatment modalities, as well as important refinements in their use, this disease is among the leading causes of morbidity and mortality in many parts of the world. In fact, the next decade is anticipated to bring over 20 million new cases per year globally, about half of whom will die from their disease. This indicates a need for better strategies to deal with cancer. One way to go forward is to draw lessons from ancient ethnopharmacological wisdom and to evaluate the plant biodiversity for compounds with potential antineoplastic activity. This approach has already yielded many breakthrough cytotoxic drugs such as vincristine, etoposide, paclitaxel, and irinotecan. The Republic of Suriname (South America), renowned for its pristine and highly biodiverse rain forests as well as its ethnic, cultural, and ethnopharmacological diversity, could also contribute to these developments. This chapter addresses the cancer problem throughout the world and in Suriname, extensively deals with nine plants used for treating cancer in the country, and concludes with their prospects in anticancer drug discovery and development programs.

Keywords: cancer, Suriname, medicinal plants, traditional uses, phytochemistry, pharmacology, anticancer activity

1. Introduction

1.1 Generalities

Cancer is a generic term to describe over 200 distinct disease forms that, nonetheless, share three distinguishing characteristics, namely uncontrolled cellular proliferation, invasion of the abnormal cells into adjacent tissues, and their spread to distant organs via blood and lymph vessels [1]. The biological events fundamental to the development of cancer involve the transformation of normal cells to a precancerous lesion which subsequently progresses to a malignant tumor in a multistage process [1]. These changes are the result of the interaction between an individual's genetic make-up and external agents including physical, chemical, and biological carcinogens [2].

Recognized physical carcinogens are ultraviolet and ionizing radiation which have been linked to skin cancer as well as leukemia and a number of solid tumors, respectively [2]. Well-studied chemical carcinogens are asbestos that has mainly been associated with lung cancer and mesothelioma; components of tobacco smoke which have been linked not only to breast and lung cancer but also to a host of other malignancies; aflatoxins produced by certain molds in improperly stored staple commodities which have been related to liver cancer; and the drinking water contaminant arsenic that has particularly been associated with lung, bladder, and kidney cancer [2]. Examples of biological carcinogens are the human papillomavirus, the hepatitis B virus, the hepatitis C virus, and the Epstein-Barr virus, the causative factors of cervical cancer, liver cancer, and certain lymphomas, respectively; the stomach bacterium *Helicobacter pylori* that has been implicated in the development of stomach cancer; and certain fish-parasitic flatworms associated with cholangiocarcinoma and urinary bladder cancer [2].

Molecular insights have revealed that the development of cancer—including its capacity to proliferate in an uncontrolled fashion, escape apoptosis, invade neighboring tissues, and disseminate to distant organs—involves aberrations in molecular networks that include oncogenes, tumor suppressor genes, and repair genes [1]. These changes occur in a multistep manner and often take place over many years [1]. This is an important reason that cancer usually manifests at older age, when sufficient carcinogenic mutations have accumulated to cause cancer and innate defense and cellular repair mechanisms have become less effective [1].

1.2 Worldwide epidemiology

According to GLOBOCAN 2018 estimates of cancer incidence and mortality produced by the International Agency for Research on Cancer, cancer will represent the leading cause of death throughout the world in the twenty-first century [3]. In 2018, there were an estimated 18.1 million new cancer cases and 9.6 million cancer deaths globally [3]. Lung cancer and female breast cancer were the most commonly diagnosed malignancy (each 11.6% of total overall cases), followed by cancer of colon and rectum (10.2%), prostate (7.1%), stomach (5.7%), and liver (4.7%) [3]. The most deadly cancers in that year were lung, colorectal, stomach, liver, and breast cancer accounting for 18.4, 9.2, 8.2, 8.2, and 6.6%, respectively, of the total number of cancer fatalities [3]. The most frequent cancers in males were lung, prostate, colorectal, stomach, and liver cancer with incidence rates of 14.5, 13.5, 10.9, 7.2, and 6.3%, respectively, and mortality rates of 22.0, 6.7, 9.0, 9.5, and 10.2%, respectively [3]. And in females, the most common cancers were those of the breast, colon and rectum, lung, and cervix uteri, with incidence rates of 24.2, 9.5, 8.4, and 6.6%, respectively, and mortality rates of 15.0, 9.5, 13.8, and 7.5%, respectively [3].

There were substantial variations among countries with respect to the most frequently diagnosed cancers and the leading causes of cancer death [3]. For instance, for many cancers, incidence rates were generally two- to threefold higher in industrialized countries than in transitioning economies [3]. However, differences in mortality were smaller, as relatively more patients in developing countries died from their disease, probably because of low screening rates as well as less advanced screening services and diagnostic methods in these regions [3]. Furthermore, cancers related to a westernized lifestyle such as lung, breast, and colorectal cancer were (much) more common in industrialized regions than in developing/

transitioning regions, even though these neoplasms were among the most common malignancies in both regions [3]. On the other hand, oral cancer and cervical cancer were much more frequent in (certain) developing/transitioning countries than in industrialized countries [3]. These differences are probably for an important part attributable to differences in associated risk factors and screening facilities, respectively, resulting in the former malignancy accounting for almost 50% to the burden of cancer in south-central Asia [4] and the latter occurring at incidence rates between 13.0 and 43.1 per 100,000 in Central America, South America, and the Caribbean, as well as in the parts of Africa [5].

1.3 Treatment modalities

The treatment modalities for cancer depend on the type of cancer as well as its stage and grade [6]. Some cases require only one form of treatment, but most patients need a combination of therapeutic modalities such as surgery with chemotherapy and/or radiation therapy. Surgery is applied for removing localized solid tumors or debulking large solid tumors in order to improve the efficacy of, for instance, chemotherapy [6]. Radiation therapy—external beam radiation therapy, brachytherapy, or systemic radioisotope therapy—uses high doses of radiation to kill cancer cells by damaging their DNA [6]. Chemotherapy is a systemic treatment with mostly combinations of antineoplastic drugs and is intended to kill cancer cells by stopping or slowing their growth or division, but it is also applied as an adjuvant to prevent disease recurrence after surgery or radiation therapy and as a neoadjuvant therapy to decrease the size of a tumor before surgery or radiation therapy [6].

Other cancer treatment modalities are immunotherapy, hormonal therapy, and angiosuppressive therapy. Immunotherapy can make use of adoptive cell transfer involving the infusion of engineered autologous or allogeneic T cells into a patient which can attack the cancer directly; monoclonal antibodies directed at cancer cell-specific antigens; or immunomodulating substances such as cytokines and Bacillus Calmette-Guérin vaccine which stimulate the immune system in a more general way [6]. Hormonal therapy slows or stops the growth of hormone-dependent tumors such as breast and prostate cancers, or reduces or prevents the symptoms in patients suffering from these cancers who do not qualify for surgery or radiation therapy [6]. Hormonal therapy can also be used in the adjuvant or neoadjuvant setting [6]. Angiosuppressive or antiangiogenic therapy interrupts the angiogenic signals that a tumor emits to its surroundings for recruiting a blood supply and causes tumors to shrink [6].

Despite this respectable array of antineoplastic agents and therapeutic modalities most cancers remain fatal, particularly when detected at an advanced stage. This implies a need for more efficacious forms of treatment of neoplastic disease. Many efforts are being dedicated to this goal, including improved early diagnosis, the development of highly specific targeted therapies, and the identification of more efficacious antineoplastic drugs. It is generally agreed that the application of ancient wisdom and folk medicine represents an important strategy to discover and develop new anticancer drugs [7–10]. This approach has led to breakthrough anticancer drugs such as the tubulin-interfering agents vincristine from the periwinkle plant *Catharanthus roseus* (L.) G. Don (Apocynaceae) [11] and paclitaxel from the Pacific yew *Taxus brevifolia* Peattie 1950 (Taxaceae) [12]; the topoisomerase I and II inhibitors irinotecan [13] and etoposide [14], respectively, from *Podophyllum* plant species (Berberidaceae) and the Chinese happy tree *Camptotheca acuminata* Decne. (Nyssaceae), respectively; as well as a host of other plant-derived compounds [7, 10]. Notably, almost half of the anticancer drugs that have been granted approval in the United States of America between 1981 and 2014 were from natural origin [9].

So far, only a relative handful of the plant kingdom has been evaluated for pharmacologically active plant substances with potential efficacy against cancer. Therefore, it is likely that further exploration of the rain forests along with other less explored environments such as deserts, tundras, as well as freshwater and marine ecosystems [15], will help identify many structurally novel and mechanistically unique compounds for fighting cancer. This chapter first reviews a few aspects of cancer throughout the world, then focuses on cancer in the Republic of Suriname, subsequently addresses in detail nine medicinal plants that are used for treating cancer in the country, and concludes with some remarks about their potential usefulness against this disease.

2. Background on Suriname

2.1 Geography, population, demographics, and economy

The Republic of Suriname is situated in the north-eastern part of South America adjacent to the Atlantic Ocean and has a land area of roughly 165,000 km^2 (**Figure 1**). The population of about 570,000 is among the ethnically most varied in the world, comprising Amerindians, the original inhabitants; Maroons, the immediate descendants of enslaved Africans shipped from western Africa between the seventeenth and the nineteenth century; Creoles, a generic term referring to anyone having one or more African ancestors; the descendants from indentured laborers attracted from China, India, and Java (Indonesia) between the second half of the nineteenth century and the first half of the twentieth century; as well as immigrants from various European, South American, and Caribbean countries [16].

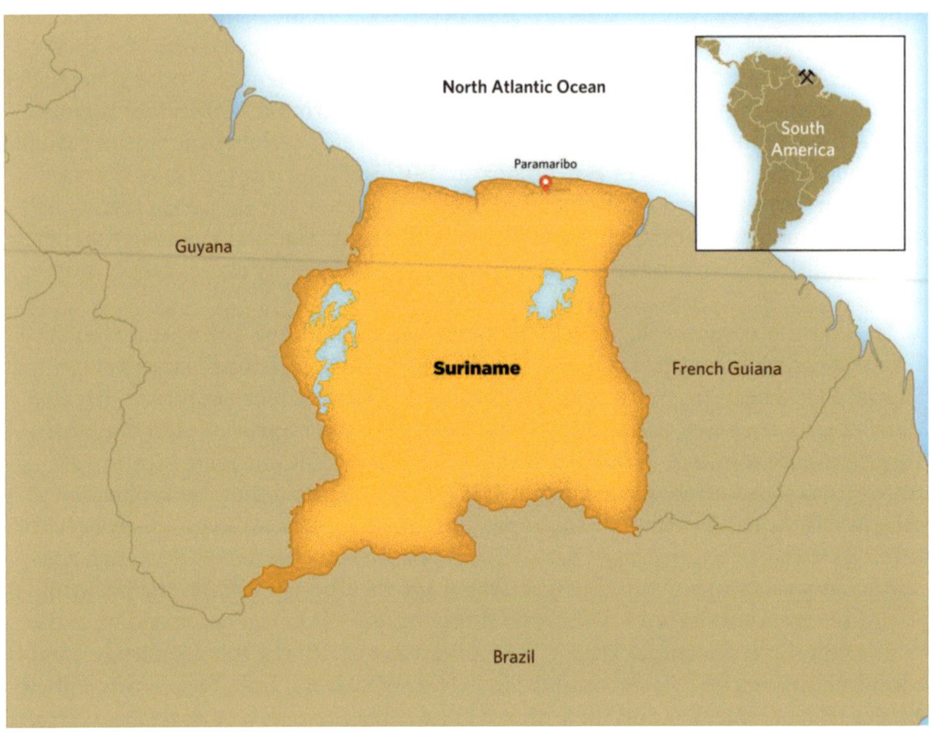

Figure 1.
Location of Suriname with respect to its neighboring countries French Guiana, Brazil, and Guyana, as well as its position in South America (insert) (from: https://goo.gl/images/F77jgS).

Suriname can be characterized as a demographically transitioning country with declining mortality and infertility rates as well as a growing and aging population. These changes are for an important attributable to considerable progress in health care, nutrition, sanitation, and drinking water quality; the eradication of various infectious diseases; as well as improvements in average living and working conditions, education, and income [17, 18]. The result was a decline of the death rate from 24 per 1000 in 1923 to 6 per 1000 in 2011 and the attainment of an average life expectancy of 70 years in 2011 [17].

The country's most important economic means of support are crude oil drilling as well as gold and bauxite mining [19]. These activities, together with agriculture, fisheries, forestry, and ecotourism, have substantially contributed to Suriname's gross domestic income (GDI) in 2014 of USD 5.21 billion and the average *per capita income* in that year of USD 9325 [19]. This positions Suriname on the World Bank's list of upper-middle income economies [20].

2.2 Health care

Suriname spends about 5.7% of its GDI—which amounted to USD 589 *per capita* in 2014—to health care [21]. This sum covers the health costs for the economically weakest individuals; insurance for government employees and employees of government-related companies; import and distribution of essential pharmaceuticals; vaccination programs; maternal and child health care; programs to fight parasitic and microbial diseases; dental care for schoolchildren; services for dermatological diseases, sexually transmitted diseases, and HIV/AIDS; as well as a Kidney Dialyses Center and a Blood Bank [21].

Primary health care in Suriname is offered by the government-subsidized Regional Health Services and Medical Mission, as well as approximately 250 general practitioners. The Regional Health Services run 43 community health centers staffed with physicians and nurses, covers the entire coastal area, and offers basic laboratory testing as well as curative and preventive services including cervical cancer screening and dental, prenatal, and obstetric care. The Medical Mission is a nongovernmental organization that provides health services to people living in Suriname's hinterland. The clinics are staffed with community health workers who are supervised by general practitioners who travel back and forth on a regular basis.

Secondary care is provided by two private and two government-supported hospitals in Paramaribo and one public hospital in the western district of Nickerie. Medical emergencies can turn around-the-clock to the First-aid Stations of the Academic Hospital Paramaribo and the Saint Vincentius Hospital Suriname. The Academic Hospital Paramaribo also functions as training facility for both general practitioners and medical specialists. All hospitals have modern clinical laboratory facilities as well as radiology services at their disposal. There are, in addition, four private clinical laboratories and three private radiology clinics. Diagnostic imaging including computed tomography and magnetic resonance imaging is possible at two private clinics and the Academic Hospital Paramaribo. This hospital also provides tertiary care at a Thorax Center, a Neurology High-Care Unit, a Neonatal Care Unit, and a Radiotherapy Center.

3. Cancer in Suriname

3.1 Epidemiology

As in many other low- and middle-income countries, there is no population-based cancer registry in Suriname. The occurrence of cancer in the country is estimated from data on the histopathologically confirmed cases at the Pathologic Anatomical Laboratory of the Academic Hospital Paramaribo that functions as the country's cancer-based registry. This institution reported for 2014 a crude incidence rate of 133 per 100,000 population with the most common cancers being breast, colorectal, prostate, and cervical cancer [22]. An earlier publication [23] mentioned an average of 70 per 100,000 population for the period 1980–2000, suggesting an almost twofold increase in the occurrence of cancer in Suriname since the turn of the century.

Cancer mortality in Suriname has been registered since 1958. In the period between 1962 and 1970, the average death rate due to cancer was 60 per 100,000 per year [24]. This figure had risen to approximately 72 in 2011, ranking cancer as the second most common cause of mortality in the country, after cardiovascular diseases [25]. The top five causes of cancer mortality in that year were prostate, lung, rectum-sigmoid, female breast, and cervical cancer [25]. Most of the fatalities in females were attributable to breast and cervical cancer, while prostate cancer was the leading cause of cancer death in males [25].

3.2 Allopathic forms of cancer treatment in Suriname

Suriname has no national guidelines for the screening, diagnosis, and treatment of cancer, and structured screening programs for breast, cervical, and colon cancer are nonexistent. For these reasons, a comprehensive national cancer control plan has been developed [22] that will be executed in the short term by the Ministry of Health.

Still, primary prevention programs such as mandatory vaccination against the hepatitis B virus (since 2011) and the availability of a HPV vaccine for young girls (implemented in 2013) may help reduce the cancer burden in the country. This may also be achieved by early detection services such as screening for cervical and breast cancer, even though these facilities are in general utilized on an *ad hoc* basis. Cervical cancer screening occurs upon referral and is done at the Lobi Foundation, a nongovernmental organization for reproductive preventive services, using cytology (Pap smear) or visual inspection with acetic acid. Unfortunately, the coverage of this program is below 20% and thus has probably little impact on cervical cancer mortality [26]. Mammography, breast ultrasound, and fine needle aspiration for the assessment of breast lesions are since 2009 possible at two private clinics and two hospitals. Stereotactic (mammogram-guided) breast biopsy has been available since 2018 at the Academic Hospital Paramaribo. Cancer-specific evaluations such as testing for hormone receptors and tumor markers, are carried out at the Pathologic Anatomical Laboratory of this hospital.

Surgery, radiation therapy, and chemotherapy as standard therapeutic modalities for cancer are all available in Suriname. Surgical treatment is offered by all four hospitals in Paramaribo. Radiation therapy has been available since 2012 and is performed by two radiation oncologists. Chemotherapy is delivered by two oncologists and two gynecologic oncologists. If diagnostic or therapeutic services are not available in Suriname, patients can be transferred to health centers abroad provided that they have a good prognosis and are younger than 70 years. More than half of the selected patients are treated in Bogotá, Columbia. All costs are covered by the Surinamese Ministry of Health through the State Health Foundation [21].

3.3 Traditional forms of cancer treatment in Suriname

All ethnic groups in Suriname have preserved their own specific identity including their particular forms of traditional medicine, probably as a means of strengthening the ethnic identity after their relocation to their new homeland [27, 28]. Not surprisingly, the use of various traditional medicinal systems—involving, among others, Indigenous, African, and Chinese traditional medicine, Indian Ayurveda, as well as Indonesian Jawa—is deeply rooted in Suriname [27, 28]. Furthermore, Suriname's large biodiversity provides ample and readily available raw material that can be processed into ethnopharmacological plant-based preparations [29]. As a result, many diseases including cancer are often treated with such medications instead of, or in conjunction with, allopathic forms of treatment [30] despite the availability of affordable and accessible modern health care throughout the entire country.

This holds true for, for instance, patients who are motivated by aversion of "chemical" drugs with attendant adverse or side effects and those whose philosophy about life is not compatible with the use of allopathic medicine or who have reservations about the viewpoints of allopathic medicine [31]. Others prefer traditional treatments because these modalities would improve conventional therapies and represent gentler means of managing their disease when compared to allopathic medicines [32]. Still other patients, particularly those with advanced disease or cancer that, from a medical standpoint, can no longer be treated, resort to traditional medicines as an ultimate means to improve their situation [33]. And cultural beliefs, traditional values, and certain perceptions of health and disease may entice some people to choose for a familiar traditional therapy rather than a "western" therapy [34, 35].

4. Plants for treating cancer in Suriname

Hereunder, nine plants that are used in Suriname for treating cancer have in detail been assessed for their presumed activity against this disease. The plants have been selected after consulting a number of comprehensive publications describing various aspects of medicinal plants in the country [36–43]. Several of these plants such as the graviola *Annona muricata* L. (Annonaceae), *Aloe vera* (L.) Burm.f. (Asphodelaceae), the bitter melon *Momordica charantia* L. (Cucurbitaceae), the neem tree *Azadirachta indica* A.Juss., 1830 (Meliaceae), *Moringa oleifera* Lam. (Moringaceae), several subspecies and varieties of the black nightshade *Solanum nigrum* L. (Solanaceae), as well as the noni *Morinda citrifolia* L. (Rubiaceae) have elaborately been dealt with in the literature. This led us to decide to leave these plants out of the current chapter and address a number of less well-known plants, which *prima facie* may not qualify for evaluation for their anticancer potential (**Table 1**).

4.1 Annonaceae—*Annona squamosa* L.

The sugar apple *A. squamosa* (**Figure 2**) is probably native to the tropical parts of South America and the Caribbean but is now widely cultivated for its flavorful fruit in many other tropical and subtropical regions throughout the world. Unripe fruits as well as seeds and leaves contain toxic alkaloids with effective vermicidal and insecticidal properties [44]. For these reasons, the seed oil is commonly used to treat head lice [44]. *A. squamosa* preparations are also used against gastrointestinal ailments, urinary tract infections, irregular menstrual flow, and cancer [42, 43, 45]. The therapeutic efficacy of some of these applications may be attributed to acetogenins, terpenes and terpenoids, as well as alkaloids [45, 46].

The seed oil as well as the essential oils from the pericarp, the leaves, and the stembark of *A. squamosa* displayed anticancer activity against a broad range of human cancer cell lines [47–62] as well as H22 hepatoma implanted into laboratory

Family	Species (vernacular names in English; Surinamese)	Part(s) used	Active constituent(s)	References
Annonaceae	*Annona squamosa* L. (sugar-apple; kaner'apra)	Oil from seed, pericarp, leaf, stembark	Annonaceous acetogenins, terpenes/terpenoids, alkaloids	[47–67]
Asteraceae	*Cyanthillium cinereum* (L.) H.Rob. (little ironweed; doifiwiwiri)	Whole plant	Sesquiterpene lactones	[74–79]
Asteraceae	*Eclipta prostrata* (L.) L. (false daisy; luwisa wiwiri)	Leaf, aerial parts, whole plant	Terthiophenes/thiophenes, saponins, triterpenoids, coumestans, flavonoids	[84–94]
Fabaceae	*Abrus precatorius* L., 1753 (crab's eye; kokriki)	Seed, leaf	Abrin, phenolics, flavonoids	[100–110]
Fabaceae	*Tephrosia sinapou* (Buch.) Chev. (Surinam poison; bumbi)	Root, leaf, aerial parts, stem	Benzil derivatives, coumestan derivatives, flavones/flavonoids, phenols	[118–131]
Loranthaceae	*Phthirusa stelis* (L.) Kuijt (bird vine; pikin fowru doti)	Whole plant, stem, leaf	Peptides, alkynic fatty acids, lectins, triterpenes, glycosides, flavonoids	[135–148]
Rubiaceae	*Uncaria guianensis* (Aubl.) J.F. Gmel. (cat's claw; popokainangra)	Stembark	Oxindole alkaloids	[157–162]
Simaroubaceae	*Quassia amara* L. (bitterwood; kwasibita)	Stem, leaf	Quassinoids, canthin alkaloids	[171–178]
Zingiberaceae	*Zingiber officinale* (ginger; gember, dyindya)	Rhizome	Gingerols, shogaols	[187–203]

Table 1.
Plants with anticancer activity addressed in this chapter, parts preferentially used, presumed constituents with anticancer and chemoprotective activity, and references supporting these activities.

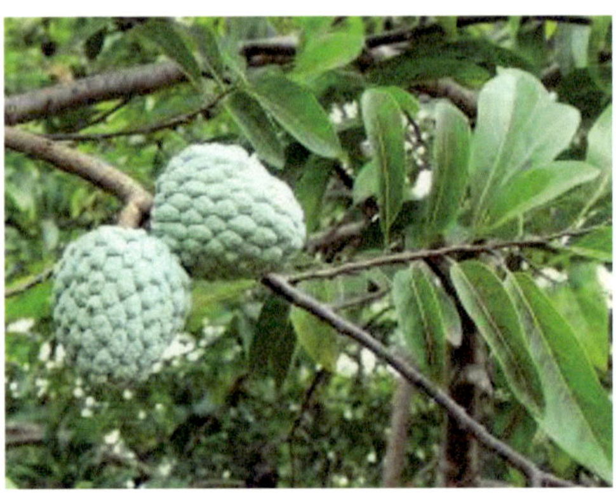

Figure 2.
The sugar apple Annona squamosa L. (Annonaceae) (from: https://goo.gl/images/Lh5g7Z).

mice [51, 60–63]. The anticancer effects have particularly been attributed to annonaceous acetogenins in the seed oil [47–53, 59] as well as annonaceous acetogenins, terpenes, and terpenoids, and alkaloids in pericarp, leaves, and stembark [56–58, 60–62]. Interestingly, the acetogenin squamoxinone-D displayed selective cytotoxicity against the (drug-resistant) SMMC 7721/T cell line [59], and annonaceous acetogens were highly active in H22 hepatoma-bearing laboratory mice [64].

The antitumor activities have in some cases been associated with cycle arrest effects and apoptotic events [54, 60–62] as indicated by the increased caspase-3 activity, the downregulation of antiapoptotic genes, and the fragmentation of the nuclear DNA [54, 60]. The mechanism underlying these events presumably involves the generation of oxidative stress [54]. This supposition is based on the enhanced generation of intracellular reactive oxygen species and the decreased levels of intracellular glutathione species noted in cultured human cells undergoing apoptosis following exposure to *A. squamosa* seed oil [54, 60].

Notably, leaf and stembark extracts protected Swiss albino mice and Syrian golden hamsters from the mutagenic effects of the alkylating agent cyclophosphamide [65] or the potent laboratory carcinogen 7, 12 dimethylbenz(a) anthracene (DMBA) [66], respectively. Furthermore, aqueous and ethanolic stembark extracts decreased lipid peroxidation and potentiated antioxidant activities in an animal model of oral carcinogenesis [67]. These observations suggest that *A. squamosa* also possesses chemopreventive properties.

4.2 Asteraceae—*Cyanthillium cinereum* (L.) H.Rob.

The little ironweed *C. cinereum*, also known as *Vernonia cinerea* (L.) Less. (**Figure 3**), is native to the tropical parts of Africa and Asia but has become naturalized in various other tropical regions including those in South America and the Caribbean. The plant is traditionally used for treating genitourinary disorders, gastrointestinal complaints, and respiratory ailments; to stimulate perspiration in malaria patients; against childhood conditions including bed-wetting; and to fight cancer [42, 43, 68]. *C. cinereum* seeds yield vernonia oil that contains vernolic acid [69], a natural epoxy fatty acid that may serve as a renewable starting material for manufacturing adhesives, paints, dyes, coatings, composites, and plastics [70].

Pharmacological and phytochemical studies have shown a wide range of bioactive compounds such as (a) sesquiterpene lactone(s), which may lend credit to the traditional uses [68]. Two clinical trials found *C. cinereum* preparations efficacious in smoking cessation [71], while one study reported encouraging results with a

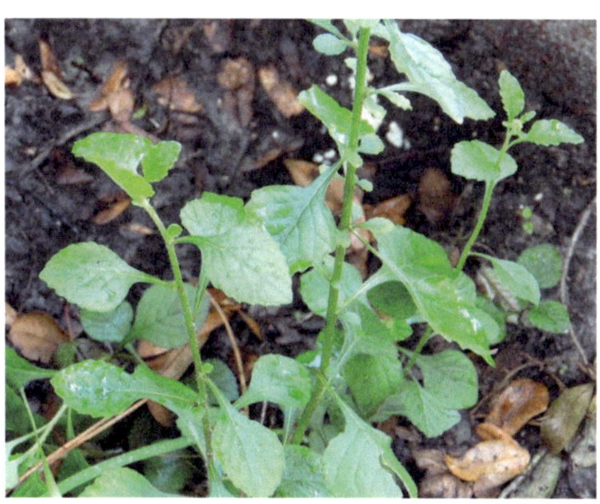

Figure 3.
The little ironweed Cyanthillium cinereum (L.) H.Rob. (Asteraceae) (from: https://goo.gl/images/Lh5g7Z).

herbal *C. cinereum*-containing preparation in patients with type 2 diabetes mellitus [72]. However, the clinical evidence available at this moment is insufficiently sound to support these applications [73].

Support for anticancer activity of *C. cinereum* came from the potent cytotoxicity of an extract from the whole plant against various drug-sensitive and multidrug-resistant human tumor cell lines [74–76]. The whole-plant extract caused the cells to apoptose and sensitized them to common cytotoxic drugs [76]. Furthermore, such an extract as well as the sesquiterpene lactone vernolide A stimulated the activity of cytotoxic T lymphocytes and natural killer cells and enhanced antibody-dependent cellular cytotoxicity and antibody-dependent complement-mediated cytotoxicity in tumor-bearing BALB/c mice by increasing the secretion of interleukin-2 and interferon-γ [77]. This suggests that (this) sesquiterpene lactone may play an important role in the anticancer activity of *C. cinereum* [68, 78].

Other indications for anticancer activity of *C. cinereum* preparations were the inhibitory effects of a 70%-methanol whole-plant extract on the *in vitro* proliferation, invasion, migration, and matrix metalloproteinase activation of B16F-10 murine melanoma cells [79]. The extract also prevented the formation of lung metastases by the B16F-10 cells in C57BL/6 mice, lowered vascular-endothelial growth factor (VEGF) levels in the animals, and substantially increased their life span when compared to untreated controls [79]. Together, these observations raise the possibility that *C. cinereum* may exert its anticancer activity by boosting the immune system, suppressing angiogenesis, and inhibiting drug transport mechanisms in addition to direct cytotoxicity.

4.3 Asteraceae—*Eclipta prostrata* (L.) L.

The false daisy *E. prostrata*, also known as *E. alba* (L.) Hassk. or *E. erecta* L. (**Figure 4**), is probably native to either Asia or the Americas but is now commonly encountered in subtropical and tropical regions throughout the world. It has become an invasive weed in many parts of the tropics, which is particularly due to its ability to grow fast and flower early. The tender leaves and young shoots are consumed as a vegetable but may also serve as a source for the synthesis of titanium dioxide nanoparticles (nano-TiO2) [80]. Nano-TiO2 is widely employed to provide whiteness and opacity to paints, plastics, papers, inks, food colorants, and toothpastes; for the production of cosmetics and skin care products such as sun blocks because of its ability to protect the skin from UV rays while remaining transparent on the skin; and as an additive in antifogging coatings and self-cleaning windows because of its photocatalytic sterilizing properties [81].

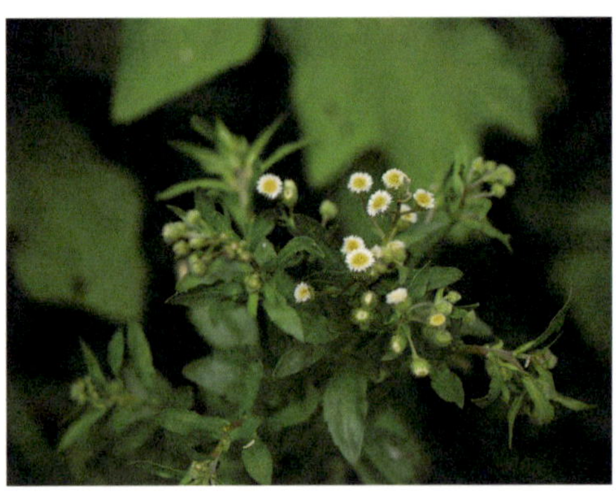

Figure 4.
The false daisy Eclipta prostrata (L.) (Asteraceae) (from: https://goo.gl/images/YGw37Z).

E. prostrata is an important herb in Indian traditional medicine and is used for treating a host of conditions such as skin wounds and certain skin disorders; toothache; hair loss and graying hair; gastrointestinal complaints; uterine disorders; microbial infections; as well as cancer [42, 43, 82]. Some of these claims may be attributable to the presence in the plant of various bioactive constituents including coumestans, thiophene derivatives, terthiophenes, flavonoids, as well as triterpenoids and their glycosides such as eclalbasaponins [82, 83].

Converging lines of evidence suggest that *E. prostrata* preparations and some of their constituents may elicit anticancer activity through multiple mechanisms including direct cytotoxicity, angiosuppression, and chemoprevention. The former possibility is supported by the growth inhibitory effects of crude extracts of the plant in a variety of drug-sensitive and drug-resistant cell lines [84–87] while causing apoptosis in some cases [87, 88]. Also, an orally administered methanolic leaf extract exerted encouraging anticancer activity against Ehrlich ascites carcinoma in Swiss albino mice [89], and a hydroalcoholic extract reversed multidrug resistance in an animal model of liver cancer induced by diethylnitrosamine and 2-acetylaminofluorene [86]. Furthermore, terthiophenes, thiophenes, saponins, triterpenoids, coumestans, and flavonoids isolated from the aerial parts exhibited cytotoxicity against cultured SKOV3 human ovarian cancer cells [90]; an eclalbasaponin I-containing fraction from the aerial parts and the saponin dasyscyphin-C isolated from the leaves inhibited the *in vitro* proliferation of SMMC-7721 human hepatocarcinoma and HeLa human cervical carcinoma cells, respectively [85, 91]; and eclalbasaponin II induced cytotoxicity as well as apoptotic and autophagic cell death in human ovarian cancer cell lines [92].

That *E. prostrata* may also exhibit angiosuppressive activities can be derived from the inhibitory effect of the juice from the whole plant on invasion, migration, and adhesion of a variety of cancer cell types and endothelial cells in the chick chorioallantoic membrane assay [93]. And indications for chemopreventive actions of this plant were provided by the growth inhibitory effect of a coumastan-containing methanolic whole-plant extract in an experimental skin cancer in mice [94]. This presumably occurred by restoring endogenous antioxidant defense mechanisms, enhancing immunosurveillance, silencing cell cycle progression signals, and inducing stable expression of p53 [94].

4.4 Fabaceae—*Abrus precatorius* L., 1753

The crab's eye or rosary pea *A. precatorius* (**Figure 5**) is a slender, woody, climbing plant that grows twisting around trees, shrubs, and hedges and probably originates from India. However, due to its severely invasive capacity, this plant is now commonly encountered in many tropical and subtropical parts of the world. Its deep roots are very difficult to remove, and its aggressive growth, hard-shelled seeds, and ability to sucker make it very difficult to eradicate and to prevent re-infestation. The brightly red colored seeds are used to make necklaces and other ornaments as well as percussion instruments in various cultures. However, they are very toxic because of their high content of the toxalbumin abrin, and ingestion of a single well-chewed seed can be fatal [95].

The sweet-tasting leaves of the plant are used in West Tropical Africa to sweeten foods [96]. These parts of the plant along with the seeds (after denaturing abrin at high temperatures [97]) are also used in various traditional medicinal systems for treating or preventing tetanus, inflammation, snake bites, rabies, and leukoderma; as aphrodisiacs; as oral contraceptives and abortifacients; and for treating cancer [42, 98].

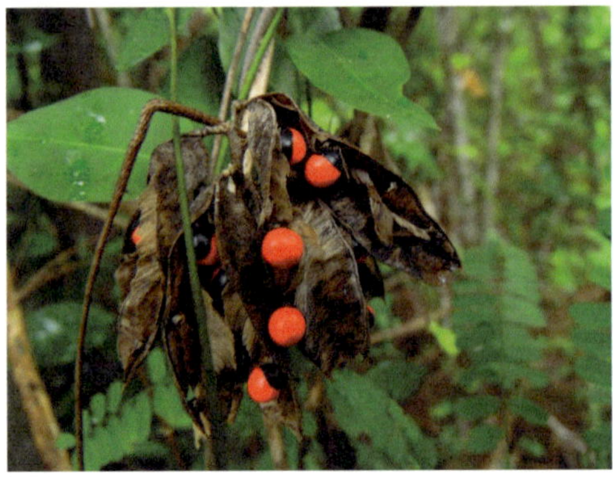

Figure 5.
The crab's eye Abrus precatorius L., 1753 (Fabaceae) (from: https://goo.gl/images/8VobSd).

Pharmacological studies with preparations from *A. precatorius* seeds and leaves revealed that many of their biological activities may be attributable to abrin [98]. This compound consists of a dimer with a B subunit that facilitates its entry into cells by binding to plasma membrane-associated transport proteins, after which the A subunit inactivates the 26S subunit of ribosomes, preventing protein synthesis [99]. One molecule of abrin is able to inactivate up to 1500 ribosomes per second [95], indicating its powerful inhibitory effect on protein synthesis. On the other hand, this mechanistic feature of abrin presents the opportunity of inhibiting the proliferation of cancerous cells which characteristically have a higher metabolic turnover when compared to normal cells.

Indeed, protein-rich extracts or peptide fractions from *A. precatorius* seeds and ethanol, ethyl acetate, and water extracts from the leaves potently inhibited the proliferation of several tumor cell lines [100–104] without affecting the growth of normal murine peritoneal macrophages [102]. The cytotoxic effects were accompanied by upregulation of particularly p21 and p53 levels [104] and clear signs of apoptosis occurring through the mitochondrial pathway [101]. The seed preparations also inhibited the growth of several tumor types implanted into laboratory rodents [105–108]. And direct injection of abrin into a murine Meth-A sarcoma growing in syngeneic BALB/c mice led to regression of the tumor [109]. The anticancer effects might be related to the antioxidant activities of phenolics and flavonoids in the extracts [102, 104].

Importantly, administration of Meth-A tumor cells which had been treated *in vitro* with abrin, induced strong antitumor immunity of the mice [109]. This suggests that the antitumor effects of abrin were also produced by boosting the immune system. Support for this presumption came from the immunopotentiating and immunostimulatory properties of abrin [107, 110] and the behavior of *Abrus* agglutinin as a B cell and T cell stimulator [111].

4.5 Fabaceae—*Tephrosia sinapou* (Bucholz) A.Chev.

The Surinam poison *T. sinapou*, also known as *T. toxicaria* (Swartz) Pers. (**Figure 6**), is native to parts of Central America, the Caribbean, and tropical South America. The plant is mainly known for its high content of the isoflavonoids rotenone and tephrosin in its black roots and seeds, which are used as a fish poison by the Amazon Indigenous peoples [112, 113]. Particularly rotenone is also highly toxic to insects and pests [112, 113]. For this reason, Guyana hinterland peoples use the root sap or the leaf juice externally against head lice [112]. These preparations are also used to ward off evil spirits and for treating eczema, snakebites, syphilis,

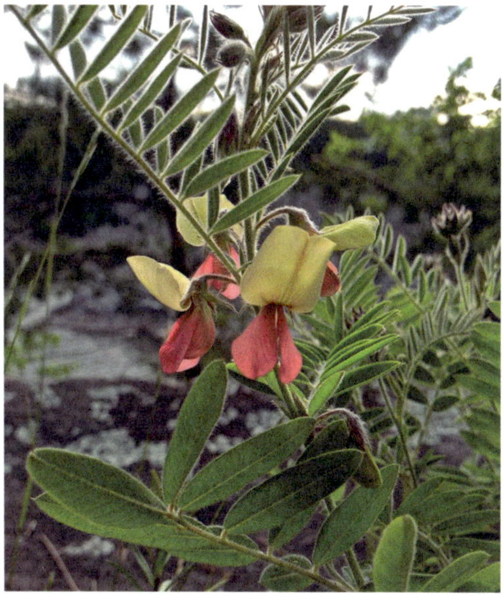

Figure 6.
The Suriname poison Tephrosia sinapou (Bucholz) A.Chev. (Fabaceae) (from: https://goo.gl/images/q6BZZN).

and gonorrhea, as well as skin ulcers associated with AIDS and cancer [42, 43, 114]. These health benefits have particularly been ascribed to the rotenoids and other flavonoids in roots, leaves, and aerial parts of the plant [115–117].

Indications for anticancer activity of *Tephrosia* preparations were provided by the cytotoxic effects of extracts from parts of *T. calophylla* Bedd., *T. persica* Boiss., *T. purpurea* (L.) Pers., *T. villosa* (L.) Pers., and *T. vogelii* Hook F. against human carcinoma cell lines and brine shrimp cultures [118–124]. In some cases, the cytotoxic effects were accompanied by signs of apoptotic cell death [118]. Comparable anticancer effects were produced by benzil and coumestan derivatives from a *T. calophylla* root extract [125]; flavonoids from parts of *T. calophylla*, *T. pulcherrima* (Baker) Gamble, and *T. pumila* (Lam.) Pers. [126]; phenol- and flavonoid-rich methanolic extracts from the leaves of *T. purpurea* and the aerial parts of *T. apollinea* (Delile) DC. [124, 127]; and a prenylated flavone from the aerial parts of *T. apollinea* [128]. Notably, the high flavonoid content of the aerial parts of *T. apollinea* has also been associated with potent anti-angiogenic activity in an *ex vivo* rat aortic ring assay [127].

There are also indications for cancer chemopreventive activity of *Tephrosia* preparations. Thus, flavonoids from an ethyl acetate-soluble extract of *T. sinapou* stem selected for potential cancer chemopreventive properties in an *in vitro* assay for quinone reductase induction, inhibited the formation of preneoplastic lesions induced by DMBA in a mouse mammary organ culture [129]. Furthermore, *T. purpurea* extracts substantially reduced the formation of skin lesions in Swiss albino mice treated with the potent tumor promoter phorbol 12-myristate 13-acetate (PMA) following treatment with DMBA [130]. The extract also inhibited the development of hepatocellular carcinoma in Wistar rats treated with the carcinogenic and mutagenic compound N-nitrosodiethylamine [131].

4.6 Loranthaceae—*Phthirusa stelis* (L.) Kuijt

The bird vine *P. stelis* (**Figure 7**) is, like many of its relatives in the plant family Loranthaceae (commonly known as mistletoes), a small flowering plant that grows

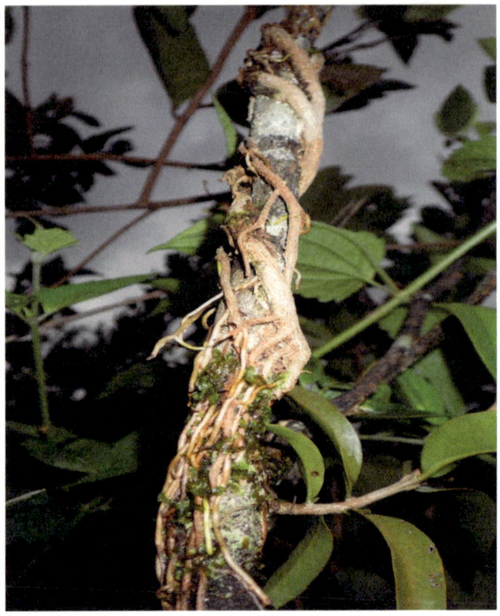

Figure 7.
The bird vine Phthirusa stelis (L.) Kuijt (Loranthaceae) (from: https://goo.gl/images/J9D1zG).

hemiparasitically on the branches of trees and shrubs. It is encountered in various Southern and Middle American countries between Costa Rica and Bolivia where it often constitutes a serious pest on cultivated trees of economic importance such as rubber, orange, cocoa, and bread fruit trees [132]. *P. stelis* is mostly spread by bird droppings, hence the abovementioned Surinamese vernacular name of "*pikin fowru doti*" meaning small birds' excrement.

None of the parts of the plant have edible uses. However, the viscous layer of its fruits has been suggested to represent a potential source of natural rubber [133]. *P. stelis* preparations are traditionally used to treat oral candidiasis in children; leukorrhea; problems of the female reproductive system; tonsillitis; and skin problems such as scabies [42, 43, 134]. The plant is also used as a chemopreventive substance and by cancer patients for whom no other options are available, presumably because of its hemiparasitic, cancer-like lifestyle, which would signal its usefulness for these purposes [43].

Indications for anticancer activity of *P. stelis* are scant, being limited to the cytotoxic effects of small polypeptides of 3–5 kDa isolated from dried dichloromethane or ethanol whole-plant extracts in cultured U-937 GTB human histiocytic lymphoma cells [135]. This finding is in line with the identification of (larger) cytotoxic peptides in the Loranthaceae species *Helicanthus elastica* (Desr.) Dans. [136] and *Ligaria cuneifolia* (Ruiz & Pav.) van Tiegh. [137]. Other phytochemicals in Loranthaceae species with *in vitro* anticancer activity are alkynic fatty acids in *Scurrula atropurpurea* (BL.) Dans. [138]; lectins in *Viscum album coloratum* Kom. [139]; the triterpene moronic acid in *Phoradendron reichenbachianum* (Seem.) Oliv. [140]; glycosides in *Macrosolen globosus* (Roxb.) Tiegh. [141], *Loranthus tanakae* Franch. & Sav. (Loranthaceae) [142], and *Viscum coloratum* (Kom.) Nakai [143]; and flavonoids in *L. cuneifolia* [144].

Crude extracts from stem or leaves of *Scurrula oortiana* (Korth.) Danser [145], leaves of *Dendrophthoe pentandra* (L.) Miq. [146], and stem *of Elytranthe parasitica* (L.) Danser [147] also exerted cytotoxic effects. In addition, the alkynic fatty acids from *S. atropurpurea* potently inhibited *in vitro* tumor cell invasion [148], and extracts from the stem or leaves of *S. oortiana* increased tumor cell sensitivity to TNF-α-mediated lysis [145].

4.7 Rubiaceae—*Uncaria guianensis* (Aubl.) J.F. Gmel.

The cat's claw *U. guianensis* (**Figure 8**) is indigenous to the Amazonian parts of Paraguay, Brazil, Bolivia, Peru, Ecuador, Colombia, Venezuela, and the Guyanas. Preparations from its stembark and leaves have a long history of traditional medicinal use and are particularly employed for treating osteoarthritis and rheumatoid arthritis [42, 43, 149]. Pharmacological studies with extracts from *U. guianensis*—and with those from other closely related species, mainly *U. tomentosum* (Willd. ex Schult.) DC—indeed showed anti-inflammatory activities [150]. These effects have primarily been attributed to pentacyclic oxindole alkaloids [149–152]. Clinical studies with an *U. guianensis* stembark extract or a highly purified pentacyclic oxindole alkaloids fraction from *U. tomentosum* reported some benefits in patients with osteoarthritis of the knee [153–155]. However, the overall clinical data are insufficient to draw a firm conclusion about the anti-inflammatory efficacy of *Uncaria* preparations [156].

No studies have been carried out on the anticancer activity of *U. guianensis*. However, studies with the oxindole alkaloids from *U. tomentosa* stembark showed notable anticancer activity against human cancer cell lines [157–160] and a mouse model [159] which was in some cases accompanied by apoptosis [157]. In addition, *Uncaria* preparations may possess immunomodulatory and chemopreventive properties besides direct cytotoxic activity. The former assumption is supported by the involvement of anti-inflammatory processes rather than cytotoxic events in the antitumor activity of a hydroethanolic *U. guianensis* stembark extract in 4 T1 mammary tumor-bearing BALB/c mice [161]. The latter supposition stems from the changes in expression patterns of critical proto-oncogenes and tumor suppressor genes in DMBA-treated CBA/Ca mice following administration of Claw of Dragon tea (CoD™ tea), a mixture of the stembarks from *U. guianensis*, *U. tomentosa*, and the trumpet-tree *Tabebuia avellanedae* Lorentz ex Griseb. (Bignoniaceae) [162].

A clinical trial with a dried extract of *U. tomentosa* stembark reported improved overall quality of life, social functioning, and fatigue in patients with advanced solid tumors, but there were no improvements in biochemical and inflammatory markers or tumor responses [163]. Another trial found a decrease in the occurrence of neutropenia caused by the 5-fluorouracil-doxorubicin-cyclophosphamide combination in patients with breast cancer [164]. However, a third study found no effect of oral tablets containing a dried ethanolic *U. tomentosa* stembark on the most prevalent adverse events caused by the 5-fluorouracil-oxaliplatin regimen in colorectal cancer patients [165].

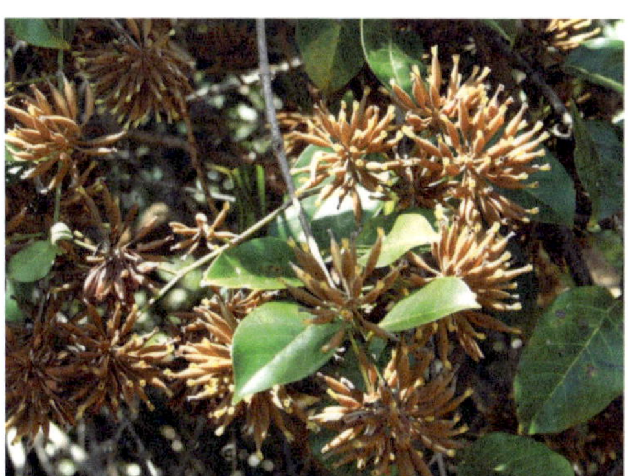

Figure 8.
The cat's claw Uncaria guianensis (Aubl.) J.F. Gmel. (Rubiaceae) (from: https://goo.gl/images/7ezTTN).

4.8 Simaroubaceae—*Quassia amara* L.

The bitterwood *Q. amara* (**Figure 9**) is native to South and Central America but is now also cultivated in various other tropical and subtropical regions throughout the world. In Suriname, the plant has been named "kwasibita" (Kwasi's bitter) after the freedman Kwasi or Quassi (1692–1787) who was the first to broadly apply the remarkable medicinal properties of the hardwood for treating malaria fevers [28]. The plant contains triterpene quassinoids, secondary metabolites that are among the bitterest in nature [166]. These compounds are almost exclusively encountered in members of the Simaroubaceae and are a taxonomic marker of this plant family [166]. They constitute basic ingredients of Angostura bitters, concentrated alcoholic preparations produced by the House of Angostura in Trinidad and Tobago, which are key ingredients of cocktails such as gin-based drinks.

The quassinoids quassin, neoquassin, bruceantin, and simalikalactones D and E have been associated with a host of pharmacological activities including antimalarial, insecticidal, anti-inflammatory, antimicrobial, and antianorectic activities [166–168]. Other *Q. amara* phytochemicals with a broad pharmacological spectrum are canthin-6-one alkaloids, which displayed antiviral, antiparasitic, antibacterial, anti-inflammatory, and cytotoxic activities [166, 168, 169]. Notably, a 4%-*Quassia* cream containing both groups of phytochemicals has been found safe and effective in the management of rosacea [170].

There is ample evidence that *Q. amara* preparations and some of its constituents also possess anticancer activity. For instance, crude stem or leaf extracts, quassimarin- and/or similikalactone-enriched fractions, partially purified quassinoid-containing fractions, as well as quassimarin, similikalactones, and canthin alkaloids displayed substantial cytotoxicity against human carcinoma cell lines [171–174] as well as P-388 lymphocytic leukemia inoculated into laboratory mice [171]. Importantly, the quassinoids did not affect the viability of nontumorogenic African green monkey Vero kidney cells [173] and produced anticancer effects at lower concentrations than those required for antimalarial effects [172, 173]. Comparable results were found with quassinoids and/or canthin alkaloids from other members of the Simaroubaceae family [175–178]. Markedly, the quassinoids and canthin alkaloids also prevented the activation of Epstein-Barr virus early antigen by PMA [175] and inhibited the activity of CYP1A1, a cytochrome P450 isoform with presumed carcinogen-activating properties [179]. These observations suggest that these compounds may also possess chemopreventive properties.

Based on this large body of preclinical data, several *Q. amara* constituents have undergone clinical evaluation in patients with advanced solid and hematological

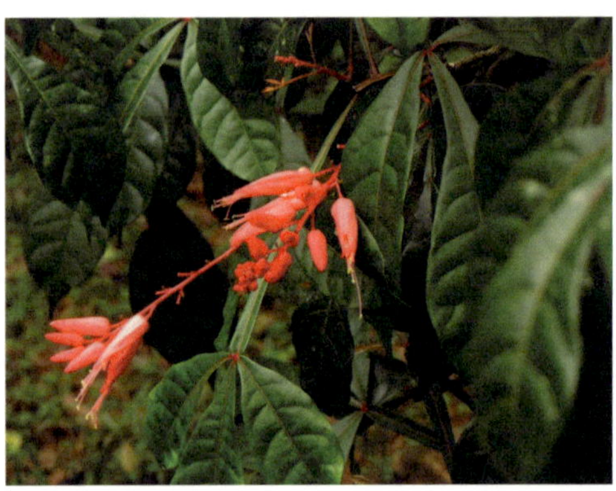

Figure 9.
The bitterwood Quassia amara L. (Simaroubaceae) (from: https://goo.gl/images/d5ZqEd).

malignancies. Unfortunately, the results from phase 1 and phase 2 studies with bruceantin—as well as Fructus bruceae oil obtained from the dried ripe fruits of *Brucea javanica* (L.) Merr.—were uniformly disappointing, showing no meaningful anticancer activity but substantial toxicity [180–182].

4.9 Zingiberaceae—*Zingiber officinale* Roscoe

The ginger *Z. officinale* (**Figure 10**) is presumably native to the Indian subcontinent and other Southern Asian regions. This plant was probably introduced in Suriname by Javanese indentured laborers around the beginning of the twentieth century [28, 38]. The rhizome is extensively used as a hot and fragrant kitchen spice in many cuisines and to prepare various hot and cold beverages. This part of the plant also has many long-standing traditional uses [43, 183]. The essential oil from the rhizomes is topically applied as an analgesic, while preparations from powdered fresh or dried rhizomes are orally or topically used for treating, among others, respiratory complaints; obesity; microbial infections; vertigo, travel sickness, morning sickness, as well as nausea and vomiting associated with surgery and chemotherapy; and cancer [43, 183].

These claims are supported by the pharmacological activities displayed by particularly gingerols (such as zingerone and zingeberol) and shogaols in the rhizomes. Gingerols are the main compounds in the volatile oil of fresh ginger rhizomes and are responsible for their characteristic fragrance [184]. They are thermally labile and easily undergo dehydration reactions to form the corresponding shogaols, which convey the typical pungent taste of dried ginger during cooking [184]. Both gingerols and shogaols exhibited pharmacological activities which supported the traditional uses of *Z. officinale* [185, 186].

A host of data supports that gingerols and shogaols possess both anticancer and chemopreventive activities. Evidence for the former suggestion came from their inhibitory effects on the proliferation, cell cycle progression, and viability of human carcinoma cell lines [187–197] and tumors implanted into laboratory animal [198, 199]. Suggestions for chemopreventive activities of these compounds came from their inhibitory effects on the development of cancer in animals treated with laboratory carcinogens [199–203]. Both activities may be mediated by multiple mechanisms including inhibition of invasion through activation of the nuclear receptor peroxisome proliferator-activated receptor γ (PPAR-γ) [197]; downregulation of matrix metalloproteinase 9 transcription [204]; suppression of tumor angiogenesis [191, 194]; deactivation of aberrant cell cycle-regulating elements [189, 200]; and interference with microtubule integrity [190, 196].

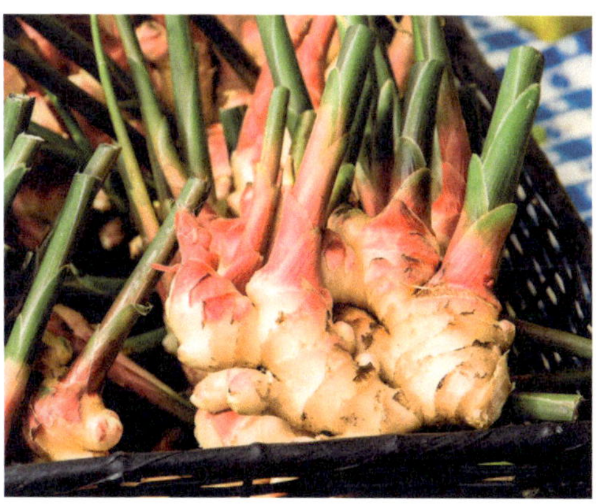

Figure 10.
The ginger Zingiber officinale Roscoe (Zingiberaceae) (from: https://goo.gl/images/Tr2fgV).

All these observations have led to the consideration of *Z. officinale* preparations for treating cancer as well as cancer-related complications such as chemotherapy-induced nausea and vomiting. So far, however, there is no scientific proof of clinical efficacy against either cancer [205] or nausea and vomiting resulting from chemotherapy or surgery [206].

5. Concluding remarks

The nine plants addressed in this chapter have a long traditional use in Suriname against various conditions including neoplastic disease and indeed showed some evidence of anticancer activity. However, in all cases, the evidence was limited to preclinical models and was not sufficient to support claims of clinical efficacy. However, this does not necessarily mean that these plants and their active constituents should be discarded as failed compounds. Some may constitute useful parts of an integrative medical approach for treating or preventing cancer. Others—including many mentioned in this chapter—may boost the immune system or improve overall health, well-being, and quality of life. And still others may help relieve some of the symptoms of cancer such as fatigue or reduce the side effects of chemotherapy and radiotherapy.

Converging lines of evidence lend support to these suppositions. Firstly, several phenolic compounds such as curcumin from the turmeric *Curcuma longa* L. (Zingiberaceae) and apigenin from the celery *Apium graveolens* L. (Apiaceae) may directly or indirectly exert cytotoxic and apoptotic effects by stimulating autophagy [207, 208]. Other plant phenols such as luteolin in celery, thyme, green peppers, and chamomile tea; epigallocatechin-3-gallate in Chinese green tea; and resveratrol in the skin of grapes, blueberries, raspberries, and mulberries have shown promise in the treatment and prevention of cancer [209–211]. These compounds are able to inactivate molecular signals and transcription pathways essential for cancer cells, scavenge harmful free radicals, and inhibit tumor angiogenesis, respectively [209–211].

Secondly, mistletoe extracts may alleviate cancer-related fatigue [212]; preparations from the holy basil *Ocimum sanctum* L. (Lamiaceae) may avert radiation-induced clastogenesis [213]; those based on *A. vera* may prevent or treat radiation-induced oral mucositis [214]; and the gingerols and shogaols in *Z. officinale* may reduce the cardiotoxicity of doxorubicin [215]. These compounds may exercise their protective effects through their anti-inflammatory, immune-modulating, free radical-scavenging, antioxidant, and/or metal-chelating properties [212–215].

Furthermore, recent advances in analytical and computational techniques as well as the introduction of innovative technologies such as predictive computational software may help employ apparently "useless" anticancer compounds in novel ways. For instance, the rejected tubulin-binding maytansines from *Maytenus* species (Celastraceae) may have found a new use as "warheads" attached to specific antitumor monoclonal antibodies in order to precisely attack tumor tissues while causing little toxicity [216]. And the discarded topoisomerase I inhibitor lapachol from the stembark of the Surinam greenheart *Handroanthus serratifolius* (Vahl) S.O. Grose—also known as *Tabebuia serratifolia* (Vahl) G. Nicholson (Bignoniaceae)—is attracting renewed attention following reports that its inhibitory effect on melanoma cell proliferation may involve interference with glycolysis and decreasing ATP levels [217].

Likewise, the therapeutic index of gingerols in the treatment of breast cancer may improve when formulated as a PEGylated nanoliposomal form, allowing for high specificity, improved bioavailability, slow release, and low systemic toxicity [218]. And structural modifications of quassinoids on the basis of, for instance, (quantitative) structure-activity relationships, may produce more potent and less toxic analogues [219, 220]. These and many other examples support continued assessment of the plants and their bioactive compounds dealt with in the current chapter for their usefulness against cancer. If only one of these compounds would reach the clinic, the efforts invested in their evaluation would have been worthwhile.

Conflict of interest

The authors declare that no conflict of interest exists.

Author details

Dennis R.A. Mans[1]* and Euridice R. Irving[2]

1 Department of Pharmacology, Faculty of Medical Sciences, Anton de Kom University of Suriname, Paramaribo, Suriname

2 Department of Medical Skills Education, Faculty of Medical Sciences, Anton de Kom University of Suriname, Paramaribo, Suriname

*Address all correspondence to: dennismans16@gmail.com

References

[1] Idikio HA. Human cancer classification: A systems biology-based model integrating morphology, cancer stem cells, proteomics, and genomics. Journal of Cancer. 2011;**2**:107-115

[2] Yadav M, Chatterjee P, Tolani S, Kulkarni J, Mulye M, Chauhan N, et al. A Nexus model of cellular transition in cancer. Biological Research. 2018;**51**:23. DOI: 10.1186/s40659-018-0173-8

[3] Bray F, Ferlay J, Soerjomataram I, Siegel RL, Torre LA, Jemal A. Global cancer statistics 2018: GLOBOCAN estimates of incidence and mortality worldwide for 36 cancers in 185 countries. CA: A Cancer Journal for Clinicians. 2018;**0**:1-31

[4] Shield KD, Ferlay J, Jemal A, Sankaranarayanan R, Chaturvedi AK, Bray F, et al. The global incidence of lip, oral cavity, and pharyngeal cancers by subsite in 2012. CA: A Cancer Journal for Clinicians. 2017;**67**:51-64

[5] Catarino R, Petignat P, Dongui G, Vassilakos P. Cervical cancer screening in developing countries at a crossroad: Emerging technologies and policy choices. World Journal of Clinical Oncology. 2015;**6**:281-290

[6] Akulapalli Sudhakar A. History of cancer, ancient and modern treatment methods. Journal of Cancer Science and Therapy. 2009;**1**:i-iv. DOI: 10.4172/1948-5956.100000e2

[7] Cragg GM, Newman DJ. Natural products: A continuing source of novel drug leads. Biochimica et Biophysica Acta. 2013;**1830**:3670-3695

[8] Mans DRA. From forest to pharmacy: Plant-based traditional medicines as sources for novel therapeutics. Academia Journal of Medicinal Plants. 2013;**1**:101-110

[9] Newman DJ, Cragg GM. Natural products as sources of new drugs from 1981 to 2014. Journal of Natural Products. 2016;**79**:629-661

[10] Iqbal J, Abbasi BA, Mahmood T, Kanwal S, Ali B, Shah SA, et al. Plant-derived anticancer agents: A green anticancer approach. Asian Pacific Journal of Tropical Biomedicine. 2017;**7**:1129-1150

[11] Van Der Heijden R, Jacobs DI, Snoeijer W, Hallard D, Verpoorte R. The Catharanthus alkaloids: Pharmacognosy and biotechnology. Current Medicinal Chemistry. 2004;**11**:607-628

[12] Kingston DG, Newman DJ. Taxoids: Cancer-fighting compounds from nature. Current Opinion in Drug Discovery & Development. 2007;**10**:130-144

[13] Legarza K, Yang LX. Novel camptothecin derivatives. In Vivo. 2005;**19**:283-292

[14] Baldwin EL, Osheroff N. Etoposide, topoisomerase II and cancer. Current Medicinal Chemistry. Anti-Cancer Agents. 2005;**5**:363-372

[15] Cragg GM, Newman DJ, Weiss RB. Coral reefs, forests, and thermal vents: The worldwide exploration of nature for novel antitumor agents. Seminars in Oncology. 1997;**24**:156-163

[16] Algemeen Bureau voor de Statistiek/Censuskantoor. Suriname in cijfers 2013/05. Resultaten achtste (8ste) volks- en woningtelling in Suriname (volume 1) (General Bureau of Statistics/Census The Office Suriname in numbers 2013/05. Results of the Eight General Census of Suriname). Demografische en sociale karakteristieken en migratie (Demographic and social characteristics and migration). Paramaribo: Algemeen Bureau voor de Statistiek; 2013

[17] Oehlers GP, Lichtveld MY, Brewster LM, Algoe M, Irving ER. Health life in Suriname (chapter 6). In: Hassankhan MS, Roopnarine L, White C, Mahase R, editors. Legacy of Slavery and Indentured Labour. Historical and Contemporary Issues in Suriname and the Caribbean. New Delhi: Manohar; 2016. pp. 111-150

[18] Eersel MGM, Vreden SGS, van Eer ED, Mans DRA. Fifty years of primary health care in the rainforest: Temporal trends in morbidity and mortality in indigenous Amerindian populations of Suriname. Journal of Global Health. 2018;**8**:020423. DOI: 10.7189/jogh.08.020403

[19] Algemeen Bureau voor de Statistiek. Suriname in cijfers 303-2014-04 (General Bureau of Statistics Suriname in Numbers 303-2014-04). Basis Indicatoren (Basic Indicators). Paramaribo: Algemeen Bureau voor de Statistiek; 2014

[20] The World Bank Group. Suriname [Internet]. 2018. Available from: https://data.worldbank.org/country/suriname [Accessed: 10-03-2018]

[21] Ministry of Health. Report of the Director of Health 2005-2007. Paramaribo: Ministry of Health Republic of Suriname; 2008

[22] Dams E. Suriname National Cancer Control Plan 2018-2028. Prepared for the Ministry of Health. Paramaribo: Ministry of Health Republic of Suriname; 2017

[23] Mans DRA, Mohamedradja RN, Hoeblal AR, Rampadarath R, Joe SS, Wong J, et al. Cancer incidence in Suriname from 1980 through 2000 a descriptive study. Tumori. 2003;**89**:368-376

[24] Lamur HE. The demographic evolution of Surinam, 1920-1970. A sociodemographic analysis (chapter III). In: Lamur HE, editor. Verhandelingen van het Koninklijk Instituut voor Taal-, Land- en Volkenkunde 65 (Discourses of the Royal institute for Linguistics, Land Science, and Ethnology 65). The Hague: Martinus Nijhoff; 1973. pp. 96-98

[25] Punwasi W. Causes of death in Suriname 2010-2011. Bureau Openbare Gezondheidsdienst (Bureau of Public Health). Paramaribo: Ministry of Health Republic of Suriname; 2012

[26] ER I, DRA M. Age and ethnic differences in the occurrence of cervical dysplasia, cervical cancer and cervical cancer deaths in Suriname. Translational Biomedicine. 2015;**6**:1. DOI: 10.21767/2172-0479.100001

[27] Mans DRA. "Nature, green in leaf and stem". Research on plants with medicinal properties in Suriname. Clinical and Medical Investigations. 2016;**2**:1-10

[28] Mans DRA, Ganga D, Kartopawiro J. Meeting of the minds: Traditional herbal medicine in multiethnic Suriname (chapter 6). In: El-Shemy H, editor. Aromatic and Medicinal Plants—Back to Nature. Rijeka: InTech; 2017. pp. 111-132. DOI: 10.5772/66509.

[29] Hammond DS. Forest conservation and management in the Guiana shield (chapter 1). In: Hammond DS, editor. Tropical Rainforests of the Guiana Shield. Wallingford: CABI Publishing; 2005. pp. 1-14

[30] Yue Q, Gao G, Zou G, Yu H, Zheng X. Natural products as adjunctive treatment for pancreatic cancer: Recent trends and advancements. BioMed Research International. 2017;**2017**:8412508. DOI: 10.1155/2017/8412508

[31] Marinac JS, Buchinger CL, Godfrey LA, Wooten JM, Sun C, Willsie SK. Herbal products and dietary supplements: A survey of use, attitudes,

and knowledge among older adults. The Journal of the American Osteopathic Association. 2007;**107**:13-23

[32] Sparber A, Bauer L, Curt G, Eisenberg D, Levin T, Parks S, et al. Use of complementary medicine by adult patients participating in cancer clinical trials. Oncology Nursing Forum. 2000;**27**:623-630

[33] Mansky PJ, Wallerstedt DB. Complementary medicine in palliative care and cancer symptom management. Cancer Journal. 2006;**1**:425-431

[34] Daher M. Cultural beliefs and values in cancer patients. Annals of Oncology. 2012;**23**(Suppl 3):66-69

[35] Luo T, Spolverato G, Johnston F, Haider AH, Pawlik TM. Factors that determine cancer treatment choice among minority groups. Journal of Oncology Practice/ American Society of Clinical Oncology. 2015;**11**:259-261

[36] Stephen HJM. Geneeskruiden van Suriname: Hun toepassing in de volksgeneeskunde en in de magie (Herbal Medicines from Suriname: Their Applications in Folk Medicine and Wizardry). Amsterdam: De Driehoek; 1979

[37] Heyde H. Surinaamse medicijnplanten (Surinamese Medicinal Plants). 2nd ed. Paramaribo: Westfort; 1987

[38] Tjong Ayong G. Het gebruik van medicinale planten door de Javaanse bevolkingsgroep in Suriname (The Use of Medicinal Plants by the Javanese in Suriname). Paramaribo: Instituut voor de Opleiding van Leraren; 1989

[39] Slagveer JL. Surinaams Groot Kruidenboek: Sranan Oso Dresie (Surinamese Herbal Medicines). Paramaribo: De West; 1990

[40] Sedoc NO. Afrosurinaamse natuurgeneeswijzen: Bevattende meer dan tweehonderd meest gebruikelijke geneeskrachtige kruiden (Afro-Surinamese Natural Remedies: Over Two Hundred Commonly Used Medicinal Herbs). Paramaribo: Vaco Press; 1992

[41] Raghoenandan UPD. Etnobotanisch onderzoek bij de Hindoestaanse bevolkingsgroep in Suriname (An ethnobotanical investigation among hindustanis in Suriname) [thesis]. Paramaribo: Anton de Kom University of Suriname; 1994

[42] DeFilipps RA, Maina SL, Crepin J. Medicinal Plants of the Guianas (Guyana, Surinam, French Guiana). Washington, DC: Smithsonian Institution; 2004

[43] Van Andel TR, Ruysschaert S. Medicinale en rituele planten van Suriname (Medicinal and Ritual Plants of Suriname). Amsterdam: KIT Publishers; 2011

[44] Zahid M, Mujahid M, Singh PK, Farooqui S, Singh K, Parveen S, et al. *Annona squamosa* Linn. (custard apple): An aromatic medicinal plant fruit with immense nutraceutical and therapeutic potentials. International Journal of Pharmaceutical Sciences and Research. 2018;**9**:1745-1759

[45] Saha R. Pharmacognosy and pharmacology of *Annona squamosa*: A review. International Journal of Pharmacy and Life Sciences. 2011;**2**:1183-1189

[46] Oo WM, Khine MM. Pharmacological activities of *Annona squamosa*: Updated review. International Journal of Pharmaceutical Chemistry. 2017;**3**:86-93

[47] Xie H, Wei J, Liu M, Yang R. A new cytotoxic acetogenin from the seeds of

Annona squamosa. Chinese Chemical Letters. 2003;**14**:588

[48] Liaw CC, Yang YL, Chen M, Chang FR, Chen SL, Wu SH, et al. Mono-tetrahydrofuran annonaceous acetogenins from *Annona squamosa* as cytotoxic agents and calcium ion chelators. Journal of Natural Products. 2008;**71**:764-771

[49] Yang HJ, Zhang N, Chen JW, Wang MY. Two new cytotoxic acetogenins from *Annona squamosa*. Journal of Asian Natural Products Research. 2009;**11**:250-256

[50] Chen Y, Chen JW, Li X. Cytotoxic bistetrahydrofuran annonaceous acetogenins from the seeds of *Annona squamosa*. Journal of Natural Products. 2011;**74**:2477-2481

[51] Chen Y, Xu SS, Chen JW, Wang Y, Xu HQ, Fan NB, et al. Anti-tumor activity of *Annona squamosa* seeds extract containing annonaceous acetogenin compounds. Journal of Ethnopharmacology. 2012;**142**:462-466

[52] Chen Y, Chem J, Wang Y, Xu S, Li X. Six cytotoxic annonaceous acetogenins from *Annona squamosa* seeds. Food Chemistry. 2012;**135**:960-966

[53] Miao Y, Xu X, Yuan F, Shi Y, Chen Y, Chen J, et al. Four cytotoxic annonaceous acetogenins from the seeds of *Annona squamosa*. Natural Product Research. 2016;**30**:1273-1279

[54] Pardhasaradhi BV, Reddy M, Kumari AM, Ali AL, Khar A. Differential cytotoxic effects of *Annona squamosa* seed extracts on human tumor cell lines: Role of reactive oxygen species and glutathione. Journal of Biosciences. 2005;**30**:237-244

[55] Nakano D, Ishitsuka K, Kamikawa M, Matsuda M, Tsuchihashi R, Okawa M, et al. Screening of promising chemotherapeutic candidates from plants against human adult T-cell leukemia/lymphoma. Journal of Natural Medicines. 2013;**67**:894-903

[56] Li XH, Hui YH, Rupprecht JK, Liu YM, Wood KV, Smith DL, et al. Bullatacin, bullatacinone, and squamone, a new bioactive acetogenin, from the bark of *Annona squamosa*. Journal of Natural Products. 1990;**53**:81-86

[57] Hopp DC, Alali FQ, Gu ZM, McLaughlin JL. Three new bioactive bis-adjacent THF-ring acetogenins from the bark of *Annona squamosa*. Bioorganic & Medicinal Chemistry. 1998;**6**:569-575

[58] Sun L, Zhu H, Gan L, Mo J, Feng F, Zhou C. Constituents from the bark of *Annona squamosa* and their anti-tumor activity. Zhongguo Zhong Yao Z Zhi. 2012;**37**:2100-2104

[59] Vilanova NS, Morais SM, Facao MJ, Machado LM, Becilaqua CM, Costa IR, et al. Leishmanicidal activity and cytotoxicity of compounds from two Annonacea species cultivated in Northeastern Brazil. Revista da Sociedade Brasileira de Medicina Tropical. 2011;**44**:567-571

[60] Ma C, Wang Q, Shi Y, Li Y, Wang X, Li X, et al. Three new anti-tumor annonaceous acetogenins from the seeds of *Annona squamosa*. Natural Product Research. 2017;**31**:2085-2090

[61] Jou B, Remanin P. Antitumor constituents from *Annona squamosa* fruit pulp. Medicinal Chemistry Research. 2008;**17**:345-355

[62] Chen YY, Cao YZ, Li FQ, XI Z, Peng CX, Lu JH, et al. Studies on anti-hepatoma activity of *Annona squamosa* L. pericarp extract. Bioorganic & Medicinal Chemistry Letters. 2017;**27**:1907-1910

[63] Chen YY, Peng CX, Hu Y, Bu C, Guo SC, Li X, et al. Studies on chemical constituents and anti-hepatoma effects of essential oil from *Annona squamosa* L. pericarp. Natural Product Research. 2017;**31**:1308-1308

[64] Chen Y, Shi Y, Ma C, Wang X, Li Y, Miao Y, et al. Antitumor activity of *Annona squamosa*. Journal of Ethnopharmacology. 2016;**193**:362-367

[65] Yang RM, Li WM, Hu WJ, Huang WH, Zhu CY, Yu JG, et al. Anticancer effect of total annonaceous acetogenins on hepatocarcinoma. Chinese Journal of Integrative Medicine. 2015;**21**:682-688

[66] Thakkar JH, Solanki HK, Tripathi P, Patel NJ, Jani GK. Evaluation of antimutagenic potential of *Annona squamosa* leaf extract. Elixir Human Physiology. 2011;**31**:1960-1965

[67] Suresh K, Manoharn S, Blessy D. Protective role of *Annona squamosa* Linn bark extracts in DMBA induced genotoxicity. Kathmandu University Medical Journal. 2008;**6**:364-369

[68] Suresh K, Manoharan S, Panjamurthy K, Kavitha K. Chemoprotective and antilipidperoxidative efficacy *of Annona squamosa* bark extracts in experimental oral carcinogenesis. Pakistan Journal of Biological Sciences. 2006;**9**:2600-2605

[69] Joshi RK. GC/MS analysis of the essential oil of *Vernonia cinerea*. Natural Product Communications. 2015;**10**:1319-1320

[70] Jaworski J, Cahoon EB. Industrial oils from transgenic plants. Current Opinion in Plant Biology. 2003;**6**:178-184

[71] Wongwiwatthananukit S, Benjanakaskul P, Songsak T, Suwanamajo S, Verachai V. Efficacy of *Vernonia cinerea* for smoking cessation. Journal of Health Research. 2009;**23**:31-36

[72] Bin Sayeed MS, Mostofa AG, Ferdous FM, Islam MS. A randomized, placebo-controlled, crossover study of an herbal preparation containing *Vernonia cinerea* in the treatment of type 2 diabetes. Journal of Alternative and Complementary Medicine. 2013;**19**:767-771

[73] Puttarak P, Pornpanyanukul P, Meetam T, Bunditanukul K, Chaiyakunapruk N. Efficacy and safety of *Vernonia cinerea* (L.) Less. for smoking cessation: A systematic review and meta-analysis of randomized controlled trials. Complementary Therapies in Medicine. 2018;**37**:37-42

[74] Khay M, Toeng P, Mahiou-Leddet V, Mabrouki F, Sothea K, Ollivier E, et al. HPLC analysis and cytotoxic activity of *Vernonia cinerea*. Natural Product Communications. 2012;7:1259-1262

[75] Guha G, Rajkumar V, Ashok Kumar R, Mathew L. Therapeutic potential of polar and non-polar extracts of *Cyanthillium cinereum in vitro*. Evidence-based Complementary and Alternative Medicine. 2011;**2011**:784826. DOI: 10.1093/ecam/nep155

[76] Appadath Beeran A, Maliyakkal N, Rao CM, Udupa N. The enriched fraction of *Vernonia cinerea* L. induces apoptosis and inhibits multi-drug resistance transporters in human epithelial cancer cells. Journal of Ethnopharmacology. 2014;**158**(Pt A): 33-42

[77] Pratheeshkumar P, Kuttan G. Modulation of cytotoxic T lymphocyte, natural killer cell, antibody-dependent cellular cytotoxicity, and antibody-dependent complement-mediated cytotoxicity by *Vernonia cinerea* L. and vernolide-A in BALB/c mice via

enhanced production of cytokines IL-2 and IFN-γ. Immunopharmacology and Immunotoxicology. 2012;**34**:46-55

[78] Shoaib M, Shah I, Ali N, Adhikari A, Tahir MN, Shah SWA, et al. Sesquiterpene lactone! a promising antioxidant, anticancer and moderate antinociceptive agent from *Artemisia macrocephala* Jacquem. BMC Complementary and Alternative Medicine. 2017;**17**:27. DOI: 10.1186/s12906-016-1517-y

[79] Pratheeshkumar P, Kuttan G. Modulation of immune response by *Vernonia cinerea* L. inhibits the proinflammatory cytokine profile, iNOS, and COX-2 expression in LPS-stimulated macrophages. Immunopharmacology and Immunotoxicology. 2011;**33**:73-83

[80] Rajakumar G, Abdul Rahuman A, Priyamvada B, Gopiesh Khanna V, Kishore Kumar D, Sujin PJ. *Eclipta prostrata* leaf aqueous extract mediated synthesis of titanium dioxide nanoparticles. Materials Letters. 2012;**68**:115-117

[81] Tamimi H, Shishesaz MR, Farzam M, Jafari D. A review on nanoparticles of titanium dioxide: Characteristics, methods of synthesis and their application in organic coatings. International Journal of Advanced Biotechnology and Research. 2016;**7**:1226-1231

[82] Chung IM, Rajakumar G, Lee JH, Kim SH, Thiruvengadam M. Ethnopharmacological uses, phytochemistry, biological activities, and biotechnological applications of *Eclipta prostrata*. Applied Microbiology and Biotechnology. 2017;**101**:5247-5257

[83] Mithun NM, Shashidhara S, Vivek Kumar R. *Eclipta alba* (L.). A review on its phytochemical and pharmacological profile. Pharmacology. 2011;**1**:345-357

[84] Lee MK, Ha NR, Yang H, Sung SH, Kim GH, Kim YC. Antiproliferative activity of triterpenoids from *Eclipta prostrata* on hepatic stellate cells. Phytomedicine. 2008;**15**:775-780

[85] Liu QM, Zhao HY, Zhong XK, Jiang JG. *Eclipta prostrata* L. phytochemicals: Isolation, structure elucidation, and their antitumor activity. Food and Chemical Toxicology. 2012;**50**:4016-4022

[86] Chaudhary H, Dhuna V, Singh J, Kamboj SS, Seshadri S. Evaluation of hydro-alcoholic extract of *Eclipta alba* for its anticancer potential: An *in vitro* study. Journal of Ethnopharmacology. 2011;**136**:363-367

[87] Yadav NK, Arya RK, Dev K, Sharma C, Hossain Z, Meena S, et al. Alcoholic extract of *Eclipta alba* shows *in vitro* antioxidant and anticancer activity without exhibiting toxicological effects. Oxidative Medicine and Cellular Longevity. 2017;**2017**:9094641. DOI: 10.1155/2017/9094641

[88] Chauhan N, Singh D, Painuli RM. Screening of bioprotective properties and phytochemical analysis of various extracts of *Eclipta alba* whole plant. International Journal of Pharmacy and Pharmaceutical Sciences. 2012;**4**:554-560

[89] Gupta M, Mazumdera UK, Haldar PK, Kandar CC, Manikanda L, Senthil GP. Anticancer activity of *Indigofera aspalathoides* and *Wedelia calendulaceae* in Swiss albino mice. Iranian Journal of Pharmaceutical Research. 2007;**6**:141-145

[90] Kim HY, Kim HM, Ryu B, Lee JS, Choi JH, Jang DS. Constituents of the aerial parts of *Eclipta prostrata* and their cytotoxicity on human ovarian cancer cells *in vitro*. Archives of Pharmacal Research. 2015;**38**:1963-1969

[91] Khanna VG, Kannabiran K. Anticancer-cytotoxic activity of saponins isolated from the leaves of *Gymnema sylvestre* and *Eclipta alba* on HeLa cells. International Journal of Green Pharmacy. 2009;**1**:227-229

[92] Cho YJ, Woo JH, Lee JS, Jang DS, Lee KT, Choi JH. Eclalbasaponin II induces autophagic and apoptotic cell death in human ovarian cancer cells. Journal of Pharmacological Sciences. 2016;**132**:6-14

[93] Lirdprapamongkol K, Kramb JP, Chokchaichamnankit D, Srisomsap C, Surarit R, Sila-Asna M, et al. Juice of *Eclipta prostrata* inhibits cell migration *in vitro* and exhibits anti-angiogenic *activity in vivo*. In Vivo. 2008;**22**:363-368

[94] Ali F, Khan R, Khan AQ, Lateef MA, Maqbool T, Sultana S. Assessment of augmented immune surveillance and tumor cell death by cytoplasmic stabilization of p53 as a chemopreventive strategy of 3 promising medicinal herbs in murine 2-stage skin carcinogenesis. Integrative Cancer Therapies. 2014;**13**:351-367

[95] Dickers KJ, Bradberry SM, Rice P, Griffiths GD, Vale JA. Abrin poisoning. Toxicological Reviews. 2003;**22**:137-142

[96] Inglett GE, May JF. Tropical plants with unusual taste properties. Economic Botany. 1968;**22**:326-331

[97] Verma D, Tiwari SS, Srivastava S, Rawat A. Pharmacognostical evaluation and phytochemical standardization of *Abrus precatorius* L. seeds. Natural Product Sciences. 2011;**17**:51-57

[98] Garaniya N, Bapodra A. Ethnobotanical and phytopharmacological potential of *Abrus precatorius* L.: A review. Asian Pacific Journal of Tropical Biomedicine. 2014;**4**(Suppl 1):S27-S34

[99] Gadadhar S, Karande AA. Abrin immunotoxin: Targeted cytotoxicity and intracellular trafficking pathway. PLoS One. 2013;**8**(3):e58304

[100] Panneerselvam K, Lin SC, Liu CL, Liaw YC, Lin JY, Lu TH. Crystallization of agglutinin from the seeds of *Abrus precatorius*. Acta Crystallographica. Section D, Biological Crystallography. 2000;**56**:898-899

[101] Bhutia SK, Mallick SK, Stevens SM, Prokai L, Vishwanatha JK, Maiti TK. Induction of mitochondria-dependent apoptosis by *Abrus* agglutinin derived peptides in human cervical cancer cells. Toxicology In Vitro. 2008;**22**:344-351

[102] Gul MZ, Ahmad F, Kondapi AK, Qureshi IA, Ghazi IA. Antioxidant and antiproliferative activities of *Abrus precatorius* leaf extracts—An *in vitro* study. BMC Complementary and Alternative Medicine. 2013;**13**:53. DOI: 10.1186/1472-6882-13-53

[103] Lébri M, Tilaoui M, Bahi C, Achibat H, Akhramez S, Fofié YBN, et al. Phytochemical analysis and *in vitro* anticancer effect of aqueous extract of *Abrus precatorius* Linn. Der Pharma Chemica. 2015;**7**:112-117

[104] Shafi Sofi M, Sateesh MK, Bashir M, Harish G, Lakshmeesha TR, Vedashree S, et al. Cytotoxic and pro-apoptotic effects of *Abrus precatorius* L. on human metastatic breast cancer cell line, MDA-MB-231. Cytotechnology. 2013;**65**:407-417

[105] Reddy VV, Sirsi M. Effect of *Abrus precatorius* L. on experimental tumors. Cancer Research. 1969;**29**:1447-1451

[106] Bhutia SK, Mallick SK, Maiti S, Maiti TK. Antitumor and proapoptotic effect of *Abrus* agglutinin derived peptide in Dalton's lymphoma tumor model. Chemico-Biological Interactions. 2008;**174**:11-18

[107] Bhutia SK, Mallick SK, Maiti TK. In vitro immunostimulatory properties of *Abrus* lectins derived peptides in tumor bearing mice. Phytomedicine. 2009;**16**:776-782

[108] Anbu J, Ravichandiran V, Sumithra M, Chowdary SB, Kumar S, Kannadhasan R, et al. Anticancer activity of petroleum ether extract of *Abrus precatorius* on *Ehrlich ascitis* carcinoma in mice. International Journal of Pharma and Bio Sciences. 2011;**2**:24-31

[109] Shionoya H, Arai H, Koyanagi N, Ohtake S, Kobayashi H, Kodama T, et al. Induction of antitumor immunity by tumor cells treated with abrin. Cancer Research. 1982;**42**:2872-2876

[110] Ramnath V, Kuttan G, Kuttan R. Immunopotentiating activity of abrin, a lectin from *Abrus precatorius* Linn. Indian Journal of Experimental Biology. 2002;**40**:910-913

[111] Ghosh D, Bhutia SK, Mallick SK, Banerjee I, Maiti TK. Stimulation of murine B and T lymphocytes by native and heat-denatured *Abrus* agglutinin. Immunobiology. 2009;**214**:227-234

[112] Van Andel T. The diverse uses of fish-poison plants in northwest Guyana. Economic Botany. 2000;**54**:500-512

[113] Fukami J, Shishido T, Fukunaga K, Casida JE. Oxidative metabolism of rotenone in mammals, fish, and insects and its relation to selective toxicity. Journal of Agricultural and Food Chemistry. 1969;**17**:1217-1226

[114] Qureshi R, Bhatti GR, Memon RA. Ethnomedicinal uses of herbs from northern part of NARA desert, Pakistan. Pakistan Journal of Botany. 2010;**42**:839-851

[115] Vasconcelos JN, Lima JQ, de Lemos TLG, Oliveira MCF, Almeida MMB, Andrade-Neto M, et al. Estudo químico e biologico de Tephrosia toxicaria Pers. (Chemical and biological study of Tephrosia toxicaria Pers.). Quím Nova. 2009;**32**:382-386

[116] Touqeer S, Saeed MA, Ajaib M. A review on the phytochemistry and pharmacology of genus *Tephrosia*. Phytopharmacology. 2013;**4**:598-637

[117] Chen Y, Yan T, Gao C, Cao W, Huang R. Natural products from the genus *Tephrosia*. Molecules. 2014;**19**:1432-1458

[118] Adinarayana K, Jayaveera KN, Madhu Katyayani B, Mallikarjuna Rao P. Growth inhibition and induction of apoptosis in estrogen receptor positive and negative human breast carcinoma cells by *Tephrosia calophylla* roots. Pharmaceutical Chemistry Journal. 2009;**3**:35-41

[119] Gulecha V, Sivakuma T. Anticancer activity of *Tephrosia purpurea* and *Ficus religiosa* using MCF 7 cell lines. Asian Pacific Journal of Tropical Medicine. 2011;**4**:526-529

[120] Nondo RS, Mbwambo ZH, Kidukuli AW, Innocent EM, Mihale MJ, Erasto P, et al. Larvicidal, antimicrobial and brine shrimp activities of extracts from *Cissampelos mucronata* and *Tephrosia villosa* from coast region, Tanzania. BMC Complementary and Alternative Medicine. 2011;**11**:33-37

[121] Shanmugapriya R, Umamaheswari G, Thirunavukkarasu P, Renugadevi G, Ramanathan T. Cytotoxic effect of *Tephrosia purpurea* extracts on HeLa cervical cancerous cell line. Inventi Rapid: Molecular Pharmacology 2011;**2**. Article ID "Inventi:mp/49/11"

[122] Subhadra S, Kanacharalapalli VR, Ravindran VK, Parre SK, Chintala S, Thatipally R. Comparative toxicity assessment of three *Tephrosia* species on *Artemia salina* and animal cell lines.

Journal of Natural Pharmaceuticals. 2011;**2**:143-148

[123] Khalighi-Sigaroodi F, Ahvazi M, Hadjiakhoondi A, Taghizadeh M, Yazdani D, Khalighi-Sigaroodi S, et al. Cytotoxicity and antioxidant activity of 23 plant species of Leguminosae family. Iranian Journal of Pharmaceutical Research. 2012;**11**:295-302

[124] Padmapriya R, Gayathri L, Ronsard L, Akbarsha MA, Raveendran R. *In vitro* antiproliferative effect of *Tephrosia purpurea* on human hepatocellular carcinoma cells. Pharmacognosy Magazine. 2017;**13**(Suppl 1):S16-S21

[125] Ganapaty S, Srilakshmi GVK, Pannakal ST, Rahman H, Laatsch H, Brun R. Cytotoxic benzil and coumestan derivatives from *Tephrosia calophylla*. Phytochemistry. 2009;**70**:95-99

[126] Ganapaty S, Srilakshmi GVK, Thomas PS, Rajeswari NR, Ramakrishna S. Cytotoxicity and antiprotozoal activity of flavonoids from three *Tephrosia* species. Journal of Natural Remedies. 2009;**9**:202-208

[127] Hassan LE, Ahamed MB, Majid AS, Baharetha HM, Muslim NS, Nassar ZD, et al. Correlation of antiangiogenic, antioxidant and cytotoxic activities of some Sudanese medicinal plants with phenolic and flavonoid contents. BMC Complementary and Alternative Medicine. 2014;**14**:406. DOI: 10.1186/1472-6882-14-406

[128] Hassan LEA, Iqbal MA, Dahham SS, Tabana YM, Ahamed MBK, Majid AMSA. Colorectal, prostate and pancreas human cancers targeted bioassay-guided isolations and characterization of chemical constituents from *Tephrosia apollinea*. Anti-Cancer Agents in Medicinal Chemistry. 2017;**17**:590-598

[129] Jang DS, Park EJ, Kang YH, Hawthorne ME, Vigo JS, Graham JG, et al. Potential cancer chemopreventive flavonoids from the stems of *Tephrosia toxicaria*. Journal of Natural Products. 2003;**66**:1166-1170

[130] Saleem M, Ahmed S, Alam A, Sultana S. *Tephrosia purpurea* alleviates phorbol ester-induced tumor promotion response in murine skin. Pharmacological Research. 2001;**43**:135-144

[131] Hussain T, Siddiqui HH, Fareed S, Vijayakumar M, Rao CV. Chemopreventive evaluation of *Tephrosia purpurea* against N-nitrosodiethylamine-induced hepatocarcinogenesis in Wistar rats. The Journal of Pharmacy and Pharmacology. 2012;**64**:1195-1205

[132] Bright EO, Okusanya BA. Infestation of economic plants in Badeggi by *Tapinanthus dodoneifolius* (DC) Danser and *Tapinanthus globiferus* (A. Rich) Van Tiegh. Nigerian Journal of Weed Science. 1998;**11**:51-56

[133] Roth I, Lindorf H. South American Medicinal Plants. Botany, Remedial Properties and General Use. Berlin: Springer Verlag; 2002

[134] Yazbek PB, Tezoto J, Cassas F, Rodrigues E. Plants used during maternity, menstrual cycle and other women's health conditions among Brazilian cultures. Journal of Ethnopharmacology. 2016;**179**:310-331

[135] Lindholm P. Cytotoxic compounds of plant origin—Biological and chemical diversity. [PhD thesis]. Uppsala: Faculty of Pharmacy; 2005

[136] Mary KT, Girija K, Ramadasan K. Partial purification of tumour-reducing principle from *Helicanthis elasticus* (Fam. Loranthaceae). Cancer Letters. 1994;**81**:53-57

[137] Fernandez T, Wagner ML, Varela BG, Ricco RA, Hajos SE, Gurni AA,

et al. Study of an Argentine mistletoe, the hemiparasite *Ligaria cuneifolia* (R. et P.) Tiegh. (Loranthaceae). Journal of Ethnopharmacology. 1998;**62**:25-34

[138] Winarno H. Antiproliferative activity of octadeca-8,10,12-triynoic acid against human cancer cell lines. Benia Biologi. 2009;**9**:343-348

[139] Yoon TJ, Yoo YC, Kang TB, Shimazaki K, Song SK, Lee KH, et al. Lectins isolated from Korean mistletoe (*Viscum album coloratum*) induce apoptosis in tumor cells. Cancer Letters. 1999;**136**:33-40

[140] Rios MY, Salina D, Villarreal ML. Cytotoxic activity of moronic acid and identification of the new triterpene 3,4-seco-olean-18-ene-3,28-dioic acid from *Phoradendron reichenbachianum*. Planta Medica. 2001;**67**:443-446

[141] Sadik G, Islam R, Rahman MM, Khondkar P, Rashid MA, Sarker SD. Antimicrobial and cytotoxic constituents of *Loranthus globosus*. Fitoterapia. 2003;**74**:308-311

[142] Kim YK, Kim YS, Choi SU, Ryu SY. Isolation of flavonol rhamnosides from *Loranthus tanakae* and cytotoxic effect of them on human tumor cell lines. Archives of Pharmacal Research. 2004;**27**:44-47

[143] Zhao YL, Wang XY, Sun LX, Fan RH, Bi KS, Yu ZG. Cytotoxic constituents of *Viscum coloratum*. Zeitschrift für Naturforschung. Section C. 2012;**67**:129-134

[144] Cerdá Zolezzi P, Fernández T, Aulicino P, Cavaliere V, Greczanik S, Caldas Lopes E, et al. *Ligaria cuneifolia* flavonoid fractions modulate cell growth of normal lymphocytes and tumor cells as well as multidrug resistant cells. Immunobiology. 2005;**209**:737-749

[145] Murwani R. Indonesian tea mistletoe (*Scurrula oortiana*) stem extract increases tumour cell sensitivity to tumour necrosis factor alpha (TNFalpha). Phytotherapy Research. 2003;**17**:407-409

[146] Elsyana V, Bintang M, Priosoeryanto BP. Cytotoxicity and antiproliferative activity assay of clove mistletoe (*Dendrophthoe pentandra* (L.) Miq.) leaves extracts. Advances in Pharmacological Sciences. 2016;**2016**:3242698. DOI: 10.1155/2016/3242698

[147] Kumar N, Biswas S, Mathew AE, Varghese S, Mathew JE, Nandakumar K, et al. Pro-apoptotic and cytotoxic effects of enriched fraction of *Elytranthe parasitica* (L.) Danser against HepG2 hepatocellular carcinoma. BMC Complementary and Alternative Medicine. 2016;**16**:420

[148] Ohashi K, Winarno H, Mukai M, Shibuya H. Preparation and cancer cell invasion inhibitory effects of C16-alkynic fatty acids. Chemical and Pharmaceutical Bulletin (Tokyo). 2003;**51**:463-466

[149] Heitzman ME, Neto CC, Winiarz E, Vaisberg AJ, Hammond GB. Ethnobotany, phytochemistry and pharmacology of *Uncaria* (Rubiaceae). Phytochemistry. 2005;**66**:5-29

[150] Sandoval M, Okuhama NN, Zhang XJ, Condezo LA, Lao J, Angeles FM, et al. Anti-inflammatory and antioxidant activities of cat's claw (*Uncaria tomentosa* and *Uncaria guianensis*) are independent of their alkaloid content. Phytomedicine. 2002;**9**:325-337

[151] Lee KK, Zhou BN, Kingston DG, Vaisberg AJ, Hammond GB. Bioactive indole alkaloids from the bark of *Uncaria guianensis*. Planta Medica. 1999;**65**:759-760

[152] Laus G. Advances in chemistry and bioactivity of the genus *Uncaria*. Phytotherapy Research. 2004;**18**:259-274

[153] Miller MJ, Mehta K, Kunte S, Raut V, Gala J, Dhumale R, et al. Early relief of osteoarthritis symptoms with a natural mineral supplement and a herbomineral combination: A randomized controlled trial [ISRCTN38432711]. Journal of Inflammation (London). 2005;**2**:11

[154] Mehta K, Gala J, Bhasale S, Naik S, Modak M, Thakur H, et al. Comparison of glucosamine sulfate and a polyherbal supplement for the relief of osteoarthritis of the knee: A randomized controlled trial [ISRCTN25438351]. BMC Complementary and Alternative Medicine. 2007;**7**:34

[155] Mur E, Hartig F, Eibl G, Schirmer M. Randomized double blind trial of an extract from the pentacyclic alkaloid-chemotype of *Uncaria tomentosa* for the treatment of rheumatoid arthritis. The Journal of Rheumatology. 2002;**29**:678-681

[156] Del Grossi Moura M, Lopes LC, Biavatti MW, Kennedy SA, de Oliveira E, Silva MC, et al. Oral herbal medicines marketed in Brazil for the treatment of osteoarthritis: A systematic review and meta-analysis. Phytotherapy Research. 2017;**31**:1676-1685

[157] Bacher N, Tiefenthaler M, Sturm S, Stuppner H, Ausserlechner M, Kofler R. Oxindole alkaloids from *Uncaria tomentosa* induce apoptosis in proliferating, G0/G1-arrested and bcl-2-expressing acute lymphoblastic leukaemia cells. British Journal of Haematology. 2006;**132**:615-622

[158] Garcia Prado E, Garcia Gimenez MD, De la Puerta Vazquez R, Espartero Sanchez JL, Saenz Rodriguez MT. Antiproliferative effects of mitraphylline, a pentacyclic oxindole alkaloid of *Uncaria tomentosa* on human glioma and neuroblastoma cell lines. Phytomedicine. 2007;**14**:280-284

[159] García Giménez D, García Prado E, Sáenz Rodríguez T, Fernández Arche A, De la Puerta R. Cytotoxic effect of the pentacyclic oxindole alkaloid mitraphylline isolated from *Uncaria tomentosa* bark on human Ewing's sarcoma and breast cancer cell lines. Planta Medica. 2010;**76**:133-136

[160] Pilarski R, Filip B, Wietrzyk J, Kuras M, Gulewicz K. Anticancer activity of the *Uncaria tomentosa* DC. preparations with different oxindole alkaloid composition. Phytomedicine. 2010;**17**:1133-1139

[161] Urdanibia I, Michelangeli F, Ruiz MC, Milano B, Taylor P. Anti-inflammatory and antitumoural effects of *Uncaria guianensis* bark. Journal of Ethnopharmacology. 2013;**150**:1154-1162

[162] Budán F, Szabó I, Varjas T, Nowrasteh G, Dávid T, Gergely P, et al. Mixtures of *Uncaria* and *Tabebuia* extracts are potentially chemopreventive in CBA/Ca mice: A long-term experiment. Phytotherapy Research. 2011;**25**:493-500

[163] De Paula LC, Fonseca F, Perazzo F, Cruz FM, Cubero D, Trufelli DC, et al. *Uncaria tomentosa* (cat's claw) improves quality of life in patients with advanced solid tumors. Journal of Alternative and Complementary Medicine. 2015;**21**:22-30

[164] Araújo MCS, Farias ILG, Gutierres J, Dalmora SL, Flores N, Farias J, et al. *Uncaria tomentosa*—Adjuvant treatment for breast cancer: Clinical trial. Evidence-based Complementary and Alternative Medicine. 2012;**2012**:676984. DOI: 10.1155/2012/676984

[165] Farias ILG, Araújo MCS, Farias JG, Rossato LV, Elsenbach LI, Dalmora SL, et al. *Uncaria tomentosa* for reducing side effects caused by chemotherapy in CRC patients:

Clinical trial. Evidence-based Complementary and Alternative Medicine. 2012;**2012**:892182. DOI: 10.1155/2012/892182

[166] Alves IABS, Miranda HM, Soares LAL, Randau KP. Simaroubaceae family: Botany, chemical composition and biological activities. Revista Brasileira de Farmacognosia. 2014;**24**:481-501

[167] Almeida MMB, Arriaga AMC, Santos AKL, Lemos TLG, Braz-Filho R, Vieira IJC. Ocorrência e atividade biológica de quassinóides da última década (Occurrence and biological activity of quassinoids in the last decade). Quimica Nova. 2007;**30**:935-951

[168] Vikas B, Akhil BS, Suja SR, Sujathan K. An exploration of phytochemicals from Simaroubaceae. Asian Pacific Journal of Cancer Prevention. 2017;**18**:1765-1767

[169] Showalter HDH. Progress in the synthesis of canthine alkaloids and ring-truncated congeners. Journal of Natural Products. 2013;**76**:455-467

[170] Diehl C, Ferrari A. Superiority of *Quassia amara* 4% cream over metronidazole 0.75% cream in the treatment of rosacea: A randomized, double-blinded trial. Journal of Clinical and Cosmetic Dermatology. 2017;**1**. DOI: 10.16966/2576-2826.117

[171] Kupchan SM, Streelman DR. Quassimarin, a new antileukemic quassinoid from *Quassia amara*. The Journal of Organic Chemistry. 1976;**41**:3481-3482

[172] Kitagawa I, Mahmud T, Yokota K, Nakagawa S, Mayumi T, Kobayashi M, et al. Indonesian medicinal plants. XVII. Characterization of quassinoids from the stems of *Quassia indica*. Chemical and Pharmaceutical Bulletin (Tokyo). 1996;**44**:2009-2014

[173] Cachet N, Hoakwie F, Bertani S, Bourdy G, Deharo E, Stien D, et al. Antimalarial activity of simalikalactone E, a new quassinoid from *Quassia amara* L. (Simaroubaceae). Antimicrobial Agents and Chemotherapy. 2009;**53**:4393-4398

[174] Houël E, Bertani S, Bourdy G, Deharo E, Jullian V, Valentin A, et al. Quassinoid constituents of *Quassia amara* L. leaf herbal tea. Impact on its antimalarial activity and cytotoxicity. Journal of Ethnopharmacology. 2009;**126**:114-118

[175] Murakami C, Fukamiya N, Tamura S, Okano M, Bastow KF, Tokuda H, et al. Multidrug-resistant cancer cell susceptibility to cytotoxic quassinoids, and cancer chemopreventive effects of quassinoids and canthin alkaloids. Bioorganic & Medicinal Chemistry. 2004;**12**:4963-4968

[176] Rivero-Cruz JF, Lezutekong R, Lobo-Echeverri T, Ito A, Mi Q, Chai HB, et al. Cytotoxic constituents of the twigs of *Simarouba glauca* collected from a plot in southern Florida. Phytotherapy Research. 2005;**19**:136-140

[177] Jiang XM, Zhou Y. Canthin-6-one alkaloids from *Picrasma quassioides* and their cytotoxic activity. Journal of Asian Natural Products Research. 2008;**10**:1009-1012

[178] Usami Y, Nakagawa-Goto K, Lang JY, Kim Y, Lai CY, Goto M, et al. Antitumor agents. 282. 2′-(R)-O-acetylglaucarubinone, a quassinoid from *Odyendyea gabonensis* as a potential anti-breast and anti-ovarian cancer agent. Journal of Natural Products. 2010;**73**:1553-1558

[179] Shields M, Niazi U, Badal S, Yee T, Sutcliffe MJ, Delgoda R. Inhibition of CYP1A1 by quassinoids found in *Picrasma excelsa*. Planta Medica. 2009;**75**:137-141

[180] Wiseman CL, Yap HY, Bedikian AY, Bodey GP, Blumenschein GR. Phase II trial of bruceantin in metastatic breast carcinoma. American Journal of Clinical Oncology. 1982;**5**:389-391

[181] Arseneau JC, Wolter JM, Kuperminc M, Ruckdeschel JC. A Phase II study of bruceantin (NSC-165, 563) in advanced malignant melanoma. Investigational New Drugs. 1983;**1**:239-242

[182] Shan GY, Zhang S, Li GW, Chen YS, Liu XA, Wang JK. Clinical evaluation of oral Fructus bruceae oil combined with radiotherapy for the treatment of esophageal cancer. Chinese Journal of Integrative Medicine. 2011;**17**:933-936

[183] Grant KL, Lutz RB. Alternative therapies: Ginger. American Journal of Health-System Pharmacy. 2000;**57**:945-947

[184] An K, Zhao D, Wang Z, Wu J, Xu Y, Xiao G. Comparison of different drying methods on Chinese ginger (*Zingiber officinale* Roscoe): Changes in volatiles, chemical profile, antioxidant properties, and microstructure. Food Chemistry. 2016;**197**(Part B:1292-1300

[185] Rahmani AH, Shabrmi FM, Aly SM. Active ingredients of ginger as potential candidates in the prevention and treatment of diseases via modulation of biological activities. International Journal of Physiology, Pathophysiology and Pharmacology. 2014;**6**:125-136

[186] Gupta R, Singh PK, Singh R, Singh RL. Pharmacological activities of *Zingiber officinale* (ginger) and its active ingredients: A review. International Journal of Innovation Science and Research. 2016;**4**:1-18

[187] Lee E, Surh YJ. Induction of apoptosis in HL60 cells by pungent vanilloids, [6]-gingerol and [6]-paradol. Cancer Letters. 1998;**134**:163-168

[188] Keum YS, Kim J, Lee KH, Park KK, Surh YJ, Lee JM, et al. Induction of apoptosis and caspase-3 activation by chemopreventive [6]-paradol and structurally related compounds in KB cells. Cancer Letters. 2002;**177**:41-47

[189] Park YJ, Wen J, Bang S, Park SW, Song SY. [6]-Gingerol induces cell cycle arrest and cell death of mutant p53-expressing pancreatic cancer cells. Yonsei Medical Journal. 2006;**47**:688-697

[190] Ishiguro K, Ando T, Maeda O, Ohmiya N, Niwa Y, Kadomatsu K, et al. Ginger ingredients reduce viability of gastric cancer cells via distinct mechanisms. Biochemical and Biophysical Research Communications. 2007;**362**:218-223

[191] Rhode J, Fogoros S, Zick S, Wahl H, Griffith KA, Huang J, et al. Ginger inhibits cell growth and modulates angiogenic factors in ovarian cancer cells. BMC Complementary and Alternative Medicine. 2007;**7**:44. DOI: 10.1186/1472-6882-7-44

[192] Kim JS, Lee SI, Park HW, Yang JH, Shin TY, Kim YC, et al. Cytotoxic components from the dried rhizomes of *Zingiber officinale* Roscoe. Archives of Pharmacal Research. 2008;**31**:415-418

[193] Lee SH, Cekanova M, Baek SJ. Multiple mechanisms are involved in 6-gingerol-induced cell growth arrest and apoptosis in human colorectal cancer cells. Molecular Carcinogenesis. 2008;**47**:197-208

[194] Brown AC, Shah C, Liu J, Pham JT, Zhang JG, Jadus MR. Ginger's (*Zingiber officinale* Roscoe) inhibition of rat colonic adenocarcinoma cells proliferation and angiogenesis *in vitro*. Phytotherapy Research. 2009;**23**:640-645

[195] Sang S, Hong J, Wu H, Liu J, Yang CS, Pan MH, et al. Increased growth inhibitory effects on human cancer cells and anti-inflammatory potency of shogaols from *Zingiber officinale* relative to gingerols. Journal of Agricultural and Food Chemistry. 2009;**57**:10645-10650

[196] Gan FF, Nagle AA, Ang X, Ho OH, Tan SH, Yang H, et al. Shogaols at proapoptotic concentrations induce G(2)/M arrest and aberrant mitotic cell death associated with tubulin aggregation. Apoptosis. 2011;**16**:856-867

[197] Tan BS, Kang O, Mai CW, Tiong KH, Khoo AS, Pichika MR, et al. 6-Shogaol inhibits breast and colon cancer cell proliferation through activation of peroxisomal proliferator activated receptor gamma (PPARgamma). Cancer Letters. 2013;**336**:127-139

[198] Surh YJ, Park KK, Chun KS, Lee LJ, Lee E, Lee SS. Antitumor promoting activities of selected pungent phenolic substances present in ginger. Journal of Environmental Pathology, Toxicology and Oncology. 1999;**18**:131-139

[199] Kim M, Miyamoto S, Yasui Y, Oyama T, Murakami A, Tanaka T. Zerumbone, a tropical ginger sesquiterpene, inhibits colon and lung carcinogenesis in mice. International Journal of Cancer. 2009;**124**:264-271

[200] Lee E, Park KK, Lee JM, Chun KS, Kang JY, Lee SS, et al. Suppression of mouse skin tumor promotion and induction of apoptosis in HL-60 cells by *Alpina oxyphylla* Miquel (Zingiberaceae). Carcinogenesis. 1998;**19**:1337-1381

[201] Jeong CH, Bode AM, Pugliese A, Cho YY, Kim HG, Shim JH, et al. [6]-Gingerol suppresses colon cancer growth by targeting leukotriene A4 hydrolase. Cancer Research. 2009;**69**:5584-5591

[202] Wu H, Hsieh MC, Lo CY, Liu CB, Sang S, Ho CT, et al. 6-Shogaol is more effective than 6-gingerol and curcumin in inhibiting 12-O-tetradecanoylphorbol 13-acetate induced tumor promotion in mice. Molecular Nutrition & Food Research. 2010;**54**:1296-1306

[203] Vinothkumar R, Sudha M, Nalini N. Chemopreventive effect of zingerone against colon carcinogenesis induced by 1,2-dimethylhydrazine in rats. European Journal of Cancer Prevention. 2014;**23**:361-371

[204] Ling H, Yang H, Tan SH, Chui WK, Chew EH. 6-Shogaol, an active constituent of ginger, inhibits breast cancer cell invasion by reducing matrix metalloproteinase-9 expression via blockade of nuclear factor-kappa B activation. British Journal of Pharmacology. 2010;**161**:1763-1777

[205] Núñez-Sánchez MA, González-Sarrías A, Romo-Vaquero M, García-Villalba R, Selma MV, Tomás-Barberán FA, et al. Dietary phenolics against colorectal cancer—From promising preclinical results to poor translation into clinical trials: Pitfalls and future needs. Molecular Nutrition & Food Research. 2015;**59**:1274-1291

[206] Marx WM, Teleni L, McCarthy AL, Vitetta L, McKavanagh D, Thomson D, et al. Ginger (*Zingiber officinale*) and chemotherapy-induced nausea and vomiting: A systematic literature review. Nutrition Reviews. 2013;**71**:245-254

[207] Lin SR, Fu YS, Tsai MJ, Cheng H, Weng CF. Natural compounds from herbs that can potentially execute as autophagy inducers for cancer therapy. International Journal of Molecular Sciences. 2017;**18**:pii: E1412. DOI: 10.3390/ijms18071412

[208] Ruela-de-Sousa RR, Fuhler GM, Blom N, Ferreira CV, Aoyama H, Peppelenbosch MP. Cytotoxicity of apigenin on leukemia cell lines:

Implications for prevention and therapy. Cell Death & Disease. 2010;**1**:e19. DOI: 10.1038/cddis.2009.18

[209] Tuorkey MJ. Molecular targets of luteolin in cancer. European Journal of Cancer Prevention. 2016;**25**:65-76

[210] Yang CS, Wang H. Cancer preventive activities of tea catechins. Molecules. 2016;**21**:pii: E1679

[211] Dybkowska E, Sadowska A, Świderski F, Rakowska R, Wysocka K. The occurrence of resveratrol in foodstuffs and its potential for supporting cancer prevention and treatment. A review. Roczniki Państwowego Zakładu Higieny. 2018;**69**:5-14

[212] Bock PR, Hanisch J, Matthes H, Zänker KS. Targeting inflammation in cancer-related-fatigue: A rationale for mistletoe therapy as supportive care in colorectal cancer patients. Inflammation & Allergy Drug Targets. 2014;**13**:105-111

[213] Baliga MS, Rao S, Rai MP, D'souza P. Radioprotective effects of the Ayurvedic medicinal plant *Ocimum sanctum* Linn. (holy basil): A memoir. Journal of Cancer Research and Therapeutics. 2016;**12**:20-27

[214] Baharvand M, Jafari S, Mortazavi H. Herbs in oral mucositis. Journal of Clinical and Diagnostic Research. 2017;**11**:ZE05-ZE11

[215] Yu J, Wang C, Kong Q, Wu X, Lu JJ, Chen X. Recent progress in doxorubicin-induced cardiotoxicity and protective potential of natural products. Phytomedicine. 2018;**40**:125-139

[216] Chen H, Lin Z, Arnst KE, Miller DD, Li W. Tubulin inhibitor-based antibody-drug conjugates for cancer therapy. Molecules. 2017;**22**:1281. DOI: 10.3390/molecules22081281

[217] Shankar Babu M, Mahanta S, Lakhter AJ, Hato T, Paul S, Naidu SR. Lapachol inhibits glycolysis in cancer cells by targeting pyruvate kinase M2. PLoS One. 2018;**13**:e0191419. DOI: 10.1371/journal.pone.0191419

[218] Khalili M, Akbarzadeh A, Chiani M, Sepideh T. The effect of nanoliposomal and pegylated nanoliposomal forms of 6-gingerol on breast cancer cells. Research Journal of Recent Sciences. 2013;**2**:29-33

[219] Cuendet M, Pezzuto JM. Antitumor activity of bruceantin: An old drug with new promise. Journal of Natural Products. 2004;**67**:269-272

[220] Guo Z, Vangapandu S, Sindelar RW, Walker LA, Sindelar RD. Biologically active quassinoids and their chemistry: Potential leads for drug design. Frontiers in Medicinal Chemistry. 2009;**4**:285-308

Chapter 7

Therapeutic Use of Some Romanian Medicinal Plants

Adina-Elena Segneanu, Claudiu Cepan, Ioan Grozescu, Florentina Cziple, Sorin Olariu, Sonia Ratiu, Viorica Lazar, Sorin Marius Murariu, Silvia Maria Velciov and Teodora Daniela Marti

Abstract

Romanian traditional medicine has an extremely old history. The Dacian knowledge of the curative properties of medicinal plants was documented by Herodotus, Hippocrates, Galen, and Dioscorides. It must be emphasized that modern chemical screening has confirmed the therapeutic properties of the medicinal plants used by the Dacians. More interesting is that Dacians used many of these herbs for different dishes. Practically, for Dacians, food was medicine. Recent research on some Romanian medicinal plants has highlighted their pharmacognostical importance. It is known that currently, the importance and dynamics of the research on medicinal plants in the area of drug discovery continues to increase worldwide. The main reason is not only the high efficiency of secondary metabolites in case of serious diseases (cancer, viral infections, malaria, etc.) but also the minimization of the side effects of the synthetic drugs.

Keywords: Dacians, phytotherapy, secondary metabolites

1. Introduction

Phytotherapy has always played an essential role in the development of humanity. Traditional medicine still continues to have major importance in many areas of the world, especially in low-income regions [1–7].

Although in developed countries, alternative medicine has been outdated by modern medical techniques, at present, there is a growing trend toward natural remedies. The importance of medicinal plants emerges from the fact that worldwide, almost 50% of existing synthetic medicaments are derived from natural extracts [2–7].

The main ancient medicinal systems are considered to be: Ayurvedic, Greek, and Chinese medicine [8, 9]. However, there are very few documents about Dacian medicine, considered by their contemporaries and later by archeological evidence as highly advanced [8, 10–21].

In traditional Romanian medicine, almost all the natural remedies taken from the Dacians are found [8, 10–23].

2. Romanian medicinal plants

Romanian phytotherapy is an important part of our natural and cultural heritage. In this respect, it should be emphasized that in the flora of Romania, there are about 4000 plant species, of which over 20% are medicinal plants. Scientific research has confirmed the therapeutic properties of almost 50% of Romanian medicinal plants and about 25% plants are already used to obtain botanical products on large scale [2, 4, 5, 12, 23].

Between the Romanian people and traditional medicine, there was always a very deep connection. Basically, through the entire evolution of Romanians, healing herbs played an important role. Daco-Getic civilization was considered as the most evolved society at that time in Europe [10, 12, 18]. The Dacian's vast knowledge about healing plants has been certified by several personalities of those times (Herodotus, Discorides, Tucidide, Pseudo-Apuleius, Ovid, Virgil, etc.) [10, 12, 13, 17, 18]. The Dacian's knowledge about medicine, surgery, phytotherapy, and astronomy was confirmed by historical documents and archeological evidence [11, 12, 18].

In fact, the life philosophy of our ancestors proves to be more current than ever. In this regard, it must be mentioned that the Dacians knew the psychosomatic concept and the interdependence between the psychological and the somatic factors that triggered different affections [10–13, 18]. This is not only extremely interesting but at the same time extremely rare for that time period. It must be underlined that psycho-somatic medicine was recognized as a branch of medicine only many centuries later.

According to the Dacians, the human body represents a complex energy system which maintains the physical body [10, 12, 18].

Our ancestors believed that there was a perfect balance between man and nature. Each plant or tree is a being to be respected. Thus, plant harvesting must take place only at a certain time of year, when the plant is mature and the concentration of active principles is maximal. For instance, Herb Robert (*Geranium robertianum*) is collected on the morning of August 15 [11, 12, 16, 18].

Plant name	Main secondary metabolites identified	Therapeutic effect	References
Dandelion	Flavonoids, phenols, fatty acids	Hepatoprotective, diuretic, anti-inflammatory, antitumoral [82]	[4, 5, 12, 15, 16, 19, 23, 66, 82]
Daisy	Saponins, triterpenes, anthocyanins, polyphenols, flavonoids	Antimicrobial, neuroprotective, cicatrizating effect, emollient, anti-inflammatory, antioxidant, hypolipidemic, hemostatic	[4, 5, 12, 15, 16]
Allheal	Tannins, sterols, phenolic acids, alkaloids	Astringent, hemostatic agent, cicatrizating effect	[4, 5, 12, 15, 16]
Borango	Fatty acids, alkaloids	Anti-inflammatory, antitumoral, antidiabetes, cardioprotective, immunomodulatory agent	[4, 5, 12, 15, 16, 78]
Hogweed	Coumarine, lignans, flavonoids	Neuroprotective, antioxidant, anticancer, antimicrobial, antidiabetic, antiviral, and anti-inflammatory	[4, 5, 12, 15, 16, 79]
Fat grass (Dacian name: Iaca)	Vitamins (A, C, B), fatty acids (omega 3), proteins, saponins, phenolic acids, coumarine, flavonoids, coenzyme Q10, alkaloids	Cicatrizating effect, wound healing, antibacterial, antipyretic, depurative, diuretic, regenerative	

Table 1.
Main bioactive compounds of some healing herbs included in Dacian's diet.

Dacian medicinal plant	Scientific name of plant	Dacian therapeutic recommendation
Aniarsexe	*Onobrychis viciifolia* (*Fabaceae*)	Diuretic, abscess, sudorific
Ionits	*Aconitum napellus* (*Ranunculaceae*)	Astringent, antidote (snake bite), poison for arrows
Sopitis	*Aristolochia clematitis*	Analgesic, contraceptive, anti-inflammatory
Dacina	*Adonis vernalis* (Ranunculaceae)	Diuretic, analgesic, cardiotonic
Boudathla	*Anchusa officinalis* (Boraginaceae)	Sudorific, diuretic, anti-inflammatory effect, respiratory infections
Cinouboila	*Bryonia alba L.* (Cucurbitaceae)	Antibacterial, depigmentation effects, antiepileptic, snake bite antidote (viper venom), headaches, anti-inflammatory, analgesic, induce abortion, wet cough, hemostatic agent, induce lactation
Coadama	*Alisma plantago-aquatica L.* (*Alismataceae*)	Astringent, dermatologic diseases (irritation, inflammations)
Coicolida	*Physalis alkekengi L.* (*Solanaceae*)	Hepatoprotective, diuretic, laxative, edema
Dielleina	*Hyoscyamus niger L.* (*Solanaceae*)	Analgesic, hallucinogenic, hypnotic, anti-inflammatory, antitussive, hemostatic, antibacterial, antipyretic, toothache, sedative, psychomotricity
Diesema	*Verbascum phlomoides L.* (*Scrophulariaceae*)	Astringent, diarrhea, antitussive, antispastic, toothache, analgesic, cicatrizating effect, expectorant, anti-inflammatory
Doctila	*Ajuga chamaepitys L.* (*Lamiaceae*)	Liver disease, sciatica pain relief
Duodela	*Achillea millefolium L.* (*Asteraceae*)	Anti-inflammatory, gallbladder relief, antiasthmatic, hemorrhoids, stimulating appetite, detoxifying, sedative, analgesic, antiviral, liver diseases, cicatrizating effect, antitussive digestive diseases
Dyn	*Urtica dioica L.* (*Urticaceae*)	Wound healing, anti-inflammatory, antitumoral, abscess, hemostatic, aphrodisiac, expectorant, cicatrizating effect, antimicrobial, detoxifying, disinfectant
Guoleta	*Lithospermum arvense L.* (*Boraginaceae*)	Nephrolithiasis, diuretic
Malva	*Mallow sylvestris* (*Malvaceae*)	Anti-inflammatory activity, cicatrizating effect, laxative, respiratory disorders
Mendruta	*Veratrum album* (*Melanthiaceae*)	Anti-inflammatory, antispastic, antibacterial (dysentery), hypotensive

Dacian medicinal plant	Scientific name of plant	Dacian therapeutic recommendation
Mizela	*Thymus vulgaris L.* (*Lamiaceae*)	Anti-inflammatory, antiasthmatic, increase fertility, anthelmintic, antiedema
Priadila	*Clematis vitalba L.* (*Ranunculaceae*).	Diuretic, analgesic, antiepileptic, antitussive, hair growth, dizziness
Propodila	*Potentilla reptans L.* (*Rosaceae*)	Toothache, anti-inflammatory for diseases of oral and pharyngeal cavity, antiviral, detoxifying, antipyretic, cicatrizating effect
Riborasta	*Arctium lappa* (*Asteraceae*)	Anti-inflammatory, disinfectant, antimicrobial, cicatrizating effect, detoxifying effect
Salia	*Datura stramonium L.* (*Solanaceae*)	Anti-inflammatory, diuretic, menstrual induction, psychomotricity
Sciare	*Dipsacus pilosus L.* (*Caprifoliaceae*)	Anti-inflammatory, hemorrhoids, anal fissures, antivral
Stirsozila	*Erythraea centaurium Pers.* (*Gentianaceae*)	Cicatrizating effect, wound healing, biliary dyskinesia, menstrual induction, anti-inflammatory, analgesic, induce abortion, eye infections, sedative
Tendila	*Mentha piperita L.* (*Lamiaceae*)	Snake bite treatment, diuretic, anti-inflammatory, anthelmintic, detoxifying, antispastic
Usazila	*Cynoglossum officinale L.* (*Boraginaceae*)	Hair growth, laxative, cicatrizating effect, wound healing

Table 2.
A brief overview of most popular Dacian medicinal plants.

Herb name	Scientific name of plant	Main chemical composition	Biological activity
Aniarsexe (Sparceta)	*Onobrychis viciifolia* (*Fabaceae*)	Tanins, flavons, proteins, minerals (Cu, Ca, P)	Anti-inflammatory, detoxifying action, urinary diseases, sexual dysfunctions, hypoglycemic, anticholesterolemic, etc. [4, 5, 26]
Cinouboila	*Bryonia alba* (*Cucurbitaceae*)	Flavonoids,cucurbitacins, sterols, lectins, aminoacids, etc.	Wound healing, hemostatic, diuretic, antispasmodic, anti-inflammatory, hepatoprotective, antiatherosclerotic agent, rheumatism, antitumoral activity [4, 5, 27–29]
Wolfsbane	*Aconitum napellus* (*Ranunculaceae*)	Aconite (alkaloid)	Antirheumatic, analgesic, neuralgia, respiratory tract disorders, anti-inflammatory activity, etc. [4, 5, 30–32]
Pheasant's eye	*Adonis vernalis* (*Ranunculaceae*)	Flavons, quinones, saponins, coumarins, etc.	Sedative, diuretic, cardiotonic effect [83, 84]
Mallow	*Mallow sylvestris* (*Malvaceae*)	Phenols, terpenoids, flavonoids, vitamins (A,B,C,E), minerals (Fe, Zn, Ca, Se, K, Mg), mucilage, inulin	Anti-inflammatory activity, asthma, respiratory diseases, antimicrobial, kidney infections, wound healing, dermatological diseases (eczema, acne), antioxidant, hepatoprotective, anticancer [4, 5, 34, 35, 82]
Budathla (ox tongue)	*Anchusa officinalis* (*Boraginaceae*)	Flavonoids, polyphenols, choline, allantoin	Antioxidant, antimicrobial, wound healing, emollient, antitumoral, expectorant, diuretic, analgesic, etc. [4, 5, 36]
Common water-plantain	*Alisma plantago-aquatica* (*Alismataceae*)	Terpenoids, phenolic acids, sterols, alkaloids,	Antibacterial, antialergic anti-cholesterolemic, diaphoretic, diuretic, hypoglycemic, hypotensive [36]
Winter cherry	*Physalis alkekengi* (*Solanaceae*)	Alkaloids (solanină şi fisolină), vitamins (C), glucocorticoids, lycopene	Diuretic, laxative, anti-inflammatory activity, sedative, hepatoprotective, analgesic, antiseptic [37–39]
Black henbane	*Hyoscyamus niger L.* (*Solanaceae*)	Alkaloids (hyoscyamine, scopolamine and atropine), flavonoids, lignans, phenols, coumarin, saponins, glycosides	Sedative, analgesic, antispasmodic, hypnotic, hallucinogenic, hypotensive, antimicrobial [4, 5, 40]
Mullein	*Verbascum phlomoides L.* (*Scrophulariaceae*)	Phenols, terpenes, sterols, fatty acids, alkaloids, glycosides	Anti-inflammatory activity, wound healing, antispasmodic, anthelmintic, expectorant, antifungal effect, diuretic [41–43]
Yellow bugle	*Ajuga chamaepitys L.* (*Lamiaceae*)	Tanins, alkaloids, anthocyanins, sterols, terpenes, glycosides, essential acids	Diuretic, anti-inflammatory activity, tonic, anti-microbial, antioxidant activity, antirheumatic, anthelmintic, antifungal effect [44–46]

Herb name	Scientific name of plant	Main chemical composition	Biological activity
Yarrow	*Achillea millefolium* L. (*Asteraceae*)	Flavonoids, choline, sterols, vitamin K, volatile oils, tanins	Anti-inflammatory activity, hemostatic, wound healing, analgesic, disinfectant, antispasmodic, gastroprotective, astringent, hypotensive, antitumoral [4, 5, 47, 48]
Stinging nettle	*Urtica dioica* L. (*Urticaceae*)	Coumarine, sterols, terpenoids, carotenoids (β-carotene lutein and lycopene) fatty acids, poly-phenols, amino acids, chlorophyll, vitamins (A,C,B D,E,F,K,P), tannins, carbohydrates, sterols polysaccharides, isolectins, minerals (Fe, Ca, Zn, Co, Na, Cr, I, S, Cu), lignans	Diuretic, anemia, laxative, anti-inflammatory, antiallergic, antimicrobial, hypoglycemic, anti-histamine effect, hemostatic [4, 5, 49]
Gromwell	*Lithospermum canescens* (*Boraginaceae*)	Phenolic acids, flavonoids, vitamins, sterols, phenols, allantoin	Sedative, anti-inflammatory, antipyretic, diuretic, antiseptic, colargol, antipruritic, contraceptive [4, 5, 50]
False hellebore	*Veratrum album* (*Melanthiaceae*)	Alkaloids, fatty acids, sterols, amino acids	Antithrombotic activity, hypotensive, anti-inflammatory, hypoglycemic [4, 5, 51, 52]
Thyme	*Thymus vulgaris* L. (*Lamiaceae*)	Terpene, flavonoids, antiviral, essential oils, tanins	Anti-inflammatory, antitussive, antiseptic, antimicrobial, astringent, antihelmintic, tonic, carminative, disinfectant [4, 5, 53–55]
Old man's beard	*Clematis vitalba* L (*Ranunculaceae*)	Terpenoids, saponins, volatile acids, alkaloids	Diuretic, diuretic, analgesic, diuretic, anti-tumor, anti-inflammatory agent, antipyretic, antirheumatic [4, 5, 56–58]
Creeping cinquefoil	*Potentilla reptans* L. (*Rosaceae*)	Tanins, flavonoids, terpenes, anthocyanins, phenolic acids	Anti-inflammatory, antimicrobial activity, hypoglycemic hepatoprotective, anticancer effect, spasmolytic [4, 5, 59–61]
Burdock	*Arctium lappa* (*Asteraceae*)	Tanins, minerals (K), vitamins (B), volatile oils, phenolic acids	Hypoglycemic, detoxifying, anticancer, anti-inflammatory, antimicrobial, antiseptic, regenerating activity, hair growth, hepatoprotective, diuretic, anticancer, antidiabetic, antiviral activities, hypolipidemic [4, 5, 62, 63]
Jimson weed	*Datura stramonium* L. (*Solanaceae*)	Alkaloids (atropine, scopolamine), saponins, lignins, sterol, tannins, flavonoids, carbohydrates, proteins	Analgesic, antiasthmatic activities, antimicrobial, wound healing, purgative [4, 5, 64]

Herb name	Scientific name of plant	Main chemical composition	Biological activity
Teasel	*Dipsacus pilosus L.* (*Caprifoliaceae*)	Phenolic acids, terpene	Stomatologic, analgesic, blood circulation, anti-inflammatory, powerful remedy for Lyme disease [65]
Centaury	*Erythraea centaurium Pers.* (*Gentianaceae*)	Terpenoids, phenolic acids, flavonoids, xanthones, volatile oils, coumarine, fatty acids, polysaccharides	Tonic, purgative, sedative, antipyretic, antihelmintic, anti-inflammatory, analgesic and diuretic properties, antidiabetic activity antimicrobial activity, gastroprotective, carbohydrate and lipid metabolism [4, 5, 67–69]
peppermint	*Mentha piperita L* (*Lamiaceae*)	Volatile oils, flavonoid glycosides	Astringent, analgesic, antiseptic, antioxidant, antispasmodic, cardioprotective, antiviral, bacteriostatic, anthelmintic, anti-protozoal, immunomodulatory, antiparasitic, carminative, antiemetic, antiallergic, antitumoral [4, 5, 23, 70, 71]
Birthwort	*Aristolochia clematitis* (*Magnoliiflorae*)	Terpenoids, alkaloids, tanins, flavonoids, glycosides, saponine, fatty oils, minerals, sterols	Aphrodisiac, immunomodulatory, cicatrisant, wound healing, dermatological diseases (eczema, acne), analgesic, antitumoral, depurative, anti-inflammatory [4, 5, 24, 73, 74, 76]
Houndstongue	*Cynoglossum officinale L.* (*Boraginaceae*)	Pyrrolizidine alkaloids	Antibacterial, antihemorrhagic, antiseptic, diuretic, anti-hyperlipidaemic, antidiabetic activity, diuretic, anti-inflammatory, and non-central analgesic activities [4, 5, 72, 73]

Table 3.
Biological activity of main groups of natural compounds identified in Dacian medicinal plants.

Their complex information about therapeutic botanicals was appreciated as being very impressive and different ancient historical texts [8, 10–13, 17, 18, 20, 21]. In the first pharmacopoeia, Discorides mentioned over 700 different medical plants and about 6% were presented as Dacian origin [8, 10–13, 17, 18, 20, 21].

Complementary to phytotherapy, various products of mineral origin were used, of which the most well known are: limestone powder (hemostatic effect), volcanic tuff (healing effect), etc.

Thermal springs are used as natural remedies for bone diseases or circulatory system disorders. In this respect, they were highly appreciated the waters of Geoagiu Bath, known by the Dacians as Germisara [11–13, 18].

Fumigations of cannabis were used as anesthetic and analgesic, mainly in labor and childbirth.

Also, Dacians paid special attention to medical preventive measures. Thus, they treated the clothing with extracts of lavender (*Lavandula angustifolia*) [4, 5, 24]

Herb name	Scientific name of plant	Chinese medicine	Indian medicine/other medicine systems
Aconite	*Aconitum napellus*	Fever treatment and skin irritation [31, 32]	
Water-plantain	*Alisma plantago-aquatica*	Antitumor, antimicrobial, anti-inflammatory, immunomodulatory agent [36]	—
Birthwort	*Aristolochia clematitis*	Antispasmodic, antidote (snake venom), analgesic [73, 74, 76, 77]	
Black henbane	*Hyoscyamus niger*	Analgesic, antispasmodic [40].	—
Old man's beard	*Clematis vitalba L*	Anti-inflammatory, analgesic, antipyretic, diuretic	—
Burdock	*Arctium lappa*	Anti-inflammatory, cicatrizating effect, wound healing [62]	—
Jimson weed	*Datura stramonium*	—	Anti-inflammatory, analgesic, cicatrizating effect, wound healing, antipyretic [64]

Table 4.
Some examples of Dacian medicinal plants recognized and used in the traditional medicine of other peoples.

and wormwood (*Artemisia absinthium*) [4, 5, 25]. Scientific screenings of these two plants have highlighted the fact that lavender has antibacterial properties and wormwood is a disinfecting agent [11–13, 18].

Moreover, the inclusion of different healing herbs in the Dacian diet once again reveals their profound knowledge on plant's active principles. Basically, for Dacians, food was more than a way to ensure daily nutrient needs, it was mainly a medicine per se. In this regard, we can remember some of the most commonly used healing herbs in Dacian and later Romanian cuisine: malva (*Althaea officinalis*), stinging nettle (*Urtica dioica* L.), dandelion (*Taraxacum officinalis*), daisy (*Bellis perennis*), allheal (*Prunella vulgaris*), thyme (*Thymus vulgaris* L.), borange (*Boranga officinalis*), hogweed (*Heracleum sphondylium*), and fat grass (*Portulaca oleracea*) [8, 10–21, 23].

In fact, modern studies have identified in these natural products different secondary metabolites with high biological activity [9, 24–83]. The main bioactive compounds and their therapeutic effect are summarized in **Table 1**.

The Dacian's botanical preparations were quite diverse from decocts, infusions, oilments, plant mixtures to fumigations. This proves the Dacians knew how to extract or capitalize on the active principles of the healing plants [8, 10–21].

Table 2 summarized some of these plants used by Dacians and their therapeutic recommendations.

It is quite remarkable that Dacian's therapeutic recommendations were corroborated by thorough scientific studies on those medicinal plants [8–21, 24–84]. This is further evidence of the fact that the Dacians had in-depth knowledge of phytotherapy, for which they were also appreciated by the great scientists of antiquity.

Table 3 summarized the main phytochemicals identified in Dacian healing herbs and their biological activity.

Another aspect to be mentioned is the fact that the Dacian medicinal plants are also found in other important traditional medicinal systems, such as Chinese or Hindu medicine (**Table 4**).

Herb name	Other uses of Dacian herbs
Mallow	Edible plant, cosmetic industry [81]
Stinging nettle	Edible plant, cosmetic industry [4, 5, 51]
Burdock	Edible plant [62]
Centaury	Cosmetic industry [4, 5, 67–69]
Mint	Cosmetic industry, food industry [4, 5, 23, 67, 69, 70]
Thyme	Cosmetic industry, food industry [4, 5, 53–55]

Table 5.
Modern applications of Dacian healing plants.

Currently, some the Dacian healing herbs are appreciated worldwide for their nutritional values and even have found modern applications in several sectors of the industry (**Table 5**).

3. *Aristolochia clematitis*: chemical screening of main phytoconstituients

Aristolochia clematitis is a highly regarded herb in traditional medicine and at the same time controversial due to the latest research that revealed the potential carcinogenic effect of aristolochic acid [73, 74, 76, 77, 85].

In an effort to identify the secondary metabolites from *Aristolochia clematitis*, the plant extract was analyzed in two different solvents (methanol and water). The plant material (*Aristolochia clematitis* leaves, young stems, and flowers) was obtained from a collection taken in 2017 in Timis, Romania. Plant sample was identified at Victor Babes University of Medicine and Pharmacy Timisoara. The botanical material was dried and then finely ground in a ball mill. Separation of the main constituents from different parts of the botanical material was done using two different polar solvents: water and methanol. A plant sample (2 g) was placed in a 100-mL volumetric flask containing 45 mL of solvent. The resulting mixture was sonicated for 50 min at 40°C, with a frequency of 50 kHz. Then, the solution was filtered through a 0.25-μm pore size filter. Thus, four birthwort fractions were prepared: B_1 (water extract from leaves and stems), B_2 (methanol extract from flowers), B_3 (water extract from leaves), and B_4 (methanol extract from stems). Identification of the main compounds from the birthwort fractions, B_1, B_2, B_3, and B_4, was performed using TOF-MS method.

4. TOF-MS analysis

The mass spectra of birthwort fractions: B_1–B_4 (acquired in positive ion mode, in a mass range of 100–3000 m/z) are presented in **Figure 1a–d**.

The results gained through mass spectrometry confirmed the presence of aristolochic acid in all four samples analyzed (m/z detected: 294, 293, 308, 355) among other secondary metabolites [86].

Further, thorough investigations are required to highlight:

- the maximum concentration of phytoconstituients from that called perfect moment to harvest the plant and the composition of active principles from a randomly harvest plant;
- validation of curative properties/cytotoxicity effects of plant extract depending on plant dosage (plant concentration, time, etc.).

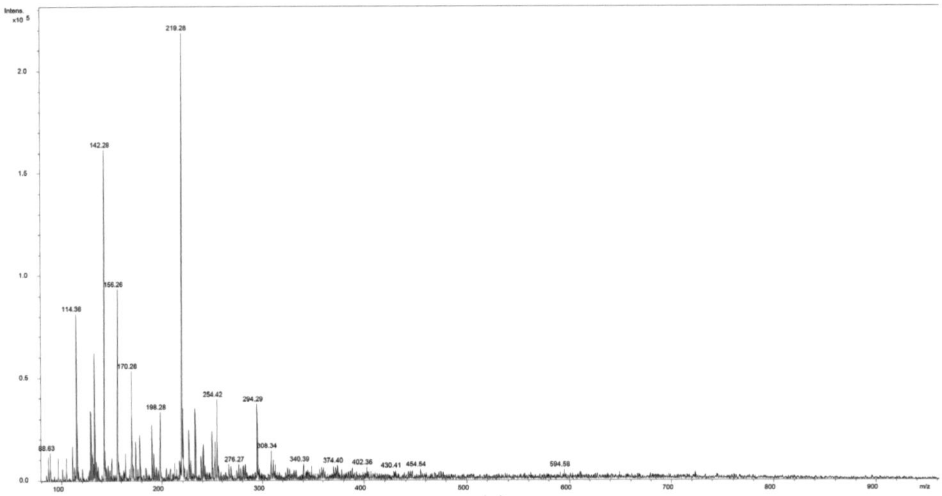
Intens.
x10 5
2.0
1.5
1.0
0.5
0.0
219.28
142.28
156.26
114.36
170.28
198.28
254.42
294.29
88.63
308.34
276.27
340.39
374.40
402.36
430.41
454.54
594.58
100
200
300
400
500
600
700
800
900
m/z

(a)

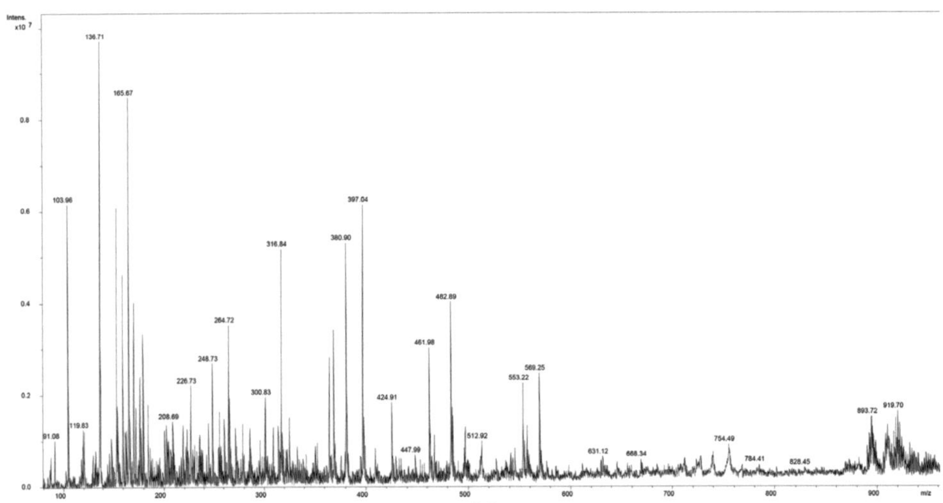
Intens.
x10 7
0.8
0.6
0.4
0.2
0.0
136.71
165.67
103.96
397.04
316.84
380.90
482.89
264.72
461.98
248.73
226.73
569.25
553.22
300.83
424.91
208.69
119.83
91.08
893.72
919.70
754.49
512.92
447.99
631.12
668.34
784.41
828.45
100
200
300
400
500
600
700
800
900
m/z

(b)

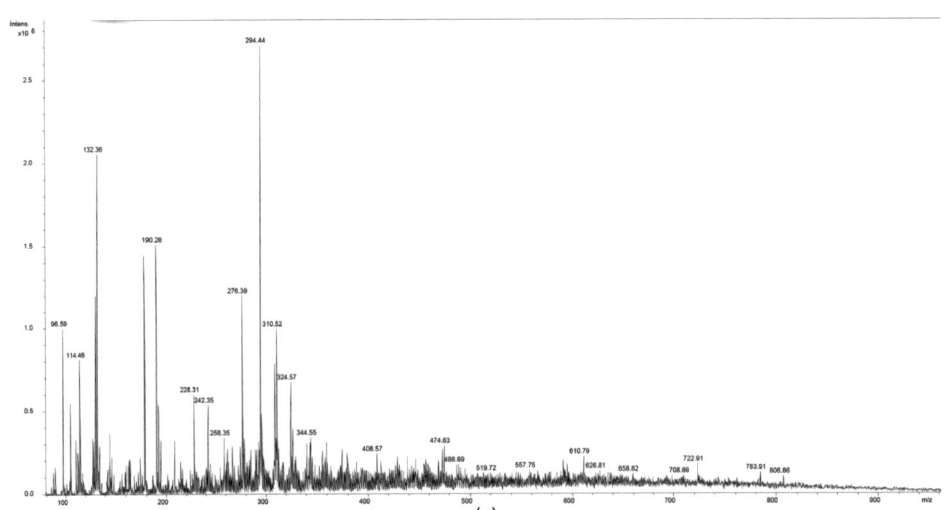
Intens.
x10 6
2.5
2.0
1.5
1.0
0.5
0.0
294.44
132.36
190.28
276.39
96.59
310.52
114.46
324.57
228.31
242.35
258.35
344.55
408.57
474.63
488.69
519.72
557.75
610.79
626.81
658.82
708.86
722.91
783.91
806.86
100
200
300
400
500
600
700
800
900
m/z

(c)

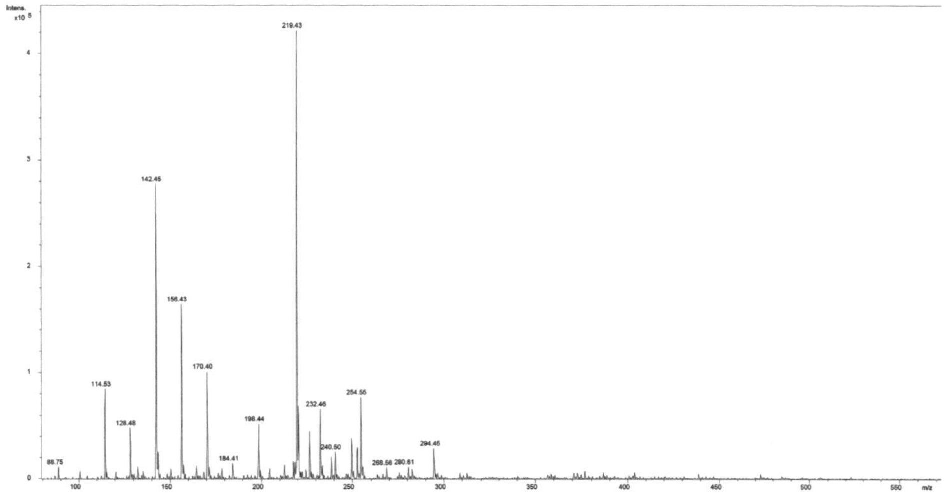
(d)

Figure 1.
Figure 1 a-d. Positive ion mode TOF-MS of of birthwort fraction B1-B4. (1a) Positive ion mode TOF-MS of of birthwort fraction B1. (1 b) Positive ion mode TOF-MS of of birthwort fraction B2. (1c)Positive ion mode TOF-MS of of birthwort fraction B3. (1d) Positive ion mode TOF-MS of of birthwort fraction B4.

5. Conclusions

Natural compounds are essential for the existence of humanity; this assertion has been demonstrated by the most modern researches which once again highlights the particular curative properties of phytochemicals isolated from medicinal plants known and appreciated since the earliest times.

Author details

Adina-Elena Segneanu[1,2*], Claudiu Cepan[3], Ioan Grozescu[2,3], Florentina Cziple[4], Sorin Olariu[5], Sonia Ratiu[5*], Viorica Lazar[6], Sorin Marius Murariu[5*], Silvia Maria Velciov[5] and Teodora Daniela Marti[6]

1 Department of Scientific Research and Academic Creation, West University of Timisoara, Romania

2 Scient Analytics, SCIENT-Research Center for Instrumental Analysis, Cromatec-Plus, Romania

3 University Politehnica Timisoara, Romania

4 Eftimie Murgu University, Romania

5 Victor Babes University of Medicine and Pharmacy, Romania

6 Vasile Goldis University of Medicine and Pharmacy, Romania

*Address all correspondence to: s_adinaelena@yahoo.com; sonienne@gmail.com and murariu.marius@umft.ro

References

[1] Segneanu AE, Cepan C, Grozescu I, Cziple F, Olariu S, Ratiu S, Lazar V, Murariu SM, Velciov SM, Marti TD. Therapetic Use of Some Romanian Medicinal Plants. London: IntechOpen; 2018. DOI: 10.5772/intechopen.82477

[2] Pârvu C. Universul Plantelor: Mică Enciclopedie. Bucuresti: Editura Enciclopedică; 1991

[3] Stanescu U, Hancianu M, Cioanca O, Aprotosoaie A, Miron A. Medicinal Plants from A to Z. Iasi: Polirom; 2014. ISBN: 978-973-46-4943-3

[4] Bujor O. The Guide of Medicinal and Aromatic Plants from A to Z. Bucuresti: Fiat Lux; 2003. ISBN: 973-9250-68-8

[5] Allen DE, Hartfield G. Medicinal Plants in Folk Tradition—An Ethnobotany of Britain & Ireland. Portland, Oregon, USA: Timber Press; 2004. ISBN: 0-88192-638-8

[6] Chikezie PC, Ojiako OA. Herbal Medicine: Yesterday, Today and Tomorrow. Alternative and Integrative Medicine. 2015;**4**:3

[7] Bhat JA, Kumar M, Bussmann RW. Ecological status and traditional knowledge of medicinal plants in Kedarnath Wildlife Sanctuary of Garhwal Himalaya, India. Journal of Ethnobiology and Ethnomedicine. 2013;**9**(1):1-18

[8] Žuškin E, Lipozenčić J, Pucarin-Cvetković J, Mustajbegović J, Schachter N, Mučić-Pučić B, et al. Ancient medicine—A review. Acta Dermatovenerologica Croatica. 2008;**16**(3):149-157

[9] Subbarayappa BV. The roots of ancient medicine: An historical outline. Journal of Biosciences. 2001;**26**(2 June):135-144

[10] Iliescu V, Popescu V, Stefan G. Izvoare Privind Istoria României (Fontes ad Historiam *Dacoromaniae pertinentes*). Vol. I. București: De la Hesiod la Itinerarul lui Antoninus; 1964

[11] Crisan IH. Medicine in Dacia. Dacica; 2007. ISBN: 978-97388076-24

[12] Herodot, The Histories. Vol. 1-2. Stiintifica; 1961

[13] Popovici R. At the Table with the Ancestors. Dacia; 2011. pp. 1-4

[14] Claudian I. Food of the Romanian People in Anthropogeography and History, Foundation for Literature and Art *King Carol II*. București. 1939

[15] Carciumaru M. Plants used by traco-geto-dacians (Attempt of synthesis) (V). Thraco-Dacica. 1987;**VIII**(1-2):171-176

[16] Dioscorides, De Materia Medica, Osbaldeston (Tess Anne). Johannesburg, South Africa: Ibidis Press; 2000. ISBN: 0-620-23435-0

[17] Desunsianu N. Dacia Preistorica. Bucuresi: Arhetip; 2002. ISBN: 9739296-33-5

[18] Paraschiv-Claudius M. The Human Natural Food Treaty. Bucuresti: Christalin; 2003. ISBN: 973-86515-0-6

[19] Bologa VL. Sinonimele "Dacice" ale Plantelor Descrise de Dioscorides pot Servi la Reconstituirea Limbii Dacice? în "Dacoromania". Cluj; 1927-1928. pp. 570-575

[20] Drăgulescu C, Drăgulescu R. Contribuţii la cunoaşterea limbii geto-dacilor. Denumirile dacice de plante. Sibiu: Editura Universităţii "Lucian Blaga"; 2000

[21] Váczy C. Nomenclatura dacică a plantelor la Dioscorides şi Pseudo –Apuleius. Acta Musei Napocensi. 1971;**VIII**:109-133

[22] Fierascu RC, Fierascu I, Ortan A, Avramescu SM, Dinu-Pirvu CE, Ionescu D. In: El-Shemy HA, editor. Romanian Aromatic and Medicinal Plants: From Tradition to Science, Aromatic and Medicinal Plants. Rijeka, Croatia: IntechOpen; 2017. DOI: 10.5772/66513

[23] Pogăciaș A. The Dacian Society—Fierce Warriors And Their Women Sources And Representations. Hiperboreea Journal. 2017;**4**(1):5-22

[24] Scarborough J. Ancient medicinal use of *Aristolochia*: Birthwort's tradition and toxicity. Pharmacy in History. 2011;**53**(1)

[25] Abroomand AP, Torabbeigi M, Sharifan A, Tehrani MS. Chemical composition and antibacterial activity of the essential oil of *Lavandula angustifolia* isolated by solvent free microwave assisted extraction and hydrodistillation. Journal of Food Biosciences and Technology, Islamic Azad University, Science and Research Branch. 2011;**1**:19-24

[26] Shirwaikar A, Khan S, Kamariya YH, Patel BD, Gajera FP. Medicinal plants for the management of post menopausal osteoporosis: A review. The Open Bone Journal. 2010;**2**:1-13

[27] Ielciu I, Frédérich M, Tits M, Angenot L, Păltinean R, Cieckiewicz E, et al. *Bryonia Alba L.* and *Ecballium elaterium* (L.) A. Rich.—Two related species of the *Cucurbitaceae* Family with important pharmaceutical potential. Farmácia. 2016;**64**:3

[28] Manvi M, Prasad Garg G. Evaluation of pharma-cognostical parameters and hepatoprotective activity in *Bryonia alba Linn*. Journal of Chemical and Pharmaceutical Research. 2011;**3**(6):99-109

[29] Attard E, Cuschieri A, Brincat MP. Morphological effects induced by *Cucurbitacin E.* on ovarian cancer cells in vitro. Journal of Natural Remedies. 2005;**5**(1):70-74

[30] Povšnar M, Koželj G, Kreft S, Lumpert M. Rare tradition of the folk medicinal use *of Aconitum spp*. is kept alive in Solčavsko, Slovenia. Journal of Ethnobiology and Ethnomedicine. 2017;**13**:45

[31] Singh MK, Vinod M, Iyer SK, Khare G, Sharwan G, Larokar YK. *Aconite*: A pharmacological update. International Journal of Research in Pharmaceutical Sciences. 2012;**3**(2):242-246

[32] Kiss T, Csupor D, Orvos P ea. Identification of diterpene alkaloids from *Aconitum napellus* subsp. firmum and GIRK channel activities of some *Aconitum* alkaloids. Fitotherapia. 2013;**90**:85-93

[33] Dipak P. A review on biological activities of common mallow (*Malva sylvestris*). Innovare Journal of Life Science. 2016;**4**(5)

[34] Sleiman NH, Daher CF. *Malva sylvestris* water extract: A potential anti-inflammatory and anti-ulcerogenic remedy. Planta Medica. 2009;**75**(9):PH10

[35] Jakovljević D, Vasić S, Stanković M, Topuzović M, Čomić L. The content of secondary metabolites and in vitro biological activity of *Anchusa officinalis L.* (Boraginaceae). Indian Journal of Traditional Knowledge. 2016;**15**(4):587-593

[36] Huang YS, Yu Q, Chen Y, Cheng M, Xie L. Phenolic constituents from *Alisma plantago-aquatica Linnaeus* and their anti-chronic prostatitis activity. Chemistry Central Journal. 2017;**11**:120

[37] Bahmani M, Rafieian-Kopaei M, Naghdi N, Mozaffari Nejad AS, Afsordeh O. *Physalis alkekengi*: A review of its therapeutic effects. Journal of Chemical and Pharmaceutical Sciences. 2016;**9**(3)

[38] Namjoyan F, Jahangiri A, Azemi ME, Arkian E, Mousavi H. Inhibitory

effects of *Physalis alkekengi* L., *Alcea rosea* L., *Bunium persicum* B. Fedtsch. and *Marrubium vulgare* L. on Mushroom Tyrosinase. Jundishapur Journal of Natural Pharmaceutical Products. 2015;**10**(1):e23356

[39] Keshtkaran R, Vessal M. Effect of the hydroalcoholic extract of winter cherry fruits (*Physalis alkekengi*) on serum lipid profile and paraoxonase activity of healthy male rats. IJMS. 2004;**29**(4)

[40] Alizadeh A, Moshiri M, Alizadeh J, Balali-Mood M. Black henbane and its toxicity—A descriptive review. AJP. 2014;**4**(5):297-311

[41] Ali N, Shah SWA, Shah I, Ahmed G, Ghias M, Khan I, et al. Anthelmintic and relaxant activities of *Verbascum thapsus* Mullein. BMC Complementary and Alternative Medicine. 2012;**12**:29

[42] Jamshidi-Kia F, Lorigooini Z, Asgari S, Saeidi K. Iranian species of *Verbascum*: A review of botany, phytochemistry, and pharmacological effects. Toxin Reviews. 2018. pp. 1-8

[43] Tatli II, Akdemir ZS. Traditional uses and biological activities of *Verbascum species*. Fabad Journal of Pharmaceutical Sciences. 2006;**31**:85-96

[44] Turkoglu S, Turkoglu I, Kahyaoglu M, Celık S. Determination of antimicrobial and antioxidant activities of Turkish endemic *Ajuga chamaepitys* (L.) *Schreber* subsp. *euphratica* P.H. Davis (*Lamiaceae*). Journal of Medicinal Plant Research. 2010;**4**(13):1260-1268

[45] Topcua G, Kokdilb G, Turkmena Z, Voelterc W, Adoud E, Kingston DGI. A new Clerodane Diterpene and other constituents from *Ajuga chamaepitys* ssp. *Laevigata*. Zeitschrift für Naturforschung. 2004;**59b**:584-588

[46] Venditti A, Frezza C, Maggi F, Lupidi G, Bramucci M, Quassinti L, et al. Phytochemistry, micromorphology and bioactivities of *Ajuga chamaepitys* (L.) *Schreb*. (*Lamiaceae*, *Ajugoideae*): Two new harpagide derivatives and an unusual iridoid glycosides pattern. Fitoterapia. 2016;**113**. DOI: 10.1016/j.fitote.2016.06.016

[47] Saeidnia S, Gohari AR, Mokhber-Dezfuli N, Kiuchi F. A review on phytochemistry and medicinal properties of the genus *Achillea*. Daru. 2011;**19**(3):173-186

[48] Lakshmi T, Geetha RV, Anitha R, Aravind KS. Yarrow (*Achillea millefolium Linn.*). A herbal medicinal plant with broad therapeutic use—A review. International Journal of Pharmaceutical Sciences Review and Research. 2011;**9**(2):136-141. Article-022

[49] Kregiel D, Pawlikowska E, Antolak H. *Urtica spp*.: Ordinary plants with extraordinary properties. Molecules. 2018;**23**:1664

[50] Dreslera S, Szymczak G, Wojcik M. Comparison of some secondary metabolite content in the seventeen species of the *Boraginaceae* family. Pharmaceutical Biology. 2017;**55**(1):691-695

[51] Mota AH. A review of medicinal plants used in therapy of cardiovascular diseases. International Journal of Pharmacognosy and Phytochemical Research. 2016;**8**(4):572-591

[52] Chandler CM, McDougal OM. Medicinal history of North American *Veratrum*. Phytochemistry Reviews. 2014;**13**(3):671-694. DOI: 10.1007/s11101-013-9328-y

[53] Prasanth RV, Kandisa RV, Varsha PV, Satyam S. Review on *Thymus vulgaris* traditional uses and pharmacological properties. Medicinal and Aromatic Plants. 2014;**3**:3

[54] Javed H, Erum S, Tabassum S, Ameen F. An overview on medicinal importance of *Thymus vulgaris*. Journal of Asian Scientific Research. 2013;**3**(10):974-982

[55] Hosseinzadeh S, Kukhdan AJ, Hosseini A, Armand R. The application of *Thymus vulgaris* in traditional and modern medicine: A review. Global Journal of Pharmacology. 2015;**9**(3):260-266

[56] Sun F, Qing H, Peigen X, Ishtiaq M, Yiyu C. Simultaneous quantification of five Triterpenoid Saponins in *Clematis L*. spp. by high-performance liquid chromatography with evaporative light scattering detection. Phytochemical Analysis. 2008;**19**:40-45

[57] Al-Taweel AM. Phytochemical and biological studies of some *Clematis species* growing in Saudi Arabia [PhD thesis]. King Saud University; 2007

[58] Yesilada E, Kupeli E. *Clematis vitalba L*. aerial part exhibits potent anti-inflammatory, antinociceptive and antipyretic effects. Journal of Ethnopharmacology. 2007;**110**:504-515

[59] Radovanovic AM, Cupara SM, Popovic SLJ, Tomovic MT, Slavkovska VN, Jankovic SM. Cytotoxic effect of *Potentilla reptans L*. rhizome and aerial part extracts. Acta Poloniae Pharmaceutica. Drug Research. 2013;**70**(5):851-854

[60] Borisova LV, Traicheva PN, Georgiev II. Optimization of biologically active substances extraction process from *Potentilla reptans L*. aerial parts. Journal of Applied Pharmaceutical Science. 2017;7(02):174-179

[61] Tomovic M, Popovic-Milenkovic M, Jankovic S. Antimicrobial activity of aqueous extracts of *Potentilla reptans* L. rhizome and aerial part. Serbian Journal of Experimental and Clinical Research. 2017:1

[62] Chan YS, Cheng LN, Wu JH, Chan E, Kwan YW, Lee SMY, et al. A review of the pharmacological effects of *Arctium Lappa* (Burdock). Inflammopharmacology. 2010;**19**(5):245-254

[63] El-Darier SM, Salama SG. *Arctium lappa* L. (Asteraceae); a new invasive highly specific medicinal plant growing in Egypt. Pyrex Journal of Plant and Agricultural Research. 2016;**2**(2):44-53

[64] Sayyed A, Shah M. Phytochemistry, pharmacological and traditional uses of *Datura stramonium L*. review. Journal of Pharmacognosy and Phytochemistry. 2014;**2**(5):123-125

[65] Ojovan A. Elements of Dacian dental medication. Journal Medicina Stomatologica. 2010;**4**(17):18-21. ISBN: 978-9975-52-006-5

[66] Šiler B, Mišić D. Biologically active compounds from the genus *Centaurium s.l.* (Gentianaceae): Current knowledge and future prospects in medicine. Studies in Natural Products Chemistry. 2016;**49**:363-397

[67] Jovanov D. Application of medicinal aromatic and spice plants *Zingiber officinale*, *Mentha piperita*, *Rubus fructicosus*, *Malva silvestris*, *Fragaria vesca*, *Sambucus nigra*, *Cornus mascula*, *Taraxacum officinale*, *Erythraea centaurium* and their phytotherapeutic action to protect against colon cancer. Agricultural Research & Technology: Open Access Journal. 2017;**9**(2):555758

[68] Stoiko L, Dakhym I, Pokotylo O, Marchyshyn S. Polysaccharides in *Centaurium erythraea Rafn*. International Journal of Research in Ayurveda and Pharmacy. 2017;**8**(Suppl 2)

[69] Singh R, Shushni MAM, Belkheir A. Antibacterial and antioxidant activities of *Mentha piperita* L. Arabian Journal of Chemistry. 2015;**8**(3):322-328

[70] Rita P, Animesh DK. An updated overview on peppermint (*Mentha piperita L.*). International Research Journal of Pharmacy. 2011;**2**(8):1-10

[71] Pfister JA, Molyneux RJ, Baker DC. Pyrrolizidine alkaloid content of houndstongue (*Cynoglossum officinale* L.). Journal of Range Management. 1992;**45**(3):254-256

[72] Joshi K. *Cynoglossum* L.—A review on phytochemistry and chemotherapeutic potential. Journal of Pharmacognosy and Phytochemistry. 2016;**5**(4):32-33

[73] Wu TS, Damu AG, Su CR, Kuo PC. Terpenoids of *Aristolochia* and their biological activities. Natural Product Reports. 2004;**2**(1):594-624

[74] Benmehdi H, Behilil A, Memmou F, Amrouche A. Free radical scavenging activity, kinetic behaviour and phytochemical constituents of *Aristolochia clematitis L.* roots. Arabian Journal of Chemistry. 2013

[75] Bhupendra K, Pooja T, Anil K, Taslimahemad K, Indraneel S. The *Artemisia genus*: A review on traditional uses, phytochemical constituents, pharmacological properties and germplasm conservation. Journal of Glycomics and Lipidomics. 2017;7:1

[76] Samsonova OE, Belous VN, Dudar YA. Medicinal plants pharmacological characterization of *Aristolochia clematitis* L. growing in the Stavropol region. Pharmaceutical Chemistry Journal. 2006;**40**(4)

[77] Asadi-Samani M, Bahmani M, Rafieian-Kopaei M. The chemical composition, botanical characteristic and biological activities of *Borago officinalis*: A review. Asian Pacific Journal of Tropical Medicine. 2014;**7**(Suppl 1):S22-S28

[78] Bahadori MB, Dinparast L, Zengin G. The genus *Heracleum*: A comprehensive review on its phytochemistry, pharmacology, and ethnobotanical values as a useful herb. Comprehensive Reviews in Food Science and Food Safety. 2016;**15**:1018-1039

[79] Iranshahy M, Javadi B, Iranshahi M, Jahanbakhsh SP, Mahyari S, Hassani FV, et al. A review of traditional uses, phytochemistry and pharmacology of *Portulaca oleracea* L. Journal of Ethnopharmacology. 2017;**205**:158-172

[80] Al-Snafi AE. The pharmaceutical importance of *Althaea officinalis* and *Althaea rosea*: A review. International Journal of PharmTech Research CODEN (USA). 2013;**5**(3):1378-1385

[81] Choi UK, Lee OH, Yim JH, Cho CW, Rhee YK, Lim SI, et al. Hypolipidemic and antioxidant effects of Dandelion (*Taraxacum officinale*) root and leaf on cholesterol-fed rabbits. International Journal of Molecular Sciences. 2010;**11**:67-78

[82] Ranfa A, Bodesmo M. An ethnobotanical investigation of traditional knowledge and uses of edible wild plants in the Umbria Region, Central Italy. Journal of Applied Botany and Food Quality. 2017;**90**:246-258

[83] Agrawal T, Vidhypeeth B. *Adonis vernalis* a useful drug. Journal of Natural & Ayurvedic Medicine. 2018;**2**(6)

[84] Butnariu M. Biodiversity of the phytoconstituents in the some plant species potentially toxic. Journal of Biodiversity and Endangered Species. 2017;**5**:1

[85] Turesky RJ, Hwa Yun B, Brennan P, Mates D, Jinga V, Harnden P, et al. Aristolochic acid exposure in Romania and implications for renal cell carcinoma. British Journal of Cancer. 2016;**114**(1):76-80

[86] Eckhardt G, Urzûa A, Cassels BK. Mass spectrometry of Aristolochic acids. Journal of Natural Products. 1983;**46**(1):92-97

Chapter 8

Medicinal Properties of Bamboos

Katarzyna B. Wróblewska, Danielle C.S. de Oliveira, Maria Tereza Grombone-Guaratini and Paulo Roberto H. Moreno

Abstract

Bamboos are described as one of the most important renewable, easily obtained, and valuable of all forest resources. These plants belong to the grasses' family (*Poaceae*), which covers about a quarter of the world's plant population, within the subfamily Bambusoideae. The estimated diversity of bamboos in the world is approximately 1400 species, distributed in 116 genera. Bamboo species have been used in Southeast Asia, as a base material to produce paper, furniture, boats, bicycles, textiles, musical instruments, and food, and their leaves have also been used as a wrapping material to prevent food deterioration since ancient times. These species accumulate biologically active components such as polyphenols and other secondary plant metabolites that might explain the use of bamboo leaves in Asian traditional medicine for the treatment of hypertension, arteriosclerosis, cardiovascular disease, and certain forms of cancer. Besides the usual secondary metabolites, bamboo extracts may contain biologically active peptides and polysaccharides that still need to be further studied for their activity and their synergistic with other metabolites. Most of the studies found in the literature are from Asian bamboo species, and the potential of the Southern American species is yet to be explored.

Keywords: bamboo, antioxidant, antimicrobial, polyphenols, triterpenes, traditional medicine

1. Introduction

Bamboos are described as one of the most important renewable, easily obtained, and valuable of all forest resources. Bamboo species have been known and used by human kind since the beginning of civilization; its use as building materials can be traced back to the pre-ceramic period 9500 years ago, while relics from bamboo mats and baskets were dated at 3300-2800 BC [1]. In Asian countries, their leaves are used as a food wrapping material to prevent food deterioration since ancient times, besides using the culms as a construction material. In this region, bamboo leaves are described in the traditional medicine for treating hypertension, arteriosclerosis, cardiovascular disease, and certain forms of cancer. These therapeutic properties are most likely mediated by their antioxidant capacity.

These plants form a large subfamily of the grasses (*Poaceae*: Bambusoideae), comprising about 1662 species distributed in 121 genera. Bamboos present a large range of functional forms found over numerous biogeographic regions, including dwarf herbaceous species in temperate climates and giant tropical woody species that can reach up to 20 m height [2]. These species can adapt and propagate in inhospitable environments, such as humid and cold mountain tops as well as the ones dry and warm [3], naturally occurring in all continents except Europe [4]. Bamboos play an important role in South American forest diversity. Brazil is the country with the greatest number of native bamboo species in the New World [5]. This means that 89% of the genera and 65% of known bamboo species (36 genera and 254 species) are distributed among the Atlantic Forest, the Cerrado, and the Amazon [6].

Bamboos have a large ecological amplitude in response to canopy disturbances and can become super dominant species after opening in natural or anthropic origin. In addition, they have a very rapid growth from the stem base to the top of the plant [7]. Currently, bamboo species are considered as one of the most available forest resources. In tropical and subtropical areas, bamboos represent approximately 20–25% of the total biomass, which contributes to their status as one of the most important renewable resources [8]. Considered a rapid atmospheric carbon sink, bamboo has also physical and mechanical properties that make it suitable to be used in the development of products normally produced with native wood or from reforestation, such as construction components, furniture industry, cables for agricultural tools, panels, and plates, among others.

Bamboo species share some common characteristics of their phenolic composition with other grasses. They contain several glycosylated flavones whose aglycones are represented by apigenin, luteolin, and tricin [9–11]. This is also the case in, for example, durum wheat (*Triticum durum*) [12] and barley (*Hordeum vulgare*) [13]. Just as in other grass species, such as corn, wheat, and rice [14], most glycosides are conjugated via a *C*-linkage to the flavone aglycone. In China, their phenolic compounds are used to make a preparation, called antioxidant of bamboo leaves (AOB), to be applied as food antioxidant whose use is sanctioned by the local Health Ministry. The AOB is composed mainly by flavonoids, lactones, and phenolic acids. The main flavonoids found in AOB are the flavone *C*-glycosides such as orientin, homoorientin, vitexin, and isovitexin [15].

2. Biological activities of bamboo species

2.1 Antioxidant potential of bamboos

The production of reactive oxygen species (ROS) is a result of normal cell metabolism; however, once the oxidative processes start to be predominant over the antioxidant, the imbalance called "oxidative stress" can be harmful to human body [16]. Oxygen's reactivity, which is under normal conditions, permits the high-energy electron transfer allowing the formation of big quantities of adenosine-5-triphosphate (ATP) by the oxidative phosphorylation and jeopardizes the cells of living organisms by attacking molecules such as proteins, lipids, or DNA [17]. Free radicals created in this process cause various genetic changes causing cancer, cardiovascular and neurological diseases, nephropathy, rheumatoid arthritis, and other disorders [18]. Plants provide an abundant source of the substances with biological activity. In case of antioxidant protection, flavonoids stand for one of the most efficient molecules combating the oxidative stress.

There are two terms describing the antioxidant efficacy: "antioxidant activity" and "antioxidant capacity," and they have different meanings. The prior expresses the kinetics of a reaction between an antioxidant and the prooxidant or radical scavenging activity, and the latter one measures the thermodynamic conversion efficiency of the reaction. The analytical methods to evaluate antioxidant activity may be divided into electron transfer (ET)-based and hydrogen atom transfer

(HAT)-based methods. ET-based methods utilize the process of the reduction in the oxidative component by the antioxidant, which leads to the change in color that can be observed [19]. Within this group, we can specify: DPPH (2,2-di(4-*tert*-octylphenyl)-1-picrylhydrazyl) method, ABTS (2,2′-azinobis-(3-ethylbenzothiazoline-6-sulfonic acid), FRAP (ferric reducing antioxidant power), and CUPRAC (cupric reducing antioxidant capacity). HAT-based assays include for instance oxygen radical absorbance capacity (ORAC) reaction, detectable by the fluorescence loss of fluorescein. More "functional" analyses count the number of lipid oxidation products like thiobarbituric acid-reactive substances (TBARS) or evaluate a desired health effect of the product [19, 20].

The majority researchers working with bamboo-derived products use DPPH, ABTS, and FRAP methods or the combination of those to evaluate the antioxidant effect of their samples, when ORAC is less common. Values are expressed in the percentage of the radical inhibition, IC_{50}, which is an inhibitory concentration (concentration needed to deactivate 50% of the radical formation) or Trolox equivalents. **Table 1** demonstrates the results grouped by the method and unit used by the authors, and **Table 2** shows IC_{50} against DPPH of the compounds isolated from the bamboo species.

The most popular method (also as per the number of results included in **Table 1**) is the certainty DPPH radical scavenging test. IC_{50} is a unit that is easy to compare because it gives an idea of the concentration, which is necessary to decrease the radical formation by 50%. The values obtained for different species of bamboo varied between 51 μg/mL for *Sasa borealis* (leaf butanolic fraction) [9] and 5300 μg/mL for *Phyllostachys nigra* (shoot water fraction) [24]. The highest antiradicalar activity was obtained in case of butanol, ethyl acetate, and ethanol fractions. Although leaf extracts seemed to be the part of the plant that provides reasonably good results, essential oils were efficient in much smaller concentrations. The essential oil from *Phyllostachys heterocycla* cv. pubescens had IC_{50} of only 2.85 μg/mL (value recalculated from μL/mL for comparison purposes if the density of an essential oil is approximately 0.9 g/mL) as reported by Jin et al. [21]. The worst in the group, but still with high activity, was an essential oil from *Phyllostachys vivax* f. *aureocaulis* N.X.Ma. (7.53 μg/mL [25]). The essential oils had their range of action like isolated compounds. For instance, isoorientin, isolated from the leaves of *Sasa borealis*, had IC_{50} determined as 9.5 μM [9], which gives 4.26 μg/mL, very close to the essential oil mentioned here.

Two from the chosen authors [10, 26] described the results for two Asian bamboo species: *Phyllostachys nigra* v. *henonis* and *Phyllostachys edulis* in the percentage of DPPH inhibition. The 20 μg/mL ethanol extract from the first species managed to suppress 40.9% of the radical formation, whereas the second one, depending on the fraction, was able to decrease it from 30.4 to 79.1% (chloroform and butanol fractions, respectively) in the concentration of 100 μg/mL. Both authors investigated in parallel the influence of the bamboo samples on lipid peroxidation. It was confirmed that the *P. nigra* scavenging effect reduced the rate of liposome peroxidation and human LDL (low-density lipoprotein) oxidation suppressing DNA modifications [10]. 3-*O*-caffeoyl-1-methylquinic acid (shown in **Table 2**), isolated from *P. edulis*, exhibited 36% of the inhibition of superoxide generation in human promyelocytic leukemia HL-60 cells [26].

The results expressed in IC_{50} for the DPPH and other methods such as ABTS, FRAP, and ORAC varied due to different mechanisms of action between prooxidant and antioxidant molecules. An ethyl acetate fraction from a Brazilian bamboo, *Merostachys pluriflora*, defined as the most active fraction from this species against DPPH (IC_{50} = 117.68 μg/mL), the second most active against ABTS cation radical (IC_{50} = 19.66 μg/mL) was also quite potent ferric reducing (IC_{50} = 51.88 μg/mL) and

Bamboo species	Sample	DPPH	ABTS	FRAP	ORAC	Ref.
Phyllostachys heterocycla cv. pubescens	Essential oil	2.85*				[21]
P. heterocycla cv. gracilis	Essential oil	4.44*				
P. heterocycla cv. heterocycla	Essential oil	3.82*				
P. kwangsiensis	Essential oil	4.93*				
Merostachys pluriflora Munro ex. C. G. Camus	Leaf ethanol	119.51	25.65	92.08	5.79	[22]
	Leaf hydromethanolic	137.37	16.30	85.73	6.18	
	Leaf ethyl acetate	117.68	19.66	51.88	2.73	
	Leaf dichloromethane	190.73	37.21	89.69	6.05	
	Culm ethanol	181.92	39.51	62.02	4.20	
	Culm hydromethanolic	413.80	47.22	108.50	9.33	
	Culm ethyl acetate	244.85	33.25	51.22	3.47	
	Culm dichloromethane	—	60.69	27.92	1.22	
	Culm hexane	296.94	94.77	145.80	9.10	
P. pubescens (Pradelle) Mazel ex J. Houz	Leaf ethanol		—			[23]
	Branch ethanol		350.60			
	Inner culm at 1 m height ethanol		373.80			
	Inner culm at 5 m height ethanol		88.50			
	Rhizome ethanol		171.50			
	Leaf water		306.70			
	Branch water		179.50			
	Inner culm at 1 m height water		231.90			
	Inner culm at 5 m height water		198.30			
	Rhizome water		266.70			
	Shoot methanol	3600.00				[24]
	Shoot chloroform	4000.00				
	Shoot ethyl acetate	800.00				
	Shoot butanolic	700.00				
	Shoot water	4700.00				
Pseudosasa amabilis McClure	Essential oil	5.29*				[25]
Pleioblastus gramineus (Bean) Nakai	Essential oil	6.50*				
P. vivax f. *aureocaulis* N.X.Ma.	Essential oil	7.53*				
Indocalamus latifolius (Keng) McClure	Essential oil	4.99*				

Bamboo species	Sample	DPPH	ABTS	FRAP	ORAC	Ref.
P. nigra (Lodd. ex Lindl.) Munro	Shoot methanol	3400.00				[24]
	Shoot Chloroform	2300.00				
	Shoot ethyl acetate	400.00				
	Shoot butanolic	800.00				
	Shoot water	5300.00				
Sasa borealis (Hack.) Makino and Shibata	Leaf butanolic	51.00				[9]

*ABTS—scavenging ABTS(2,2′-azinobis-(3-ethylbenzothiazoline-6-sulfonic acid) cation radical effect; DPPH—scavenging DPPH (2,2-di(4-tert-octylphenyl)-1-picrylhydrazyl)radical effect; FRAP—ferric reducing antioxidant power; all the values in the table are the—IC_{50} [μg/mL]—inhibitory concentration, concentration needed to diminish the production the radical/oxidized product by 50%; ORAC—oxygen radical absorbance capacity. *Values recalculated from μL/mL to μg/mL, assuming that the density of an essential oil is approximately 0.9 g/mL.*

Table 1.
Antioxidant activity of different bamboo species.

Bamboo species	Part of the plant	Isolated compound	DPPH (IC_{50})	Reference
Sasa borealis (Hack.) Makino and Shibata	Leaves	Isoorientin	9.5	[9]
		Isoorientin 2-O-α-L-rhamnoside	34.5	
		Apigenin 6-C-β-D-xylopyranosyl-8-C-β-D-glucopyranoside	161.5	
Phyllostachys edulis (Carrière) J. Houz.	Leaves	3-O-(3′-methylcaffeoyl) quinic acid	16.00	[26]
		5-O-caffeoyl-4-methylquinic acid	8.8	
		3-O-caffeoyl-1-methylquinic acid	6.9	

DPPH—scavenging DPPH (2,2-di(4-tert-octylphenyl)-1-picrylhydrazyl) radical effect; IC_{50}—inhibitory concentration, concentration needed to diminish the production of DPPH radical by 50% [μM].

Table 2.
Antioxidant activity of isolated compounds of bamboos.

oxygen radical scavenging (IC_{50} = 2.73 μg/mL) agent. On the other hand, dichloromethane culm fraction from the same plant, not so active against DPPH nor ABTS, reduced almost two times more the ferric cation in the FRAP method than the previous sample (IC_{50} = 27.92 μg/mL) and was an excellent scavenger of the oxygen radical in ORAC assay (IC_{50} = 1.22 μg/mL) [22]. No direct correlation between the results assessed by ABTS and ORAC was also found in another study, evaluating the antioxidant activity of different parts of *P. pubescens* [23].

Trolox equivalents received by two methods: DPPH and FRAP were also compared, and it was found that in case of *P. heterocycla* cv. pubescens, gracilis, Tao Kiang, and *P. aureosulcata*, leaf and shoots in both evaluations were very similar to the TE content. Additionally, the extract that was the richest in TE in DPPH assay (*P. heterocycla* leaf) had also the highest value of it in the FRAP method [27]. As per this author, the shoots of bamboo were the part of the plant with the poorest antioxidant activity.

In general, bamboos were classified as good antioxidants, which can be related to their high flavonoid and phenol contents [27]. The scavenging activity against superoxide anion and hydroxyl radical of some methanol and hot water extracts from a bamboo powder, used in Japan for different purposes, was higher than the ones received for the control—α-tocoferol and ascorbic acid [28]. A polysaccharide-rich extract from *Bambusa rutila* had hydroxyl radical scavenging activity equal to vitamin C [29], where an isoorientin and its ester, derived from a Chinese product called antioxidant of bamboo leaves (AOB), had their IC_{50} lower than vitamin E [30]. The acylation of isoorientin was performed to improve its solubility in lipidic media, however, the process did not have a positive impact on the antioxidant activity of the substance. A nutritional formulation developed from bamboo vinegar (5%) and maltodextrin (30%) had better *in vitro* antioxidant effect that tested commercial beverages [31]. In other study, it was proved that bamboo oil from *P. bambusoides*, when incubated for 20 h, had its linoleic acid scavenging rate similar to that of ascorbic acid [32].

Few studies of the functional antioxidant activity with correlated health effect were described in the literature as well. The lignophenol derivatives obtained from a wood mixture containing bamboo *P. bambusoides* demonstrated neuroprotective activity in cells influenced by hydrogen peroxide-induced apoptosis [33]. A short-term assay established that both Asp-Tyr identified and isolated from *P. pubescens* shoot fractions diminished significantly the systolic blood pressure of spontaneously hypertensive rats [34]. An extract from *Sasa senanensis*, named Absolutely Hemicellulose Senanensis (AHSS), had determined its *in vivo* activity, and it was shown that it inhibited the production of lipid peroxide by intestinal ischemia and subsequent reperfusion (I/R) injury model in rats [35].

2.2 Antimicrobial properties

Quality and safety of various products can be affected by the presence of microorganisms; therefore, antimicrobial substances are widely used in cosmetic, food, and pharmaceutical industries. In cosmetics, preservatives protect the formulation during the production and the use by the consumers [36]. In the food industry, these additives can improve organoleptic characteristics of food, such as color, smell, and taste, in addition to the protection of food during production, storage, and consumption [37]. The growing microbial resistance to existing drugs has generated the need for the pharmaceutical industry to search for new molecules that can be used as preservatives, antibiotics, and disinfectants [38]. This factor associated with the toxicity of certain additives [39] and the consumer appeals for the reduction in synthetic substances [40], encourage the search for alternative solutions. The complexity and molecular diversity of natural products make them an interesting source of new molecules [41].

The antimicrobial capacity of bamboo species was evaluated through several methodologies, resulting in different units for the presentation of the results. In **Table 3**, results are shown as minimal inhibitory concentration (MIC), which is the lowest concentration that is able to completely inhibit microbial growth.

The lower the MIC values, the more potent the substance is. To be considered as promising antimicrobial agents, natural products must have MICs below 100 μg/mL [39]. Therefore, the essential oils of *Phyllostachys kwangsiensis*, *P. heterocycla* cv. gracilis, and *P. heterocycla* cv. *Heterocycla* are the most active extracts, with MIC values ranging from 22.23 to 45.24 μg/mL for *S. aureus* and 31.76 μg/mL for *E coli*. 2,6-Dimethoxy-*p*-benzoquinone presented lower values than the essential oils; however, it is an isolated compound and not an extract. It is possible to affirm that the essential oils evaluated have an intense antimicrobial activity because their MIC values are close to those of an isolated compound.

In **Table 4**, the species were evaluated using the disk diffusion method. Three different extracts of each species were compared. All of them presented similar inhibition zones, around 7 mm. The wider inhibition zones were presented by

Bamboo species	Product	Microorganism	MIC (μg/mL)	Ref.
P. heterocycla var. *pubescens* (Pradelle) Ohwi	2,6-Dimethoxy-*p*-benzoquinone	*Escherichia coli*	400	[42]
		Bacillus subtilis	200	
		Salmonella typhimurium	400	
		Sarcina lutea	400	
		Pseudomonas aeruginosa	800	
		Staphylococcus aureus	200	
		Candida albicans	800	[43]
		Saccharomyces cerevisiae	25	
			10	
			25	
			800	
		Aspergillus niger	800	
	Chloroform/methanol extract (bark)	*Escherichia coli*	10,000	[44]
		Bacillus subtilis	5000	
		Salmonella typhimurium	10,000	
		Sarcina lutea	10,000	
P. heterocycla var. *pubescens* (Pradelle) Ohwi	Chloroform/methanol extract (bark)	*Pseudomonas aeruginosa*	50,000	[44]
		Staphylococcus aureus	2000	
	Essential oil	*Escherichia coli*	31.76*	[21]
		Staphylococcus aureus	31.76*	
P. pubescens (Pradelle) Mazel ex J. Houz.	Ethanol extract (outer culm)	*Staphylococcus aureus*	400	[23]
P. pubescens (Pradelle) Mazel ex J. Houz.	Hot water extract (leaf)	*Staphylococcus aureus*	1200	[23]
	Hot water extract (branch)	*Staphylococcus aureus*	1400	
	Hot water extract (inner culm)	*Staphylococcus aureus*	>16,000	
P. kwangsiensis W.Y. Hsiung, Q.H. Dai and J.K. Liu	Essential oil	*Escherichia coli*	31.76*	[21]
		Staphylococcus aureus	22.23*	
P. heterocycla fo. gracilis (W.Y. Hsiung ex Houz.) T.P. Yi	Essential oil	*Escherichia coli*	31.76*	
		Staphylococcus aureus	22.23*	
P. heterocycla (Carrière) Mitford cv *heterocycla*	Essential oil	*Escherichia coli*	31.76*	
		Staphylococcus aureus	45.24*	

Concentration calculated considering the density value 0.9.

Table 3.
Antimicrobial activity of bamboo extracts—MIC.

Bamboo species	Product	Inhibition zone (mm)		Ref.
		E. coli	*S. aureus*	
B. blumeana var. luzonensis Hack.	Acetone extract	7.2	9.3	[44]
	Ethanol extract	7.6	7.2	
	Hot water extract	7.4	7.4	
B. blumeana Schult. and Schult. f.	Acetone extract	6.6	7.0	
	Ethanol extract	9.8	9.3	
	Hot water extract	7.3	7.3	
B. vulgaris Schrad.	Acetone extract	7.5	6.9	
	Ethanol extract	7.5	7.8	
	Hot water extract	7.2	10.7	

Table 4.
Antimicrobial activity of bamboo extracts—inhibition zone.

Symbol	Diameter (mm)	Classification
–	<10	No activity
+	10–15	Activity
++	15–20	Good activity
+++	>20	Very good activity

Table 5.
Interpretation of inhibition zones [47].

the ethanolic extract of *Bambusa blumeana* against *E. coli* (9.8 mm) and *Bambusa vulgaris* hot water extract (10.7 mm) against *S. aureus*. However, all the extracts can be considered inactive, comparing them with the inhibition zones in **Table 5**. It is important to say that during the measurement of the diameter of the inhibition zones, the diameter of the disk is considered.

The search for bioactive compounds is not limited only to the compounds produced by a plant species. Microorganisms hosted in plant tissues and organs have become a new source of useful metabolites for the pharmaceutical, agricultural, and food industries [45, 46]. Found in various parts of plants (roots, stems, leaves, and barks), endophytic fungi colonize various species [47], and the relationship between the endophytic fungi and the host plant may be advantageous since many of them improve the growth and protect the plant against pathogens [46].

Using the agar diffusion method, some authors evaluated the antimicrobial activity of fungal strains isolated from bamboos. The antimicrobial potential of the strains was evaluated against human pathogens, and in **Table 6**, it is possible to find the main results. Isolate 130 from *P. edulis* culms and isolate B38 from the same species presented similar results, with activity ranging from good to very good for most pathogens evaluated. Nevertheless, the isolate FB16 from *P. edulis* presented the best result, with very good activity against a larger number of microorganisms.

One of the studies also evaluated the activity of fermentation products of fungal strains of *P. edulis*, and the results can be seen in **Table 7**. The product FB16 is the most active, with the biggest zones of inhibition. This behavior agrees with the results presented by the isolated fungus, as shown in **Table 6**. It is important to note that although the fermentation product FB16 presented the best result among the samples, its zones of inhibition are smaller than those presented by the isolated fungus.

Bamboo species	Isolate no.	*S. aureus*	*B. subtilis*	*L. monocytogenes*	*S. bacteria*	*E. coli*	*P. vulgaris*	*C. albicans*	*R. rubra*	Ref.
P. edulis (Carrière) J. Houz. *(Culms)*	106	+	+	–	–	NT	NT	++	–	[45]
	120	+++	+++	+	–	NT	NT	+++	++	
	127	–	+	+	+	NT	NT	+	–	
	128	+	+	–	–	NT	NT	+	+	
	130	+++	+++	++	++	NT	NT	+++	+	
P. edulis (Carrière) J. Houz.*(Seeds)*	B09	+	+	–	–	NT	NT	++	–	[47]
	B34	–	+	+	+	NT	NT	+	–	
	B35	+	+	–	–	NT	NT	+	+	
	B38	+++	+++	++	++	NT	NT	+++	+	
	ZZZ816	+++	+++	+	–	NT	NT	+++	+	
P. heteroclada Oliv.	FB16	NT	+++	+++	+++	+++	++	+++	NT	[46]
	FB43	NT	–	++	++	+	+	–	NT	
	FB06	NT	++	++	–	+	–	+	NT	
	FB21	NT	–	++	++	+	+	++	NT	

NT—not tested.

Table 6.
Antimicrobial activity of fungal isolates.

Isolate no.	Inhibition zone (mm)						Ref.
	B. subtilis	*L. monocytogenes*	*S. bacteria*	*E. coli*	*P. vulgaris*	*C. albicans*	
FB16	13.2	11.8	10.29	12.46	8.8	16	[46]
FB43	—	10.6	8.95	7.6	7.52	—	
FB06	8.66	9.1	—	7.84	—	7.66	
FB21	—	8.7	8.64	7.52	7.77	8.69	

—: not active.

Table 7.
Antimicrobial activity of fermentation products of fungal isolates from Phyllostachys heteroclada.

Despite the search for new substances with the ability to inhibit microbial growth, the presence of microorganisms is not always harmful. In some cases, certain microorganisms may contribute to human health, such as the human intestinal microbiota. It is composed of more than 400 bacterial species, and bifidobacteria and lactobacilli are the main ones [48]. They help in the digestion and synthesize bioactive compounds, besides preventing diseases, avoiding the growth of pathogenic microorganisms [49]. Through the consumption of probiotics and prebiotics, it is possible to maintain the balance of these intestinal bacteria. Probiotics are supplements containing the microorganisms of interest. Nondigestible carbohydrates that undergo fermentation by intestinal microbes are called prebiotics [48, 49].

Prebiotic activity was evaluated in bamboo shoots, since they are a rich source of polysaccharides and oligosaccharides [50]. The polysaccharides isolated from the shoots of *Gigantochloa levis* were able to stimulate the growth of *Bifidobacterium animalis*, *Bifidobacterium longum*, and *Lactobacillus acidophilus*. At the same time, they were able to reduce the growth of Salmonella sp., pathogenic bacteria [50]. Heteropolysaccharides-protein complexes from *Phyllostachys praecox* shoots were isolated, and the fractions containing these substances increased the *Bifidobacterium adolescentis* and *Bifidobacterium bifidum* counts [50]. These results suggest that bamboo shoots can be a source of probiotics.

2.3 Miscellaneous activities

Chinese traditional medicine has described the use of different parts of bamboos, such as leaves and rhizomes, to treat many diseases. Nowadays, scientific studies have demonstrated that bamboo extracts have excellent biological efficacy regarding their antioxidant activity. Theoretically, this activity might also be related for the treatment of diverse pathologies, such as resistance to free-radical, cardiovascular protection against neurodegenerative diseases, anticancer, and many others.

Bamboo shavings are a sort of Chinese traditional medicine that can be obtained from different bamboo species by scraping off the coating from bamboo stems, cutting the stems into slices, and binding them together by drying in shadowy places. A triterpenoid-rich extract of bamboo shavings was obtained from *P. nigra* var. *henonis* by superfluid carbon dioxide extraction and tested for antitumor activity. The extract showed a significant inhibitory activity against P388 and A549 cancer cell lines. The extract also presented an effective inhibitory effect on the sarcoma-loaded mice S180 model. Friedelin, the main compound in the extract, was also active on inhibiting the proliferation of four cancer lines, A375, L929, Hela, and THP-1 [51].

Bamboo extracts used as dietary supplement demonstrated a protective effect on the development of induced breast cancer by 7,12-dimethylbenz[a]anthracene

(DMBA). A crude hydroethanolic extract from *P. edulis* was incorporated into a standard rodent diet at a concentration of 5 g/kg (0.5%), and it was able to delay the onset of mammary tumor by 1 week, decreasing the tumor incidence by 44% and tumor multiplicity by 67%. The biochemical analysis indicated that the activity might be related to an increased estrogen metabolism [52].

Bamboo vinegar, a natural liquid derived from the condensation produced during bamboo charcoal production, a pyrolyzate product, has been used in agriculture and used as a food additive. This liquid is composed mainly by water and acetic acid, but it also contains a variety of phenolic compounds. A vinegar preparation produced from *P. pubescens* reduced inducible nitric oxide synthase expression and nitric oxide levels and interleukin-6 secretion using lipopolysaccharide-activated macrophages. The mechanism proposed for the anti-inflammatory effect of the vinegar involved a decrease in reactive oxygen species production and protein kinase C-α/δ activation. The main component involved in the anti-inflammatory activity was creosol (2-methoxy-4-methylphenol) in *in vivo* tests [53]. Vinegars obtained from *P pubescens*, *P. nigra*, and *P. bambusoides* were tested for protective effect against N-methyl-D-aspartate (NMDA)-induced cell death in primary cultured cortical neurons. All the preparations were able to restore cell viability when compared to untreated cells in an NMDA-induced neuronal cell death assay. Additionally, vinegars of *P. pubescens* and *P. nigra* showed a reduction of apoptosis following the exposure to NMDA, indicating them as supplements for ischemic injury treatment [54].

Besides the usual secondary metabolites, aqueous bamboo extracts contain many amino acids and polysaccharides that have not been investigated for their biological activities. Hypertension is associated with cardiovascular diseases such as arteriosclerosis, stroke, and myocardial infarction. Angiotensin converting enzyme (ACE, EC 3.4.15.1) is a dipeptidyl carboxypeptidase involved in different blood pressure regulating mechanisms. A peptide enriched *P. pubescens* shoot aqueous extract could significantly reduce systolic blood pressure, improve oxidant stress status (GSH-Px, SOD, TAC and MDA), and increase NO level in serum and NO synthase activity in kidney. This extract also decreased total cholesterol, triglyceride, and low-density lipoprotein cholesterol content and MDA level of hyperlipidemic rats. These activities were higher for crude extract rather than for the synthetic peptide used. This indicates a synergism with the phenolic compounds still present in the crude extract, such as p-coumaric acid, ferulic acid, caffeic acid, homoorientin, and orientin [55]. The antihyperlipidemic effect of these metabolites has been demonstrated later. The lipid metabolism was affected by phenolics and triterpenoids present in the inner culm water found from *Dendrocalamus giganteus* Wall. ex Munro. The freeze-dried powder obtained from this water was composed mainly of protocatechuic acid, *p*-hydroxybenzoic acid, syringic acid, friedelan-3-one, lup-20(29)-en-3-one, lup-20(29)-en-3-ol, and α-amyrin. The powder reduced the contents of triglycerides, total cholesterol, and free fatty acids in model assay with steatosis human liver cell L02 [56].

Most of the bamboo applications are related to the paper, textile, and construction industries, due to its high fiber contents. For this reason, scientists have been isolating and characterizing bamboo hemicelluloses since the 1970s. Hemicelluloses are polysaccharides found in plant cell walls that are characterized by being neither cellulose nor pectin and by having β-(1 $\rightarrow$ 4)-linked backbones with an equatorial configuration. Some of these polysaccharides are known to have an immunomodulatory activity. Hemicelluloses isolated from *P. pubescens* shavings showed *in vitro* immunomodulatory activity and significantly stimulated mouse splenocyte proliferation. All the isolated compounds markedly enhanced the phagocytosis activity and nitric oxide production of the murine macrophage

RAW264 [57]. The total polysaccharide fraction of *Sasa veitchii* (Carrière) Rehder inhibited the production of interferon gamma (IFN-γ) by not only the toll like receptors (TLRs) but also the C-type lectin receptors (CLRs) dectin-1, and dectin-2 of BWMP also inhibited the autologous production of IFN-γ in the splenocyte culture mice splenocytes in the presence of immunostimulant fungal polysaccharides [58].

3. Conclusions

Although bamboo has been used for centuries by the Traditional Chinese Medicine, this is still a group of plant under investigated regarding its medicinal properties. In Asian countries, such as China, Korea, and Japan, among others, the most used species have already been studied regarding their biological properties and chemical composition. On the other hand, in Southern American countries, where a huge bamboo diversity is available, very little has been done to access its medicinal properties.

Several species have shown an important antioxidant potential demonstrating that they can be applied in the treatment of different diseases such as anti-inflammatory, antitumor, and several other ailments involving oxidative processes. Additionally, besides the usual secondary metabolites, bamboo extracts may contain biologically active peptides and polysaccharides. The combined effect of these macromolecules with polyphenols and other metabolites may lead to multiple biological effects, such as antifree radical, antiaging, antifatigue, antibacteria, antivirus, and as a functional dietary supplement, cosmetic ingredient, and food additive.

Acknowledgements

The authors wish to thank CAPES and CNPq for the scholarships granted.

Conflict of interest

The authors declare that there is no conflict of interest.

Author details

Katarzyna B. Wróblewska[1], Danielle C.S. de Oliveira[1],
Maria Tereza Grombone-Guaratini[2] and Paulo Roberto H. Moreno[1*]

1 Department of Fundamental Chemistry, Institute of Chemistry, University of São Paulo, São Paulo, Brazil

2 Botanical Institute of São Paulo, São Paulo, Brazil

*Address all correspondence to: prmoreno@iq.usp.br

References

[1] Liese, W. Bamboo: Past, Present and Future. American Bamboo Society. 1999; Newsletter, 20

[2] Canavan S, Richardson DM, Visser V, Roux JJLR, Vorontsova MS, Wilson JRU. The global distribution of bamboos: assessing correlates of introduction and invasion. Aob Plants. 2017;**9**:1-18. DOI: 10.1093/aobpla/plw078

[3] Filgueiras TS, Santos-Gonçalves AP. A checklist of the basal grasses and bamboos in Brazil (*Poaceae*). Bamboo Science and Culture. 2004;**18**:7-18

[4] Soderstrom TR, Calderón CE. A Commentary on the Bamboo (*Poaceae*: Bambusoideae). Biotropica. 1979;**11**:161-172

[5] Judziewicz EJ, Clark LG, Londoño X, Stern MJ. American bamboos. Washington, DC, Smithsonian Institution Press; 1999. 392

[6] *Poaceae* in Lista de Espécies da Flora do Brasil. Jardim Botânico do Rio de Janeiro. 2016. Available from: http://floradobrasil.jbrj.gov.br/jabot/floradobrasil/FB193 [Accessed: 18-01-2016]

[7] González ME, Veblen TT, Donoso C, Valeria L. Tree regeneration responses in a lowland Notophagus-dominated forest after bamboo dieback in South-Central Chile. Plant Ecology. 2002;**161**:59-73. DOI: 10.1023/A:1020378822847

[8] Bansal A, Zoolagud SS. Bamboo composites: Material of the future. Journal of Bamboo and Rattan. 2002;**1**:119-130. DOI: 10.1163/156915902760181595

[9] Park H, Lim JH, Kim HJ, Choi HJ, Lee I. Antioxidant flavone glycosides from the leaves of *Sasa borealis*. Archives of Pharmacal Research. 2007;**30**(2):161-166

[10] Hu C, Zhang Y, Kitts DD. Evaluation of antioxidant and prooxidant activities of bamboo *Phyllostachys nigra* var. Henonis leaf extract in vitro. Journal of Agricultural and Food Chemistry. 2000;**48**:3170-3176. DOI: 10.1021/jf0001637

[11] Jiao J, Zhang Y, Liu C, Liu J, Wu X, Zhang Y. Separation and purification of tricin from an antioxidant product derived from bamboo leaves. Journal of Agricultural and Food Chemistry. 2007;**55**:10086-10092. DOI: 10.1021/jf0716533

[12] Cavaliere C, Foglia P, Pastorini E, Samperi R, Laganà A. Identification and mass spectrometric characterization of glycosylated flavonoids in Triticum durum plants by high-performance liquid chromatography with tandem mass spectrometry. Rapid Communications in Mass Spectrometry. 2005;**19**:3143-3158. DOI: 10.1002/rcm.2185

[13] Ferreres F, Andrade PB, Valentão P, Gil-Izquierdo A. Further knowledge on barley (*Hordeum vulgare* L.) leaves O-glycosyl-C-glycosyl flavones by liquid chromatography-UV diode-array detection-electrospray ionisation mass spectrometry. Journal of Chromatography A. 2008;**1182**:56-64. DOI: 10.1016/j.chroma.2007

[14] Brazier-Hicks M, Evans KM, Gershater MC, Puschmann H, Steel PG, Edwards R. The C-glycosylation of flavonoids in cereals. Journal of Biological Chemistry. 2009;**284**:17926-17934. DOI: 10.1074/jbc.M109.009258

[15] Zhang Y, Bao B, Lu B, Ren Y, Tie X, Zhang Y. Determination of flavone C glucosides in antioxidant of bamboo leaves (AOB) fortified foods by reversed-phase high-performance liquid chromatography with ultraviolet

diode array detection. Journal of Chromatography, A. 2005;**1065**:177-185

[16] Birben E, Sahiner UM, Sackesen C, Erzurum S, Kalayci O. Oxidative Stress and Antioxidant Defense. WAO Journal. 2012;**5**:9-19

[17] Burton GJ, Jauniaux E. Oxidative stress. Best Practice&Research Clinical Obstetrics Gynaecology. 2011;**25**(3):287-299. DOI: 10.1016/j.bpobgyn.2010.10.016

[18] Pham-huy LA, He H, Pham-huy C. Free radicals, antioxidants in disease and health. International Journal of Biomedical Sciences. 2008;**4**(2):89-96

[19] Apak R, Gorinstein S, Böhm V, Schaich KM, Özyürek M, Güçlü K. Methods of measurement and evaluation of natural antioxidant capacity/activity (IUPAC technical report). Pure and Applied Chemistry. 2013;**8**(5):957-998

[20] Pisoschi AM, Negulescu GP. Methods for total antioxidant activity determination: A review. Biochemistry and Analytical Biochemistry. 2011;**1**(1):1-10. DOI: 10.4172/2161-1009.1000106

[21] Jin YC, Yuan K, Zhang J. Chemical composition, and antioxidant and antimicrobial activities of essential oil of *Phyllostachys heterocycla* cv. *Pubescens* varieties from China. Molecules;**16**:4318-4327. DOI: 10.3390/molecules16054318

[22] Gagliano J, Grombone-guaratini MT, Furlan CM. Antioxidant potential and HPLC-DAD profile of phenolic compounds from leaves and culms of *Merostachys pluriflora*. South African Journal of Botany. 2018;**115**:24-30. DOI: 10.1016/j.sajb.2017.12.008

[23] Tanaka A, Zhu Q, Tan H, Horiba H, Ohnuki K, Mori Y, et al. Biological activities and phytochemical profiles of extracts from different parts of bamboo (*Phyllostachys pubescens*). Molecules. 2014;**19**:8238-8260. DOI: 10.3390/molecules19068238

[24] Park E-J, Jhon D-Y. The antioxidant, angiotensin converting enzyme inhibition activity, and phenolic compounds of bamboo shoot extracts. LWT—Food Science and Technology. 2010;**43**(4):655-659. DOI: 10.1016/j.lwt.2009.11.005

[25] Hu CJ, Liao HB, Yuan K, Hu JH, Lin XC. Chemical composition and antioxidant activity of essential oil of bamboo leaves from four species in China. Asian Journal of Chemistry. 2011;**23**(6):2543-2547

[26] Kweon MH, Hwang HJ, Sung HC. Identification and antioxidant activity of novel chlorogenic acid derivatives from bamboo (*Phyllostachys edulis*). Journal of Agricultural and Food Chemistry. 2001;**49**(10):4646-4655. DOI: 10.1021/jf010514x

[27] Li YX, Cheng FR, Jin YC, Yuan K. Studies on the active components and antioxidant activity of the extracts from different parts of bamboo. Asian Journal of Chemistry. 2013;**25**(11):6354-6360. DOI: 10.14233/ajchem.2013.14584

[28] Nagai T, Suzuki N, Tanoue Y, Kai N, Nagashima T. Antioxidant activities of the extracts from bamboo powder as underutilized resource. Journal of Food, Agriculture and Environment. 2009;7(2):228-232

[29] Gao YN, Tian CR, Zhao LL. Extraction, purification and antioxidant activity of polysaccharides from bamboo leaves. Journal of Forestry Research. 2012;**23**(1):139-143. DOI: 10.1007/s11676-012-0223-y

[30] Xu J, Qian J, Li S. Enzymatic acylation of isoorientin isolated from antioxidant of bamboo leaves with palmitic acid and antiradical activity

of the acylated derivatives. European Food Research and Technology. 2014: 661-667. DOI: 10.1007/s00217-014-2262-4

[31] Echavarría ACC, Yepes FJ, Torres HP. Determinación del potencial antioxidant en extractos de vinagre *Guadua angustifolia* Kunth para aplicaciones alimenticias. Determination of the antioxidant potential in *Guadua angustifolia* Kunth vinegar extracts for food applications. Revista Cubana de Plantas Medicinales. 2012;**17**(4):330-342

[32] Choi D, Cho K, Na M, Choi H, Kim Y, Lim DH, et al. Effect of bamboo oil on antioxidative activity and nitrite scavenging activity. Journal of Industrial and Engineering Chemistry. 2008;**14**:765-770. DOI: 10.1016/j.jiec.2008.06.005

[33] Akao Y, Seki N, Nakagawa Y, Yi H, Matsumoto K, Ito Y, et al. A highly bioactive lignophenol derivative from bamboo lignin exhibits a potent activity to suppress apoptosis induced by oxidative stress in human neuroblastoma SH-SY5Y cells. Bioorganic and Medicinal Chemistry. 2004;**12**(18):4791-4801. DOI: 10.1016/j.bmc.2004.07.022

[34] Liu L, Liu L, Lu B, Chen M, Zhang Y. Evaluation of bamboo shoot peptide preparation with angiotensin converting enzyme inhibitory and antioxidant abilities from byproducts of canned bamboo shoots. Journal of Agricultural and Food Chemistry. 2013;**61**:5226-5533. DOI: 10.1021/jf305064h

[35] Kurokawa T, Itagaki S, Yamaji T, Nakata C, Noda T, Hirano T, et al. Antioxidant activity of a novel extract from bamboo grass (AHSS) against ischemia-reperfusion injury in rat small intestine. Biological and Pharmaceutical Bulletin. 2006;**29**(11):2301-2303. Available from: http://www.ncbi.nlm.nih.gov/pubmed/17077533

[36] Kokura S, Handa O, Takagi T, Ishikawa T, Naito Y, Yoshikawa T. Silver nanoparticles as a safe preservative for use in cosmetics. Nanomedicine: Nanotechnology, Biology, and Medicine. 2010;**6**:570-574. DOI: 10.1016/j.nano.2009.12.002

[37] Zhang J, Gong J, Ding Y, Lu B, Wu X, Zhang Y. Antibacterial activity of water-phase extracts from bamboo shavings against food spoilage microorganisms. African Journal of Biotechnology. 2010;**9**:7710-7717

[38] Gallón AIM, Torres EC, Cabrera CG. Actividad antiséptica de vinagre de *Guadua angustifolia* Kunth. Revista Cubana de Plantas Medicinales. 2011;**16**:244-252

[39] Moreno PRH, Costa-Issa FI, Rajca-Ferreira AK, Pereira MAA, Kaneko TM. Native Brazilian plants against nosocomial infections: A critical review on their potential and the antimicrobial methodology. Current Topics in Medicinal Chemistry. 2013;**13**:3040-3078

[40] Tanaka A, Shimizu K, Kondo R. Antibacterial compounds from shoot skins of moso bamboo (*Phyllostachys pubescens*). Journal of Wood Science. 2013;**59**:155-159. DOI: 10.1007/s10086-012-1310-6

[41] Cragg GM, Newman DJ. Natural products: A continuing source of novel drug leads. Biochimica et Biophysica Acta. 2013;**1830**:3670-3695. DOI: 10.1016/j.bbagen.2013.02.008

[42] Nishina A, Hasegawa KI, Uchibori T, Seino H, Osawa T. 2,6-Dimethoxy-*p*-benzoquinone as an antibacterial substance in the bark of *Phyllostachys heterocycla* var. pubescens, a species

of thick-stemmed bamboo. Journal of Agricultural and Food Chemistry. 1991;**39**:266-269

[43] Nishina A, Uchibori T. Antimicrobial of 2,6-Dimethoxy-*p*-benzoquinone, isolated from Thick-stemmed bamboo, and its analogs. Agricultural and Biological Chemistry. 1991;**55**:2395-2398

[44] Valentino MJG, Ganado LS, Ganado MR, Undan JR. Phytochemical screening and bio assay of the anti-microbial activity of three species of bamboo in Nueva Ecija, Philippines. Advances in Environmental Biology. 2015;**9**:389-396

[45] Shen X, Zheng D, Gao J, Hou C. Isolation and evaluation of endophytic fungi with antimicrobial ability from *Phyllostachys edulis*. Bangladesh Journal of Pharmacology. 2012;7:249-257. DOI: 10.3329/bjp.v7i4.12068

[46] Zhou YK, Shen XY, Hou CL. Diversity and antimicrobial activity of culturable fungi from fishscale bamboo (*Phyllostachys heteroclada*) in China. World Journal of Microbiology and Biotechnology. 2017;**33**:104:1-7. DOI : 10.1007/s11274-017-2267-9

[47] Shen XY, Cheng YL, Cai CJ, Fan L, Gao J, Hou CL. Diversity and antimicrobial activity of culturable endophytic fungi isolated from Moso bamboo seeds. PLoS ONE. 2014;**9**:1-7. DOI:10.1371/journal.pone.0095838

[48] Azmi AFMN, Mustafa S, Hashim DM, MAnap YA. Prebiotic activity of polysaccharides extracted from Gigantochloa Levis (Buluh beting) shoots. Molecules. 2012;**17**:1635-1651. DOI: 10.3390/molecules17021635

[49] Singh SP, Jadaun JS, Narnoliya LK, Pandey A. Prebiotic oligosaccharides: Special focus on fructooligosaccharides, its biosynthesis and bioactivity. Applied Biochemistry and Biotechnology. 2017;**183**:613-635. DOI: 10.1007/s12010-017-2605-2

[50] He S, Wang X, Zhang Y, Wang J, Sun H, Wang J, et al. Isolation and prebiotic activity of water-soluble polysaccharides fractions from the bamboo shoots (*Phyllostachys praecox*). Carbohydrate Polymers. 2016;**151**:295-304. DOI: 10.1016/j.carbpol.2016.05.072

[51] Lu B, Liu L, Zhen X, Wu X, Zhang Y. Anti-tumor activity of triterpenoid rich extract from bamboo shavings (Caulis bamfusae in Taeniam). African Journal of Biotechnology. 2010;**9**:6430-6436

[52] Lin Y, Collier AC, Liu W, Berry MJ, Panee J. The inhibitory effect of bamboo extract on the development of 7,12-dimethylbenz[a]anthracene (DMBA)-induced breast cancer. Phytotherapy Research. 2008;**22**:1440-1445. DOI: 10.1002/ptr.2439

[53] Ho CL, Lin CY, Ka SM, Chen A, Tasi YL, Liu ML, Chiu YC, Hua KF. Bamboo vinegar decreases inflammatory mediator expression and NLRP3 inflammasome activation by inhibiting reactive oxygen species generation and protein kinase C-α/δ activation. PLoS ONE. 2013;**8**:1-12. DOI:10.1371/journal.pone.0075738

[54] Hong EJ, Jung EM, Lee GS, Kim JY, Na KJ, Park MJ, et al. Protective effects of the pyrolyzates derived from bamboo against neuronal damage and hematoaggregation. Journal of Ethnopharmacology. 2010;**128**:594-599. DOI: 10.1016/j.jep.2010.01.045

[55] Liu L, Liu L, Lu B, Xia D, Zhang Y. Evaluation of antihypertensive and antihyperlipidemic effects of bamboo shoot angiotensin converting enzyme inhibitory peptide in vivo. Journal of Agricultural and Food Chemistry.

2012;**60**:11351-11358. DOI: 10.1021/jf303471f

[56] Du P, Huang XJ, Wang TD, Huang SJ, Shan Y, Yu J, et al. Lipid metabolism effects of freeze-dried powder of bamboo juice on liver cell line L02 with steatosis. Advance Journal of Food Science and Technology. 2015;**9**:854-859. DOI: 10.19026/ajfst.9.1642

[57] Huang JQ, Qi RT, Pang MR, Liu C, Li GY, Zhang Y. Isolation, chemical characterization, and immunomodulatory activity of naturally acetylated hemicelluloses from bamboo shavings. Journal of Zhejiang University Science B. 2017;**18**:138-151. DOI: 10.1631/jzus.B1500274

[58] Sato W, Takeshita K, Tsuboi M, Kanamori M, Ishibashi K, Miura NN, et al. Specificity of the Immunomodulating Activity of *Sasa veitchii* (Japanese Folk Medicine Kumazasa) to Fungal Polysaccharides. International Journal of Medicinal Mushrooms. 2015;**17**:415-426

Chapter 9

Medicinal Plants for Treatment of Prevalent Diseases

Susana Oteng Mintah, Tonny Asafo-Agyei, Mary-Ann Archer, Peter Atta-Adjei Junior, Daniel Boamah, Doris Kumadoh, Alfred Appiah, Augustine Ocloo, Yaw Duah Boakye and Christian Agyare

Abstract

This chapter focuses on reviewing publications on medicinal plants used in the treatment of common diseases such as malaria, cholera, pneumonia, tuberculosis and asthma. Traditional medicine is still recognized as the preferred primary health care system in many rural communities, due to a number of reasons including affordability and effectiveness. The review concentrated on current literature on medicinal plants, highlighting on information about ethnobotany, phytochemistry and pharmacology. The search for publications on medicinal plants with scientifically proven efficacy was carried out using electronic databases such as Science Direct, Google Scholar, SciFinder and PubMed. In all, about 46 species of different families with potent biological and pharmacological activities were reviewed. All the plants reviewed exhibited potent activity confirming their various traditional uses and their ability to treat prevalent diseases.

Keywords: medicinal plants, malaria, diarrhea, tuberculosis, asthma

1. Introduction

Traditional medicine is still recognized as the preferred primary health care system in many communities, with over 60% of the world's population and about 80% in developing countries depending directly on medicinal plants for their medical purposes [1]. This is due to a number of reasons including affordability, accessibility and low cost [2].

The use of plants to cure several kinds of human diseases has a long history. Various parts of plants such as leaf, stem, bark, root, etc. are being used to prevent, allay symptoms or revert abnormalities back to normal. Since the practice of "herbal remedies" does not adhere strictly to facts accrued using scientific approaches, orthodox medicine sees "herbal medicines" as an alternative medicine. However, most of the pharmaceutical products currently dispensed by physicians have a long history of use as herbal remedies, including opium, aspirin, digitalis and quinine. Modern medicine today utilizes active compounds isolated from higher plants, and about 80% of these active ingredients indicate a positive correlation between their modern therapeutic use and the traditional uses [3].

The search for, and use of drugs and dietary supplements obtained from plants have increased in recent years. Scientist such as pharmacologists, microbiologists, botanists, and phytochemists are combing the Earth for phytochemicals and clues that could be developed into medicines for various diseases treatment. This study therefore reviewed electronic database (Google Scholar, SciFinder, PubMed, etc.) for medicinal plants that have potent activity in treating some prevalent and common ailments like malaria, diarrhea, tuberculosis, pneumonia and asthma.

2. Medicinal plants with demonstrated anti-malarial activity

Malaria is one of the world's most important parasitic disease and a leading cause of death especially in developing countries [4]. It is endemic in about 100 developing countries, leading to about 1.2 million estimated deaths each year in Africa [5], with pregnant women and children below 5 years being mostly affected [6]. A wide range of medicinal plants is employed for the treatment of malaria, since majority of the people who get infected cannot afford the existing expensive orthodox medicines [7]. The problem of resistance to existing antimalarial agents by parasite has necessitated the search for new and potent agents, and the focus of researchers is on natural products especially medicinal plants since active compounds like quinine and artemisinin were isolated from plants and have been lead compounds for antimalarial drug development [8, 9]. Various medicinal plants have been investigated for their anti-malarial activity and some with demonstrated potent *in vitro* activity have been reviewed below.

2.1 *Cryptolepis sanguinolenta*

C. sanguinolenta (Lindl.) Schlechter (Apocynaceae) is known by Ghanaians as 'Ghana quinine' and specifically by the Asantes and Ewes as 'Nibima' and 'Kadze,' respectively [10]. It is a twining and scrambling thin-stemmed shrub, indigenous to Africa, with much ethno-medicinal importance and interest in the West African sub-region [11]. It is used traditionally for the treatment of malaria, upper respiratory and urinary tract infections, diarrhea, hypertension and as cicatrizant of wounds [12, 13]. The ethanolic and aqueous extracts of *C. sanguinolenta* exhibited an *in vitro* antiplasmodial activity against multi-drug resistance *Plasmodium falciparum* (K1) strain, with all the extracts inhibiting 90% of parasite growth at concentrations below 23 μg/mL. The ethanolic roots and leaves extracts showed potent activity with IC_{50} of 0.895 ± 0.02 and 3.01 ± 0.02 μg/mL, respectively. While the aqueous roots and leaves extracts had IC_{50} of 2.32 ± 0.3 and 13.5 ± 0.7 μg/mL, respectively [14]. Evaluating the clinical efficacy of a tea bag formulation of the root of *C. sanguinolenta* in patients with uncomplicated malaria showed that within 72 h, Fifty percent (50%) of the patients had their *P. falciparum* parasitaemia cleared, and all patients, by Day 7. By Day 3, all presenting symptoms such as fever, chills, nausea and vomiting were completely no more. The overall cure rate when one tea bag of *C. sanguinolenta* was taken three times a day for 5 days was 93.5%, due to two cases of recrudescence on Days 21 and 28 [15].

2.2 *Terminalia ivorensis*

T. ivorensis A. Chev. belongs to the family Combretaceae and is commonly known as 'black afara' and by the Asantes as 'amire.' It is a large deciduous forest tree of 15–46 m high, normally grown as timber plantation in many tropical countries [16]. In traditional medicine, various parts of the plant is used to treat malaria, yellow fever, pile, stomach ulcer, wounds and other infections [17, 18]. A study by Komlaga et al. [19] revealed an active *in vitro* antiplasmodial activity of *T. ivorensis* aqueous leaf extract, against *P. falciparum* chloroquine-sensitive (3D7) and chloroquine resistant (W2) strains with IC_{50} of 0.64 ± 0.14 and 10.52 ± 3.55 μg/mL, respectively. The ethanolic stem bark extract also showed an *in vitro* antimalarial activity against chloroquine-resistant strains of *P. falciparum* with an IC_{50} of 6.949 μg/mL [20].

2.3 *Elaeis guineensis*

E. guineensis Jacq (Arecaceae), popularly known as oil palm is a monocotyledonous plant which belongs to the coccoid group of palms. It grows up to 15 m high with a lifetime of over 100 years and occurs throughout the tropical rainforest belt of West Africa [21]. *E. guineensis* is commonly used for treating gonorrhea, rheumatism, headache, wounds [22]. An *in vitro* anti-plasmodial assay revealed that, the ethanolic extract of *E. guineensis* leaves has potent antimalarial activity with IC_{50} of 1.195 μg/mL, against chloroquine-resistant *P. falciparum* [20].

2.4 *Phyllanthus emblica*

P. emblica L. of the family Euphorbiaceae is a deciduous medium-sized plant (10–18 m high), native to tropical south eastern Asia and widely distributed in most subtropical and tropical countries. It is commonly known as Indian gooseberry, rich in vitamin C, minerals and amino acids which helps to build up lost vitality and vigor [23, 24]. Various parts of the plant is used traditionally for the treatment of diarrhea, inflammation, diabetes, jaundice, cough, asthma, peptic ulcer, skin diseases, leprosy, intermittent fevers, headache, anemia, dizziness, snakebite and scorpion-sting [25]. In an SYBR green I-based fluorescence assay to assess the anti-plasmodial potential of *P. emblica*, the methanol leaf extract exhibited potent activity against CQ-sensitive (3D7) and CQ-resistant (Dd2 and INDO) strains of *P. falciparum* with IC_{50} of 3.125, 4.8 and 5 μg/mL, respectively. Also the ethyl acetate leaf extract showed activity with IC_{50} of 7.25, 15 and 9 μg/mL against 3D7, Dd2 and INDO *P. falciparum* strains, respectively [26].

2.5 *Syzygium aromaticum*

S. aromaticum (L.) Merril. & Perry, syn. *Eugenia caryophyllata*, an ancient and valuable spice is a member of the family Myrtaceae and is commonly known as clove. It is mostly used as a spice to flavor all kinds of foods and has other medicinal values including anthelmintic, anti-asthma and other allergic disorders, anti-inflammatory, antioxidant, antiviral and anti-parasitic properties [27]. A study by Bagavan et al. [26], revealed the antimalarial activity of methanol extract of *S. aromaticum* flower buds with IC_{50} of 6.25, 9.5 and 10 μg/mL against *P. falciparum* CQ-sensitive (3D7) and CQ-resistant (Dd2 and INDO) strains, respectively.

2.6 *Goniothalamus marcanii*

G. tamirensis Pierre ex Finet & Gagnep is an accepted synonym for the species and is from the family Annonaceae. It occurs naturally in tropical and subtropical parts of Southeast Asia. 80%-EtOH extracts showed an in vitro antimalarial activity (IC_{50} = 6.3 μg/mL) against the drug resistant K1 strain of *P. falciparum* [28].

2.7 *Casearia sylvestris*

C. sylvestris var. lingua (Cambess.) Eichler, (Salicaceae) is an evergreen shrub or small tree with long, slender branches and a very dense globose crown. Usually

4–6 m tall, but can grow up to 20 m high, with wide distribution throughout South America. It has been employed in traditional medicine for treating snake bites, wounds, inflammation, fevers, gastric ulcers and diarrhea [29]. The hexane extracts of *C. sylvestris* stem wood, stem bark, root bark, leaf and root wood as well as ethanol extract of the root bark, exhibited potent *in vitro* antiplasmodial activity against chloroquine-resistance FcB1/Colombia *P. falciparum* strain with IC_{50} values of 0.9 ± 0.2, 1.0 ± 0.4, 1.2 ± 0.4, 1.3 ± 0.1, 2.3 ± 0.5 and 7.7 ± 1.1 μg/mL, respectively [30].

2.8 *Cupania vernalis*

C. vernalis Cambess. (Sapindaceae) is a semi-deciduous tree with elongated and dense crown, which can grow up to 10–22 m tall. It can be found in almost all forest formations in Brazil, South America, Argentina, Uruguay, Paraguay and Bolivia. The tree serves as source of tannins and wood locally, and in traditional medicine as diuretic, stimulant, expectorant, natural surfactant, sedative and for treating stomach-ache and dermatitis [31]. The hexane and ethanol leaf extracts showed active antimalarial activity against chloroquine-resistance (FcB1/Colombia) *P. falciparum* with IC_{50} of 0.9 ± 0.3 and 6.6 ± 0.2 μg/mL, respectively [30].

2.9 *Xylopia emarginata*

X. emarginata Mart. is a species of plant in the Annonaceae family. It is native to Cerrado vegetation in Brazil. It is an evergreen tree with a very narrow, almost columnar crown which can grow up to 10–20 m tall and 30–40 cm in diameter. It usually grows in large clusters, forming a homogeneous mass. It is a species characteristic of swamp forest, and does not grow in the driest places. It is used as a condiment in food, a carminative and aphrodisiac in traditional medicine [32]. *X. emarginata* hexane root bark and stem bark extracts were able to inhibit *P. falciparum* (chloroquine-resistance FcB1/Colombia strains) with IC_{50} of 4.9 ± 0.2 and 5.2 ± 0.4 μg/mL, respectively [30].

2.10 *Xylopia aromatic*

X. aromatica (Lam.) Mart. belongs to the family Annonaceae and the accepted name is *X. xylopioides*. It is a tree native to Cerrado grassland vegetation, particularly in the states of Goiás and Minas Gerais, in eastern Brazil. It is a medium-sized tree with long, hanging branches that can make the crown look like a Christmas tree. Leaves are alternate, narrow, pointed, in a flat plane and arranged regularly along the branches. It is a common roadside and farmland species of the Pacific slope, not in the forest [33]. The root wood and root bark hexane extracts demonstrated an *in vitro* antimalarial activity against chloroquine-resistance (FcB1/Colombia) strains of *P. falciparum* with IC_{50} of 4.7 ± 0.9 and 6.8 ± 0.6 μg/mL, respectively [30].

2.11 *Aspidosperma macrocarpon*

A. macrocarpon Mart. (Apocynaceae) is a deciduous tree with an open crown growing up to 3–25 m tall and 25-35 cm in diameter. It is a timber tree, native to Brazil, Venezuela, Bolivia, Paraguay and Peru. Traditionally, it is employed in the treatment of fever [33]. The *in vitro* antiplasmodial study of the ethanol extract revealed an effective activity against *P. falciparum* (chloroquine-resistance FcB1/Colombia) with an IC_{50} of 4.9 ± 1.1 μg/mL [30].

2.12 *Azadirachta indica*

A. indica A. Juss is commonly known as neem tree or Indian lilac and belongs to the mahogany family Meliaceae. It is an evergreen, fast-growing tree that can reach a height of 15–20 m with few of them growing up to 35–40 m, but in severe drought it may shed most of its leaves or nearly all leaves. It is typically grown in tropical and semi-tropical regions. Neem is effective against certain fungi that infect humans and hence used to treat skin diseases like eczema, psoriasis [34]. The 80% methanol leaf extract showed *in vitro* anti-plasmodial activity against chloroquine and pyrimethamine sensitive, 3D7 strain, and chloroquine resistant and pyrimethamine sensitive, Dd2 strain, with IC_{50} of 5.8 and 1.7 μg/mL, respectively [35].

2.13 *Harrisonia abyssinica*

H. abyssinica Oliv. of the family Rutaceae, is a spiny, evergreen shrub that branches from the base and can become a spreading or much-branched tree. It usually grows up to 6–13 m tall and commonly found in Tropical Africa, in the areas of Sierra Leone, Cameroon, Sudan, Ethiopia, Uganda, Kenya, Angola, Zambia and Mozambique [33]. The methanolic stem bark extract inhibited chloroquine resistant *P. falciparum* strain Dd2, with IC_{50} value of 4.7 ± 0.113 while in chloroquine sensitive *P. falciparum* strain 3D7, the IC_{50} value was 10 ± 0.114 μg/mL [35].

2.14 *Maytenus senegalensis*

M. senegalensis Lam. Exell which belongs to the family Celastraceae is an African shrubs or trees widely distributed throughout Central and South America, Southeast Asia, Micronesia and Australasia, the Indian Ocean and Africa, growing up to 15 m high with spines up to 7 cm long. Traditionally, it is an anti-inflammatory herbal drug and is useful in treating toothaches [36]. The stem bark methanol extract showed anti-plasmodial activity with IC_{50} of 3.9 and 10 μg/mL when treated *in vitro* on chloroquine sensitive, 3D7 and chloroquine resistant, Dd2 strains, respectively [35].

3. Medicinal plants with demonstrated activity against *Vibrio cholera*

Cholera is an acute intestinal disease caused by a facultative anaerobic, Gram-negative, comma-shaped rod bacterium, known as *V. cholerae*. Cholera is a life threatening disease transmitted by the fecal-oral route. The organisms adhere to and colonize the small bowel within a short incubation period, where they secrete cholera enterotoxin leading to severe and watery diarrhea accompanied with vomiting, dehydration and eventually death if not treated promptly [37]. Various antibiotics have been effective for the treatment of cholera; however, the worldwide problem of microbial resistance to existing antimicrobial medicines has led to most antibiotic failure. Researchers are therefore shifting their focus to natural products, especially medicinal plant, with effective antimicrobial properties. Some medicinal plants with potent anti-cholera activity are reviewed below.

3.1 *Terminalia chebula*

T. chebula Retz. (Combretaceae) commonly known as black or chebulic myrobalan is a medium to large deciduous tree growing up to 30 m tall, with a trunk of 1 m in diameter. It leaves are oval, alternate to subopposite in arrangement and is a native to South Asia, from India and Nepal east to southwest China, Sri Lanka, Malaysia and Vietnam. Traditionally, it has been used for treatment of indigestion, diarrhea and diabetes [38]. The plant extract used to treat Cholera worked effectively against the strains of *V. cholera* the causative agent. The methanol fruit extract of *T. chebula* had strong bactericidal activity with MIC ranging from 0.125 to 1.5 mg/mL and MBC ranging from 0.25 to 2 mg/mL, against multi-drug resistance strains of *V. cholerae* (serotypes O1, O139, and non-O1, non-O139) [39].

3.2 *Syzygium cumini*

S. cumini (L.) Skeels (Myrtaceae), known as Jam is an evergreen tropical tree, native to the Indian Subcontinent, adjoining regions of Southeast Asia, China and Queensland. It Grows up to 30 m and can live more than 100 years, with a dense foliage which provides shade and is grown just for its ornamental value. The leaves are pinkish when young, and changes to dark green with a yellow midrib as they mature [40]. The seeds have traditionally been used to treat diarrhea, dysentery, piles, indigestion and diabetes. *S. cumini* methanol seed extract exhibited a bactericidal anti-cholera activity against multi-drug resistance strains of *V. cholerae* (serotypes O1, O139, and non-O1, non-O139), with MICs and MBCs ranging from 1.25–3 mg/mL [39]. Also Sharma et al. [41] reported the *in vitro* anti-vibrio activity of the ethanolic stem bark extract against different strains of *V. cholera* with MICS ranging from 2.5 to 20 mg/mL.

3.3 *Saraca indica*

S. indica auct. L. commonly known as Asoka-tree or Ashok is a plant belonging to the Detarioideae subfamily of the Fabaceae family. Asoka tree is an evergreen tree with a spreading crown which can grow up to 24 m tall and 34 cm in diameter. The original plant specimen came from Java. Some traditional uses of the plant include treatment of dyspepsia, fever, burning sensation, colic, ulcers, menorrhagia, leucorrhoea, pimples [42]. *S. indica* evoked strong bactericidal activity against different strains of multi-drug resistance *V. cholera*, with MBCs ranging from 1 to 4 mg/mL [39]. A study by Sharma et al. [41] also showed the anti-vibrio potential of the ethanolic stem bark extract, with MICs range of 2.5–10 mg/mL against 13 strains of *V. cholera*.

3.4 *Butea monosperma*

B. monosperma (Lam.) Taub. (Papilionaceae) is a native to tropical and subtropical parts of the Indian Subcontinent and Southeast Asia, ranging across India, Bangladesh, Nepal, Sri Lanka, Myanmar, Thailand, Laos, Cambodia, Vietnam, Malaysia and western Indonesia. Common names include flame-of-the-forest and bastard teak. It is a medium-sized dry season-deciduous tree, growing to 15 m tall. Leaves are pinnate, with (8–16 cm) petiole and three leaflets of 10–20 cm long. Its flowers are used in traditional medicine for the treatment of ulcer, inflammation, hepatic disorder and eye diseases [43]. The methanol flower extract showed anti-cholera activity with MIC and MBC ranging from 1.75 to 5 mg/mL against different strains of multi-drug resistance *V. cholera* [39].

3.5 *Euphorbia serpens*

E. serpens Kunth is a member of the Euphorbiaceae family. It is native to South America but it can be found on most continents as an introduced species and often a weed. This is an annual herb forming a mat of prostrate stems [44]. Purified bioactive fraction of aqueous extract of *E. serpens* exhibited an anti-Vibrio activity at a Minimum Inhibitory Concentration of 3.92 mg/mL [45].

3.6 *Acacia farnesiana*

Vachellia farnesiana, also known as *A. farnesiana* (L.) Willd, commonly known as sweet acacia or needle bush, is a species of shrub or small tree in the legume family, Fabaceae. The species grows to a height of 4.6–9.1 m and grows multiple trunks. *V. farnesiana* has been used in Colombia to treat malaria, in the Philippines the leaves are traditionally rubbed on the skin to treat skin diseases in livestock. In Malaysia, an infusion of the plant's flowers and leaves is mixed with turmeric for post-partum treatment [46]. The bark methanolic extract revealed a potent bactericidal activity against two strains of *V. cholera*, O139 (AI-1837) and O1 (569-B) with MBCs of 0.5 ± 0.1 and 0.9 ± 0.1, respectively [47].

3.7 *Artemisia ludoviciana*

A. ludoviciana (Nutt.) White sagebrush of the family Asteraceae is native to North America where it is widespread across most of the United States, Canada and Mexico. It is a rhizomatous perennial plant growing to height of 0.33–1 m. Medicinally, it is used for dermatological purposes and for treating cold [48]. The anti-cholera activity of the methanol whole plant extract was effective and bactericidal against O139 (AI-1837) and O1 (569-B) *V. cholera* strains. The minimum bactericidal concentrations against the two strains were 0.7 ± 0.2 and 1 ± 0.3, respectively [47].

3.8 *Ocimum basilicum*

O. basilicum (L.) Basil (Lamiaceae) can be found in Tropical Asia. It is a perennial growing up to 0.5 m tall and by 0.3 m in diameter. Medicinally it is used for the treatment of fever, colds, influenza, poor digestion, nausea, abdominal cramps, gastro-enteritis, migraine, insomnia, depression and exhaustion [49]. The methanol whole plant extract exhibited a bactericidal activity against *V. cholera* O139 (AI-1837) and O1 (569-B) strains with MBCs of 2 ± 0.6 and 3 ± 0.5, respectively [47].

3.9 *Opuntia ficus*

O. ficus-indica (L.) of the family Cactaceae is species of cactus that has long been domesticated. It is commonly known as prickly pear or Nopal cactus. It originated from Mexico and cultivated in other parts of the world including Mediterranean Basin, Middle East and northern Africa [50]. A study by Sánchez et al. [47], revealed the anti-cholera activity of the methanol cladode extract of *O. ficus*, with minimum bactericidal concentrations against O139 (AI-1837) and O1 (569-B) *V. cholera* strains to be 3 ± 0.05 and 3 ± 0.1, respectively.

3.10 *Lawsonia inermis*

L. inermis Linn. (Apocynaceae) commonly known in India as Henna is a flowering plant and the sole species of the genus Lawsonia. It is a tall shrub or small tree, standing 1.8–7.6 m tall, glabrous and multi-branched, with spine-tipped branchlets. The henna plant is native to northern Africa, western and southern Asia, northern Australia, and thrives well in semi-arid zones and tropical areas. It is useful medicinally for burning sensation, leprosy, skin diseases, amenorrhoea, and dysmenorrhea and as abortifacient [51]. The ethanolic leaf extract exhibited an *in vitro* anti-vibrio activity with MICs ranging from 2.5 to 10 mg/mL against 13 strains of *V. cholera* [41].

4. Medicinal plants with demonstrated anti-tuberculosis activity

Tuberculosis (TB) is an airborne infectious disease which does not only affect the lungs but also other parts of the body such as the brain and spine [52]. The main cause of TB is *Mycobacterium tuberculosis*. Other *M. tuberculosis* complex that causes TB include *M. bovis*, *M. africanum*, *M. canetti* and *M. microti* [53]. The predominant symptoms of active TB are fever, night sweat, weight loss and chronic cough with blood containing sputum. However, most TB infections are latent which may progress into active disease if left untreated [52]. Treatment of TB is very tedious and requires a long course with multiple antibiotics involved. However, this fastidious bacteria have become resistant to most antibiotics, and hence researchers are working tirelessly to come up with new and effective products especially from natural products such as medicinal plant. Some medicinal plants that have been investigated to possess active anti-tuberculosis activity are reviewed below.

4.1 *Anogeissus leiocarpa*

A. leiocarpa (Combretaceae) commonly called African birch is a tall deciduous tree which is indigenous to the savannas of tropical Africa. Traditionally, its stem and root barks are used to treat gonorrhea, worm infestation, cough, asthma and tuberculosis [54]. The susceptibility of clinical isolates of *M. tuberculosis* to the methanolic extract of *A. leiocarpa* was investigated using the broth dilution method. The results demonstrated anti-mycobacterial property (MIC 78 μg/mL). *A. leiocarpa* fraction showed an increased anti-mycobacterial activity (MIC 7.8 μg/mL) [55].

4.2 *Terminalia avicennioides*

T. avicennioides (Combretaceae) is a tree commonly found in West Africa. Its root bark, fruit and mistletoes are used traditionally to treat diarrhea, hemoptysis, sore throat, TB, asthma and cough [54]. The *in vitro* antibacterial studies using broth dilution method of methanolic extract of *T. avicennioides* showed a significant anti-mycobacterial activity (MIC 78 μg/mL) against clinical isolates of *M. tuberculosis.* The n-hexane and ethyl acetate fractions obtained from the crude methanol extract of *T. avicennioides* showed inhibitory activity (MIC 200 and 625 μg/mL, respectively) against attenuated strains of *M. bovis*. A further study of *T. avicennioides* fraction obtained demonstrated anti-mycobacterial activity (MIC 4.7 μg/mL) [55].

4.3 *Capparis brassii*

C. brassii (Capparidaceae), the narrow-leaf caper bush is distributed in the coastal forest and mixed woodland from tropical West Africa to South-East Africa. The root bark is used to treat TB in folk medicine [54]. The methanol extract of *C. brassii* has demonstrated some level of anti-mycobacterial activity (MIC 1.25 mg/mL) against clinically isolated strains of *M. tuberculosis* [55].

4.4 *Combretum* spp.

Combretum (Combretaceae) commonly called the bush willows has about 370 species of shrubs and trees, predominant in southern and tropical Africa,

Madagascar, Asia and tropical America. Traditionally, its root and stem barks are used to treat cough, bronchitis and TB [54]. The methanol extract exhibited anti-mycobacterial activity (MIC 1.25 mg/mL) against *M. tuberculosis* clinical isolates when evaluated in vitro using the broth microdilution method [55].

4.5 *Solanum torvum*

S. torvum (Solanaceae) also called turkey berry is an upright bushy and spiny perennial plant which is native to the Caribbean, southern Mexico, tropical and central America. However, it is also widely naturalized in the warmer and coastal regions of New South Wales, northern and eastern Australia, tropical Africa, Asia, Papua New Guinea, South-Eastern USA and on several pacific islands. The juice from this plant is used for the treatment of fever, sore throat, dropsy, rheumatism, gonorrhea, stomach ache, chest ailment, and asthma, while leaves and fruits can also be used to control a wide range of microbial activity [56]. The crude leave extract of *S. torvum* has demonstrated a significant inhibitory activity against two stains of *M. tuberculosis* (H37Ra and H37Rv) with MIC of 156.3 and 1250 μg/mL, respectively [57].

4.6 *Galenia africana*

G. africana (Aizoaceae) is an upright green to yellow-green aromatic woody perennial shrublet commonly found on the western and southern edges of Karoo [16]. The ethanolic extract of *G. africana* demonstrated anti-mycobacterial activity (MIC 1.2 mg/mL) against *M. tuberculosis.* A further study of flavone, 5,7,2′-trihydroxyflavone which was isolated from *G. africana* showed an increased activity (MIC 0.1 mg/mL) against *M. tuberculosis* [58].

4.7 *Allium sativum*

A. sativum (Amaryllidaceae) popularly called garlic is a bulbous plant, native to northern and eastern Iran and Central Asia [59], however, garlic can grow in the wild and in places where it has become naturalized. During World War I and II, garlic was used as an antiseptic to prevent gangrene [60]. Aside its reported nutritional value, garlic can demonstrate antimicrobial effect at temperature as high as 120°C. The aqueous and ethanolic extracts of *A. sativum* has shown anti-tuberculosis activity (MIC 0.05 and 0.1 mg/mL, respectively) against *M. tuberculosis*, H37Ra via the use of Microplate Alamar Blue Assay (MABA) [61]. A study by Gupta et al. [62] also showed the inhibitory activity of *A. sativum* against multidrug resistant isolates DKU-156 and JAL-1236, as well as sensitive *M. tuberculosis* H37Ra with percentage inhibition of 72, 72 and 63%, respectively.

4.8 *Allium cepa*

A. cepa commonly called onions is from the family Liliaceae. Onions have several pharmacological activity such as antidiabetic, antioxidant, anticancer, cardiovascular, antimicrobial and others [63]. The minimum inhibitory concentration by which the ethanolic and aqueous extracts of the tissue of *A. cepa* inhibited the growth of *M. tuberculosis* H37Ra was recorded to be 0.1 mg/mL for both extracts [61]. Another *in vitro* study showed a 79% proportion of inhibition of aqueous extract of the bulb of *A. cepa* against MDR isolate JAL-1236 [62].

4.9 *Cinnamomum verum*

C. verum, (formerly *C. zeylanicum*) of the family Lauraceae, commonly known as cinnamon tree is an evergreen small tropical plant native to Sri Lanka, it is also cultivated in Madagascar and Seychelles on commercial scale [33]. Its anti-tuberculosis activity reported by Sivakumar and Jayaraman, [61] revealed that, the aqueous and ethanolic extracts of the bark of *C. verum* exhibited anti-mycobacterial activity (MIC 0.1 and 0.2 mg/mL, respectively) against *M. tuberculosis* H37Ra.

4.10 *Acalypha indica*

A. indica popularly known as Indian nettle is from the family Euphorbiaceae. In Africa, it is distributed in Nigeria, from eastern part of Sudan to Somalia and south through DR Congo and East Africa to Southern Africa. It also occurs in South-East Asia, India, Oceania and widely in the Indian Ocean islands. Traditionally, it is used as an antifungal and antibacterial agent for both human and plant pathogens. It is also used as an expectorant to treat pneumonia and asthma [33]. The *in-vitro* study of the aqueous leave extract of *A. indica* against MDR isolate DKU-156, JAL-1236 and sensitive *M. tuberculosis* H37Rv, demonstrated 95, 68 and 68% inhibition, respectively [62].

5. Medicinal plants with demonstrated activity against pneumonia

Pneumonia is a respiratory tract infection characterized by the inflammation of one or both lungs as a results of the accumulation of pus in the alveoli. Pneumonia which can be caused by bacteria, viruses or fungi can be mild, severe or life threatening. Bacterial pneumonia can be caused by *Streptococcus pneumoniae* which is the commonest cause, *Staphylococcus aureus*, *Moraxella catarrhalis*, *Klebsiella pneumoniae*, *Haemophilus influenza*, *Chlamydophila pneumonia* and *Legionella pneumophila*. *Pneumocystis jirovecii pneumonia* (PCP) is a fungal pneumonia commonly found in immunocompromised patients. Viral pneumonia can also be caused by adenovirus, Varicella zoster, Influenza virus and respiratory syncytial virus [64, 65]. Traditionally, medicinal plants have been employed for treating pneumonia and hence the need to prove, scientifically, their folkloric uses. Researchers have investigated such plant, and below is a review on some of the reported plants with demonstrated activity.

5.1 *Echinops adenocaulos*

In Ethiopian herbal medicine, members of the genus *Echinops* from family Asteraceae are used for the treatment of diarrhea, intestinal worm infestation, hemorrhoids, migraine and different forms of infections [66]. Zamzam water extract of *E. adenocaulos* demonstrated an antibacterial activity against multidrug resistance *S. pneumoniae* with a minimum inhibitory concentration (MIC) of 0.781 mg/mL [67].

5.2 *Verbascum fruticulosum*

Various species of *Verbascum*, of the family Scrophulariaceae, have been used to treat pulmonary diseases in traditional medicine as a results of its antibacterial activity against *Klebsiella pneumonia* and *Staphylococcus aureus* [68]. The *in vitro* antimicrobial activity of aqueous extract of *V. fruticulosum* against multidrug resistant clinical isolate of *S. pneumoniae* showed a high antibacterial activity with MIC value of 0.195 mg/mL [67].

5.3 *Parietaria judaica*

P. judaica commonly known as pellitory of wall from family Urticaceae has been valued for its use as a diuretic, balm for wounds and burns and also as a soother for chronic cough in herbal medicine [69]. The micro-broth dilution method was used to study the inhibitory activity of aqueous extract of *P. Judaica.* The extract was able to inhibit multidrug resistant *S. pneumonia* at an MIC value of 3.125 mg/mL [67].

5.4 *Urtica urens*

U. urens commonly known as dwarf nettle or annual nettle from family Urticaceae is used medicinally for the treatment of pulmonary diseases [70]. A study by Saleh Fares et al. [67] on the inhibitory activity of the aqueous extract of this plant against multidrug resistant clinical isolates of *S. pneumoniae*, using micro-broth dilution method, gave an MIC of 6.25 mg/mL. This illustrates its potential to be used as medicine in the treatment pneumonia caused by multidrug resistant *S. pneumoniae.*

5.5 *Beta vulgaris*

B. vulgaris popularly known as sugar beet from family Amaranthaceae is a sugar producing plant. Sugar-producing plants contain bioactive compounds, which are active against microbes and hence are able to protect the sugar from fermenting or from undergoing any alteration [71]. The study of the antimicrobial activity of the crude ethanolic leaf (lamina and midrib) extracts as well as fractions (n-hexane and chloroform) against *K. pneumonia,* showed zones of growth inhibition at different concentrations tested. At 1 mg/12 μL, the lamina and midrib crude extracts recorded 19 and 9 mm inhibition zone. The chloroform lamina and midrib fraction recorded 12 and 14 mm at concentration 1 mg/6 μL, while at concentration 1 mg/12 μL, their inhibition zones were 15 and 20 mm, respectively. Also the n-hexane lamina and midrib fractions had 20 and 16 mm inhibition zones (1 mg/6 μL),while 36 and 32 mm zones of inhibition (1 mg/12 μL) were recorded, respectively [72].

6. Medicinal plants with demonstrated anti-asthmatic activity

Asthma is a complex inflammatory disease and congestive respiratory disorder brought about by airway narrowing. It symptoms may include episodic wheezing, cough and chest tightness resulting in airflow block. It leads to changes in the levels of eosinophils, mast cells, lymphocytes, cytokines and other inflammatory cell products. There is increased prevalence worldwide especially in industrialized countries and among children with increased morbidity and mortality rate [73, 74]. Medicinal plants have been screened for properties that enhance their activity as anti-asthmatic agents, since current medications have adverse side effects. Few of such plants with demonstrated activity are reviewed below.

6.1 *Curcuma longa*

C. longa L. is a rhizomatous herbaceous perennial flowering plant of the ginger family, Zingiberaceae. It is native to the Indian subcontinent and Southeast Asia, and requires temperatures between 20 and 30°C and a considerable amount of annual rainfall to thrive. Methanolic extracts (curcumin-II at 200 mg/kg and curcumin-I at 100 mg/kg) of the finger rhizomes of *C. longa* reduced significantly ($P < 0.01$) estimated white blood cells count in ovalbumin (OVA) sensitized Wistar rat models for both long and short term. At a higher dosage, curcumin-II (200 mg/kg) tends to protect intact mast cells from degranulation [3]. This suggests that curcumin can be used as complementary medicine in the treatment of Asthma.

6.2 *Aerva lanata*

A. lanata (L.) A. L. Juss. ex Schult (Amaranthaceae) is a perennial herb, frequently becoming more or less woody at the base. The stems can be erect to prostrate, sometimes scrambling or climbing into other plants for support. It is widespread in the tropics and subtropics of Africa through Asia to the Philippines and New Guinea. It is used traditionally for treating cough, sore throat, indigestion, wounds, and diabetics and as a vermifuge for children [75]. The ethanol extract of aerial parts of *A. lanata* at 100 μg/mL significantly ($^{***}p < 0.01$) exhibited percentage decreased contraction in the isolated goat tracheal chain preparation model. Also in clonidine induced mast cell degranulation, the extract at 30 and 60 mg/kg administered orally, showed percentage protection of 64.2 and 68.9%, respectively [76].

6.3 *Cynodon dactylon*

C. dactylon (L.) Pers, of the family Poaceae is a short-lived, prostrate, perennial grass. It is widely naturalized in the temperate to tropical zones of Europe, Africa, Asia, the Pacific and the Americas. Its habitat is along roadsides and in exposed rocky or sandy sites. It use in traditional medicine to stop bleeding in minor injuries, for weak vision and eye disorders, piles, asthma, tumors among others [77]. The findings of Savali et al. [78], indicated that isolated *C. dactylon* compound was potent and has significant ($p < 0.01$ and $p < 0.001$) inhibitory effect on compound 48/80 induced anaphylactic reaction and mast cell activation. Also, compound 48/80 induced increased level of nitric oxide in rat serum and rat peritoneal mast cells were significantly inhibited.

6.4 *Piper betle*

P. betle L. (Piperaceae) commonly referred to as Betel pepper, is an evergreen climbing shrub producing woody stems, 5–20 m long, and distributed in Southeast Asia—probably originally from Malaysia. It is traditionally used to cure cough, cold, pruritis, asthma and rheumatism [79]. Ethanol and aqueous extract of leaves at doses 100 and 200 mg/kg possesses anti-asthmatic activity on histamine induced bronchoconstriction in guinea pig and histamine induced dose dependent contraction of guinea pig tracheal chain [80].

6.5 *Lepidium sativum*

L. sativum L. (Brassicaceae) also referred to as Garden cress is a profusely-branched, erect, annual plant growing up to 80 cm tall [81]. It commonly grown in many regions of Saudi Arabia and the Eastern Province. The seeds are used to cure bronchitis, asthma, cough, and useful as abortifacient, antibacterial, aphrodisiac, diuretic, expectorant, gastrointestinal stimulant, gastroprotective, laxative and stomachic [82]. The bronchodilatory effect of ethanolic seed extract and ethyl acetate, n-butanol and methanol fractions, against histamine and acetylcholine induced acute bronchospasm in guinea pigs, exhibited significant inhibition of bronchospasm, with n-butanol fraction showing a significant ($p < 0.001$) protection comparable to the reference standards used in the study [83]. Rehman et al. [84] also confirmed the bronchodilatory effect of *L. sativum* crude extract by investigating the various pathways for its activity in airway disorders. It was revealed that, the extract's activity was mediated through a combination of anticholinergic, Ca^{++} antagonist and phosphodiesterase inhibitory pathways.

6.6 *Curculigo orchioides*

C. orchioides Gaertn. (Hypoxidaceae) is a stemless evergreen perennial herb producing a cluster of leaves from the roots and spreading to form a clump. It grows up to 50 cm tall. It ranges from East Asia—South China, Japan, Indian subcontinent, Myanmar, Thailand, Cambodia, Laos, Vietnam, Malaysia, Indonesia, Philippines, New Guinea, W. Pacific. Alcoholic extract of *C. orchioides* rhizomes at doses (100–400 mg/kg) shows mast cell stabilizing and antihistaminic activity on Compound 48/80-induced mast cell degranulation and systemic anaphylaxis [85]. Also Pandit et al. [86] established the usefulness of the ethanol extract in treating asthma, as it was reported to exhibit significant relaxant effect ($p < 0.01$) at concentrations 100 and 25 μg/mL in isolated goat tracheal chain and isolated guinea pig ileum preparations respectively. In an *in vivo* study using histamine induced bronchoconstriction in guinea pigs, egg albumin induced passive paw anaphylaxis in rats and haloperidol-induced catalepsy in mice, there was significant ($p < 0.01$) protection at lower doses. Again, maximum increase in leucocytes and lymphocytes (99%) and maximum decrease in eosinophils up to 0% at dose 375 mg/kg p.o. was reported in milk-induced total leukocytes and differential leukocyte counts.

6.7 *Casuarina equisetifolia*

C. equisetifolia L. (Casuarinaceae) also commonly known as Common Ru, is an evergreen tree with a finely branched, feathery crown usually growing from 6 to 35 m and 20–100 cm in diameter. The tree is widely planted throughout the tropics, and ranges from East Asia to Bangladesh, Myanmar, Thailand, Vietnam, Malaysia, Indonesia, Philippines, Australia and the Pacific [87]. The methanol extract of wood and bark (10–80 mcg/mL) exhibited a significant dose dependent ($p < 0.05$) antihistaminic activity by inhibiting the histamine induced contraction of trachea. The wood extract (100 mg/kg, i.p.) significantly reduced clonidine induced catalepsy ($p < 0.05$) and mast cell degranulation ($p < 0.001$) [88].

7. Conclusion

All the plants reviewed exhibited potent activity confirming their various traditional uses and their ability to treat prevalent diseases. There is therefore the need to subject these plants to further studies, by isolating active compounds which can be processed into new and potent medicines and the need to study their mechanisms of action.

Author details

Susana Oteng Mintah[1*], Tonny Asafo-Agyei[2], Mary-Ann Archer[3], Peter Atta-Adjei Junior[2], Daniel Boamah[1], Doris Kumadoh[6], Alfred Appiah[4], Augustine Ocloo[4], Yaw Duah Boakye[5] and Christian Agyare[5]

1 Department of Microbiology, Center for Plant Medicine Research, Akuapem-Mampong, Ghana

2 Plant Development Department, Center for Plant Medicine Research, Akuapem-Mampong, Ghana

3 Department of Pharmaceutics, Center for Plant Medicine Research, Akuapem-Mampong, Ghana

4 Center for Plant Medicine Research, Akuapem-Mampong, Ghana

5 Department of Pharmaceutics, Faculty of Pharmacy and Pharmaceutical Sciences, Kwame Nkrumah University of Science and Technology, Kumasi, Ghana

6 Department of Pharmacology, Faculty of Pharmacy and Pharmaceutical Sciences, Kwame Nkrumah University of Science and Technology, Kumasi, Ghana

*Address all correspondence to: somintah@cpmr.org.gh

References

[1] Shrestha PM, Dhillion SS. Medicinal plant diversity and use in the highlands of Dolakha district, Nepal. Journal of Ethnopharmacology. 2003;**86**(1):81-96

[2] Asase A, Kokubun T, Grayer RJ, Kite G, Simmonds MSJ, Oteng-Yeboah AA, et al. Chemical constituents and antimicrobial activity of medicinal plants from Ghana: *Cassia sieberiana*, *Haematostaphis barteri*, *Mitragyna inermis* and *Pseudocedrela kotschyi*. Phytotherapy Research. 2008;**22**(8):1013-1016

[3] Sarkar S, Zaidi S, Chaturvedi AK, Srivastava R, Dwivedi PK, Shukla R. Search for a herbal medicine: Anti-asthmatic activity of methanolic extract of *Curcuma longa*. Journal of Pharmacognosy and Phytochemistry. 2015;**3**:59-72

[4] Fischer PR, Bialek R. Prevention of malaria in children. Clinical Infectious Diseases. 2002;**34**(4):493-498

[5] WHO. World Malaria Report 2014. Washington, DC: World Health Organization; 2015

[6] Tabuti JRS. Herbal medicines used in the treatment of malaria in Budiope county, Uganda. Journal of Ethnopharmacology. 2008;**116**(1):33-42

[7] Zirihi GN, Mambu L, Guédé-Guina F, Bodo B, Grellier P. In vitro antiplasmodial activity and cytotoxicity of 33 West African plants used for treatment of malaria. Journal of Ethnopharmacology. 2005;**98**(3):281-285

[8] Basco LK, Mitaku S, Skaltsounis A-L, Ravelomanantsoa N, Tillequin F, Koch M, et al. In vitro activities of furoquinoline and acridone alkaloids against *Plasmodium falciparum*. Antimicrobial Agents and Chemotherapy. 1994;**38**(5):1169-1171

[9] Chiyaka C, Garira W, Dube S. Effects of treatment and drug resistance on the transmission dynamics of malaria in endemic areas. Theoretical Population Biology. 2009;**75**(1):14-29

[10] Ameyaw Y. Morpho-histological characters for the identification of *Cryptolepis sanguinolenta* (Lindl.) Schtr. International Journal ofScience and Nature. 2012;**3**(2):331-339

[11] Irvine FR. Woody plants of Ghana. In: Woody Plants of Ghana. England, UK: Oxford University Press; 1961

[12] Boye GL, Ampofo O. Proceedings of the First International Symposium on Cryptolepine. Kumasi, Ghana: University of Science and Technology; 1983

[13] Wright CW, Phillipson JD, Awe SO, Kirby GC, Warhurst DC, Quetin-Leclercq J, et al. Antimalarial activity of cryptolepine and some other anhydronium bases. Phytotherapy Research. 1996;**10**(4):361-363

[14] Paulo A, Gomes ET, Steele J, Warhurst DC, Houghton PJ. Antiplasmodial activity of *Cryptolepis sanguinolenta* alkaloids from leaves and roots. Planta Medica. 2000;**66**(01):30-34

[15] Bugyei KA, Boye GL, Addy ME. Clinical efficacy of a tea-bag formulation of *Cryptolepis sanguinolenta* root in the treatment of acute uncomplicated falciparum malaria. Ghana Medical Journal. 2010;**44**(1):3-9

[16] Burkill HM. The Useful Plants of West Tropical Africa. 2nd ed. Vol. 1. Kew: Royal Botanic Gardens; 1985

[17] Oliver-Bever BEP. Medicinal Plants in Tropical West Africa. England: Cambridge University Press; 1986

[18] Agyare C, Asase A, Lechtenberg M, Niehues M, Deters A, Hensel A. An

ethnopharmacological survey and in vitro confirmation of ethnopharmacological use of medicinal plants used for wound healing in Bosomtwi-Atwima-Kwanwoma area, Ghana. Journal of Ethnopharmacology. 2009;**125**(3):393-403

[19] Komlaga G, Cojean S, Dickson RA, Beniddir MA, Suyyagh-Albouz S, Mensah MLK, et al. Antiplasmodial activity of selected medicinal plants used to treat malaria in Ghana. Parasitology Research. 2016;**115**(8):3185-3195

[20] Annan K, Sarpong K, Asare C, Dickson R, Amponsah KI, Gyan B, et al. In vitro anti-plasmodial activity of three herbal remedies for malaria in Ghana: *Adenia cissampeloides* (Planch.) Harms., *Termina liaivorensis* A. Chev, and *Elaeis guineensis* Jacq. Pharmacognosy Research. 2012;**4**(4):225

[21] Henson IE. A brief history of the oil palm. In: Palm Oil. Amsterdam, Netherlands: Elsevier; 2012. pp. 1-29

[22] Mshana NR. Traditional Medicine and Pharmacopoeia: Contribution to the Revision of Ethnobotanical and Floristic Studies in Ghana. Accra, Ghana: Organization of African Unity/ Scientific, Technical & Research Commission; 2000. 920 p

[23] Calixto JB, Santos ARS, Filho VC, Yunes RA. A review of the plants of the genus Phyllanthus: Their chemistry, pharmacology, and therapeutic potential. Medicinal Research Reviews. 1998;**18**(4):225-258

[24] Gaire BP, Subedi L. Phytochemistry, pharmacology and medicinal properties of *Phyllanthus emblica* Linn. Chinese Journal of Integrative Medicine. 2014:1-8. DOI: 10.1007/s11655-014-1984-2

[25] Mirunalini S, Krishnaveni M. Therapeutic potential of *Phyllanthus emblica* (amla): The ayurvedic wonder. Journal of Basic and Clinical Physiology and Pharmacology. 2010;**21**(1):93-105

[26] Bagavan A, Rahuman AA, Kaushik NK, Sahal D. In vitro antimalarial activity of medicinal plant extracts against *Plasmodium falciparum*. Parasitology Research. 2011;**108**(1):15-22

[27] Mittal M, Gupta N, Parashar P, Mehra V, Khatri M. Phytochemical evaluation and pharmacological activity of Syzygium aromaticum: A comprehensive review. International Journal of Pharmacy and Pharmaceutical Sciences. 2014;**6**(8):67-72

[28] Ichino C, Soonthornchareonnon N, Chuakul W, Kiyohara H, Ishiyama A, Sekiguchi H, et al. Screening of Thai medicinal plant extracts and their active constituents for in vitro antimalarial activity. Phytotherapy Research. 2006;**20**(4):307-309

[29] Sleumer HO. Flora neotropica: Monograph number 22. Flacourtiaceae. New York New York Bot Gard Organ Flora Neotrop 499p Illus, maps, keys. Icones, Maps Geog. 1980;4

[30] De Mesquita ML, Grellier P, Mambu L, De Paula JE, Espindola LS. In vitro antiplasmodial activity of Brazilian Cerrado plants used as traditional remedies. Journal of Ethnopharmacology. 2007;**110**(1):165-170

[31] Lorenzi H. Brazilian trees. Vol. 2. Brazil: Instituto plantarum de estudos da flora; 2002

[32] Luchi AE. Fibre pits in wood of Xylopia emarginata Mart. (Annonaceae), Reserva Biológica e Estação Ecológica de Mogi-Guaçu, São Paulo State, Brazil. Hoehnea. 2016;**43**(3):517-520

[33] Fern K, Fern A, Morris R. Useful tropical plants database. Recuper http// tropical theferns info. 2014

[34] Porter AH. Neem: India's Tree of Life. BBC News; 2006. p. 17

[35] El Tahir A, Satti GMH, Khalid SA. Antiplasmodial activity of selected Sudanese medicinal plants with emphasis on *Maytenus senegalensis* (Lam.) Exell. Journal of Ethnopharmacology. 1999;**64**(3):227-233

[36] Da Silva G, Serrano R, Silva O. *Maytenus heterophylla* and *Maytenus senegalensis*, two traditional herbal medicines. Journal of Natural Science, Biology and Medicine. 2011;**2**(1):59

[37] Finkelstein RA. Cholera, Vibrio Cholerae O1 and O139, and Other Pathogenic Vibrios, Chapter 24. Univ Texas Med Branch; 1996

[38] Wu Z, Raven PH, Hong D. Flora of China. Volume 5: Ulmaceae through Basellaceae. Beijing, and Missouri Botanical Garden Press, St. Louis: Science Press; 2003

[39] Acharyya S, Patra A, Bag PK. Evaluation of the antimicrobial activity of some medicinal plants against enteric bacteria with particular reference to multi-drug resistant Vibrio cholerae. Tropical Journal of Pharmaceutical Research. 2009;**8**(3):231-237

[40] Govaerts RHA, Faden RB. World Checklist of Selected Plant Families. Kew: Royal Botanic Gardens; 2013

[41] Sharma A, Patel VK, Chaturvedi AN. Vibriocidal activity of certain medicinal plants used in Indian folklore medicine by tribals of Mahakoshal region of Central India. Indian Journal of Pharmacology. 2009;**41**(3):129

[42] Srivastava GN, Bagchi GD, Srivastava AK. Pharmacognosy of Ashoka stem bark and its adulterants. International Journal of Crude Drug Research. 1988;**26**(2):65-72

[43] Muthuswamy R, Senthamarai R. Anatomical investigation of flower of Butea monosperma lam. Ancient Science of Life. 2014;**34**(2):73

[44] Hyde MA, Wursten BT, Ballings P, Palgrave CM. Flora of Zimbabwe: Species information. *Cardiospermum halicacabum*. 2011

[45] Payne A, Mukhopadhyay AK, Deka S, Saikia L, Nandi SP. Anti-vibrio and antioxidant properties of two weeds: *Euphorbia serpens* and *Amaranthus viridis*. Research Journal of Medicinal Plant. 2015;**9**:170-178

[46] US Department of Agriculture NRCS. The Plants Database. Greensboro, NC, USA: National Plant Data Team; 2012

[47] Sánchez E, García S, Heredia N. Extracts of edible and medicinal plants damage membranes of *Vibrio cholerae*. Applied and Environmental Microbiology. 2010;**76**(20):6888-6894

[48] Turner BL. The comps of Mexico: A systematic account of the family Asteraceae (chapter 8: Liabeae and Vernonieae). Phytologia Memoirs. 2007;**12**:1-144

[49] Chevallier A. The Encyclopaedia of Medicinal Plants—A Practical Reference Guide to over 550 Key Herbs and their Medicinal Uses. London: DK Publishing; 1996

[50] Wiersema JH. Taxonomic information on cultivated plants in the USDA/ARS germplasm resources information network (GRIN). In: II International Symposium on Taxonomy of Cultivated Plants 413. 1994. pp. 109-116

[51] Warrier PK, Nambiar VPK. Indian Medicinal Plants: A Compendium of 500 Species. Vol. 5. Telangana, India: Orient Blackswan; 1993

[52] WHO. Tuberculosis Fact sheet N 104. 2015. Avaialble at: http://www.who.int/mediacentre/factsheets/fs104/en. 2015

[53] Van Soolingen D, Hoogenboezem T, De Haas PEW, Hermans PWM, Koedam MA, Teppema KS, et al. A novel pathogenic taxon of the *Mycobacterium tuberculosis* complex, Canetti: Characterization of an exceptional isolate from Africa. International Journal of Systematic and Evolutionary Microbiology. 1997;**47**(4):1236-1245

[54] Mann A, Amupitan JO, Oyewale AO, Okogun JI, Ibrahim K. An ethnobotanical survey of indigenous flora for treating tuberculosis and other respiratory diseases in Niger State, Nigeria. Journal of Phytomedicine and Therapeutics. 2007;**12**(1):1-21

[55] Mann A, Amupitan JO, Oyewale AO, Okogun JI, Ibrahim K, Oladosu P, et al. Evaluation of in vitro antimycobacterial activity of Nigerian plants used for treatment of respiratory diseases. African Journal of Biotechnology. 2008;**7**(11):1630-1636

[56] Manandhar NP. Plants and People of Nepal. Portland, Oregon: Timber Press; 2002

[57] Nguta JM, Appiah-Opong R, Nyarko AK, Yeboah-Manu D, Addo PGA, Otchere I, et al. Antimycobacterial and cytotoxic activity of selected medicinal plant extracts. Journal of Ethnopharmacology. 2016;**182**:10-15

[58] Mativandlela SPN, Meyer JJM, Hussein AA, Houghton PJ, Hamilton CJ, Lall N. Activity against *Mycobacterium smegmatis* and *M. tuberculosis* by extract of South African medicinal plants. Phytotherapy Research. 2008;**22**(6):841-845

[59] Block E. Garlic and other alliums: The lore and the science. Cambridge: Royal Society of Chemistry; 2010. pp. 454

[60] Tattelman E. Health effects of garlic. American Family Physician. 2005;**72**(1):103-106

[61] Sivakumar A, Jayaraman G. Anti-tuberculosis activity of commonly used medicinal plants of South India. Journal of Medicinal Plants Research. 2011;**5**(31):6881-6884

[62] Gupta R, Thakur B, Singh P, Singh HB, Sharma VD, Katoch VM, et al. Anti-tuberculosis activity of selected medicinal plants against multi-drug resistant *Mycobacterium tuberculosis* isolates. The Indian Journal of Medical Research. 2010;**131**(6):809

[63] Kuete V. Other health benefits of African medicinal spices and vegetables. In: Medicinal Spices and Vegetables from Africa. England: Elsevier; 2017. pp. 329-349

[64] van der Poll T, Opal SM. Pathogenesis, treatment, and prevention of pneumococcal pneumonia. Lancet. 2009;**374**(9700):1543-1556

[65] File TM Jr. Community-acquired pneumonia. Lancet. 2003;**362**(9400): 1991-2001

[66] Hymete A, Iversen T-H, Rohloff J, Erko B. Screening of *Echinops ellenbeckii* and *Echinops longisetus* for biological activities and chemical constituents. Phytomedicine. 2005;**12**(9):675-679

[67] Saleh Fares GO, Abdallah L, Almasri M, Slaileh A, Zurba Z. Antibacterial activity of selected Palestinian wild plant extracts against multidrug-resistant clinical isolate of Streptococcus pneumoniae. Journal of Pharmacy Research. 2013;**1**(10):963-969

[68] Turker AU, Camper ND. Biological activity of common mullein, a medicinal plant. Journal of Ethnopharmacology. 2002;**82**(2-3):117-125

[69] Giachetti D, Taddei E, Taddei I. Diuretic and uricosuric activity of *Parietaria judaica* L. Bollettino della Società Italiana di Biologia Sperimentale. 1986;**62**(2):197

[70] Ozkarsli M, Sevim H, Sen A. In vivo effects of Urtica urens (dwarf nettle) on the expression of CYP1A in control and

3-methylcholanthrene-exposed rats. Xenobiotica. 2008;**38**(1):48-61

[71] Srivastava R, Kulshreshtha DK. Bioactive polysaccharides from plants. Phytochemistry. 1989;**28**(11):2877-2883

[72] Hussain Z, Mohammad P, Sadozai SK, Khan KM, Nawaz Y, Perveen S. Extraction of anti-pneumonia fractions from the leaves of sugar beets *Beta vulgaris*. Journal of Pharmacy Research. 2011;**4**(12):4783

[73] Masoli M, Fabian D, Holt S, Beasley R. Program GI for A (GINA). The global burden of asthma: Executive summary of the GINA dissemination committee report. Allergy. 2004;**59**(5):469-478

[74] Braman SS. The global burden of asthma. Chest. 2006;**130**(1):4S-12S

[75] Umaramani M, Sivakanesan R. Vitamin C content of commonly eaten green leafy vegetables in fresh and under different storage conditions. Tropical Plant Research. 2015;**2**(3):240-245

[76] Kumar D, Prasad DN, Parkash J, Bhatnagar SP, Kumar D. Antiasthmatic activity of ethanolic extract of *Aerva lanata* Linn. Pharmacology Online. 2009;**2**:1075-1081

[77] Nandkarni AK. Indian Materia Medica. Vol I & II (Reprinted). Bombay: Popular Prakashan; 1982

[78] Savali AS, Biradar PR, Jirankali MC. Antianaphylactic and mast cell stabilization activity of *Cynodon dactylon*. International Journal of Pharmacy and Pharmaceutical Sciences. 2010;**2**(2):69-73

[79] Pradhan D, Suri KA, Pradhan DK, Biswasroy P. Golden heart of the nature: *Piper betle* L. Journal of Pharmacognosy and Phytochemistry. 2013;**1**(6):147-167

[80] Jawale NM, Shewale AB, Nerkar GS, Patil VR. Evalution of antihistaminic activity of leaves of *Piper betel* Linn. Pharmacology. 2009;**3**:966-977

[81] Facciola S. Cornucopia: A Source Book of Edible Plants. Vista, California: Kampong Publications; 1990

[82] Duke JA. Handbook of Medicinal Herbs. Boca Raton, Florida: CRC Press; 2002

[83] Mali R, Mahajan S, Mehta A. Studies on bronchodilatory effect of *Lepidium sativum* against allergen induced bronchospasm in Guinea pigs. Pharmacognosy Magazine. 2008;**4**(15):189

[84] Rehman N, Khan A, Alkharfy KM, Gilani A-H. Pharmacological basis for the medicinal use of *Lepidium sativum* in airways disorders. Evidence-Based Complementary and Alternative Medicine. 2012;**2012**:8

[85] Venkatesh P, Mukherjee PK, Nema NK, Bandyopadhyay A, Fukui H, Mizuguchi H. Mast cell stabilization and antihistaminic potentials of *Curculigo orchioides* rhizomes. Journal of Ethnopharmacology. 2009;**126**(3):434-436

[86] Pandit P, Singh A, Bafna AR, Kadam PV, Patil MJ. Evaluation of antiasthmatic activity of *Curculigo orchioides* Gaertn. Rhizomes. Indian Journal of Pharmaceutical Sciences. 2008;**70**(4):440

[87] Jensen M. Trees Commonly Cultivated in Southeast Asia: An Illustrated Field Guide. Vol. 38. Bangkok, Thailand: RAP Publ.; 1995. p. 93

[88] Aher AN, Pal SC, Patil UK, Yadav SK, Bhattacharya S. Evaluation of anthistaminic activity of *Casuarina equisetifolia* frost (Casuarinaceae). Pharmacology. 2009;**1**:1144-1149

Section 3

Bioactive Compounds

Chapter 10

Cytotoxic and Antitumoral Activities of Compounds Isolated from Cucurbitaceae Plants

Carlos Alberto Méndez-Cuesta, Ana Laura Esquivel Campos, David Salinas Sánchez, Cuauhtemoc Pérez González and Salud Pérez Gutiérrez

Abstract

The WHO says that annual cases of cancer will increase from 14 million in 2012 to 22 million in the next two decades. Cancer is the second cause of death in the world; in 2015, it caused 8.8 million deaths. On the other hand, it is necessary to consider that 70% of the total deaths due to this disease occur in developing countries, who have the least resources to acquire the drugs of choice for the treatment of this disease. Although there are treatments and these are effective, there are currently cases of resistance to drugs used to treat this disease, which has led to the search for new sources of drugs or compounds effective against the cancer being active; plants are the possible sources to achieve this. Cucurbitaceae is a family of plants widely distributed on the planet which has been used traditionally for the treatment of this disease and from they have been isolated different cucurbitanes. These compounds possess a wide biological activity, antidiabetic, anti-inflammatory, hepatoprotective, or cytotoxic and antitumoral effects. The aim of this review is to present 51 cucurbitacin compounds and 2 with different structures isolated from Cucurbitaceae plants with cytotoxic or antitumoral activity.

Keywords: cucurbitacin, Cucurbitaceae, cytotoxic, cancer, natural product

1. Introduction

Cancer is an abnormal growth of cells, which begin to divide without stopping and can form solid tumors. Cancer is a collection of more than 100 different diseases with genetic changes, which can be inherited or be caused by environmental exposure to chemicals, tobacco smoke, or radiation, such as UV rays from the sun.

Cancer is the second leading cause of death in the US and is responsible for approximately 1 out of every 4 deaths. Globally, nearly 1 in 6 deaths is due to cancer. Approximately, 70% of deaths from cancer occur in low- and middle-income countries. There were 14.1 million new cancer cases, 8.2 million cancer deaths, and 32.6 million people living with cancer (within 5 years of diagnosis) in 2012 worldwide, based on World Health Organization (WHO) estimates. A total of 57% (8 million) of new cancer cases, 65% (5.3 million) of cancer deaths, and 48% (15.6 million) of 5-year prevalent cancer cases occurred in less-developed regions [1, 2].

The most common treatments for cancer are surgery, chemotherapy, and radiation therapy, and in many cases, they are used in combination [3]. These treatments can be effective but can cause side effects, such as anemia, appetite loss, fatigue, and alopecia [4].

1.1 Generalities of the Cucurbitaceae family

Plants are an important source of compounds currently used in cancer chemotherapy. The Cucurbitaceae family, also called cucurbits, contains 120 genera with 825 species that are widely distributed in tropical and temperate regions [5], and those with edible fruits were the first cultivated plants in Europe and America. Many species of the Cucurbitaceae family are used as human food [6]. Most of the species in this family are annual vines, and some are lianas, thorny shrubs, or trees. The most important genera of this family are *Cucurbita* (squash, pumpkin, zucchini), *Lagenaria* (calabash), *Citrullus* (watermelon), *Cucumis* (cucumber, various melons), and *Luffa* (luffa).

1.2 Cucurbitanes of the Cucurbitaceae family with cytotoxic effects

Some cucurbitanes have been isolated from different species of the Cucurbitaceae family. These compounds exhibit an extensive range of biological actions, specifically antidiabetic, anti-inflammatory, cytotoxic, hepatoprotective, cardiovascular, and antiparasitic effects [7].

Cucurbitacins are characteristic compounds in many species of cucurbits. These compounds are tetracyclic triterpenes arising from a rearrangement of the protostane cation and are unsaturated and polyfunctional oxygenated compounds and occur most often as glycosides. They are particularly toxic and bitter chemicals, and their cytotoxicity contributes to their toxicity [8]. Cucurbitanes are found in many plants.

The most significant mechanisms of the apoptotic effects of cucurbitacins are their ability to modify the mitochondrial transmembrane potential and transcriptional activity via nuclear factors or genes and their ability to activate or inhibit pro- or antiapoptotic proteins.

Similar to other plant-derived compounds, cucurbitacins exert toxic effects in different cancer cell lines by inducing apoptosis. The main mechanism of this induction is the ability to modify the mitochondrial transmembrane potential [6].

Therefore, some compounds obtained from Cucurbitaceae could be useful scaffolds for developing new drugs. We consider it necessary to review the main chemicals from this genus with potential anticancer activity.

2. Cucurbitacins tetracyclic triterpenoids

Cucurbitacins are primarily tetracyclic triterpenoids (**Figure 1**) that compose a class of biochemical compounds contained in plants of the family Cucurbitaceae, which include the Thai medicinal plants *Trichosanthes cucumerina* L. and *T. kirilowii* Maximowicz, the leaves and fruits of the Tunisian plant *Ecballium elaterium*; the fruits of *Cucurbita pepo* cv. dayangua; the roots of *Cayaponia tayuya* (Tayuya), which has long been used in folk medicines from Brazil, Peru, and Colombia; *C. racemosa* Cong., the roots of *Hemsleya amabilis*, an ancient Chinese remedy, *Cucumis melo* L., *Momordica balsamina* L. (balsam pear), *Cucurbita andreana* (winter squash), and *Citrullus colocynthis* (bitter cucumber). Below, the most important cucurbitacins that have shown interesting cytotoxicity and anticancer activity are listed.

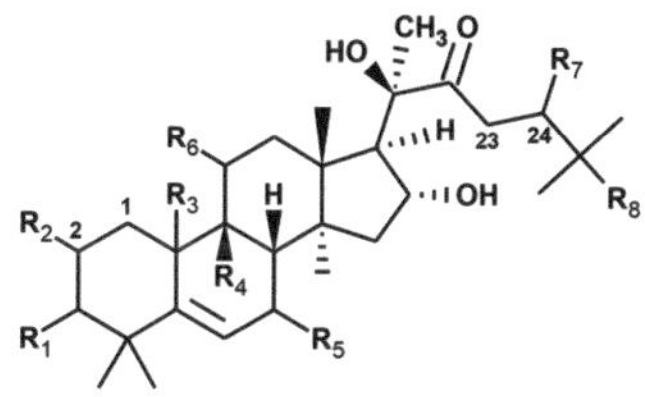

1′: R_1= Ketone, R_2= -OH(*S*), R_3= -H(*R*), R_4= -CH_3(*R*), R_5= -H, R_6= Ketone, R_7= H, R_8= -OAc, 1-2= Simple, 23-24= Double(E)
2′: R_1= Ketone, R_2= -OH(*S*), R_3= -H(*R*), R_4= -CH_3(*R*), R_5= -H, R_6= Ketone, R_7= H, R_8= -OAc, 1-2= Simple, 23-24= Simple
3′: R_1= -OH(*S*), R_2= -OH(*S*), R_3= -H(*R*), R_4= -CH_3(*R*), R_5= -H, R_6= Ketone, R_7= H, R_8= -OH, 1-2= Simple, 23-24= Simple
4′: R_1= Ketone, R_2= -OH(*S*), R_3= -H(*R*), R_4= -CH_3(*R*), R_5= -H, R_6= Ketone, R_7= H, R_8= -OAc, 1-2= Double, 23-24= Double(*E*)
5′: R_1= Ketone, R_2= -OH(*S*), R_3= -H(*R*), R_4= -CH_3(*R*), R_5= -H, R_6= Ketone, R_7= H, R_8= -OH, 1-2= Simple, 23-24= Simple
6′: R_1= Ketone, R_2= -OH(*S*), R_3= -H(*R*), R_4= -CH_3(*R*), R_5= -H, R_6= Ketone, R_7= H, R_8= -OH, 1-2= Double, 23-24= Double(*E*)
7′: R_1= Ketone, R_2= -OH(*S*), R_3= -H(*R*), R_4= -CH_3(*R*), R_5= -H, R_6= Ketone, R_7= H, R_8= -OH, 1-2= Simple, 23-24= Double(*E*)
8′: R_1= Ketone, R_2= -OH(*S*), R_3= -H(*R*), R_4= -OH(*R*), R_5= -H, R_6= Ketone, R_7= H, R_8= -OAc, 1-2= Simple, 23-24= Double(*E*)
9′: R_1= -OH(*R*), R_2= -OH(*S*), R_3= -H(*S*), R_4= -CH_3(*R*), R_5= -H, R_6= -H, R_7= -H, R_8= -OH, 1-2= Simple, 23-24= Simple
10′: R_1= Ketone, R_2= -Glucose-1-yl(*S*), R_3= -H(*R*), R_4= -CH_3(*R*), R_5= -H, R_6= Ketone, R_7= H, R_8= -(1-Ribose)Purine-6-yl, 1-2= Double, 23-24= Simple
11′: R_1= Ketone, R_2= -Glucose-1-yl(*S*), R_3= -H(*R*), R_4= -CH_3(*R*), R_5= -H, R_6= Ketone, R_7= H, R_8= -1*H*-Purine-6-yl, 1-2= Double, 23-24= Simple
12′: R_1= -OH(*S*), R_2= -OH(*S*), R_3= -H(*R*), R_4= -CH_3(*R*), R_5= -H, R_6= Ketone, R_7= H, R_8= -OAc, 1-2= Simple, 23-24= Simple
13′: R_1= -OH(*S*), R_2= -OH(*S*), R_3= -H(*R*), R_4= -CH_3(*R*), R_5= -OH(*R*), R_6= Ketone, R_7= H, R_8= -OAc, 1-2= Simple, 23-24= Double(*E*)

Figure 1.
General structure of cucurbitacin tetracyclic triterpenoid.

2.1 Cucurbitacin B (1′)

Cucurbitacin B (CuB) is an oxygenated tetracyclic triterpenoid compound (**1′**). The growth-inhibiting effect of CuB was evaluated on MCF-7 and MDA-MB-231 breast cancer cells and B16F10 melanoma cells by the MTT assay. This compound had antiproliferative effects against breast cancer cells in a dose-dependent manner, and the IC_{50} values for MCF-7 and MDA-MB-231 were 4.12 and 3.68 μM, respectively [9].

CuB potently suppressed the growth of four types of NSCLC cells (H1299, A549, HCC-827, and H661), inhibiting the proliferation of all the cell lines with IC_{50} values between 0.05 and 0.130 μM. The mean tumor volume at the end of the study in CuB-treated mice was 200 ± 111 mm^3, compared to 684 ± 321 mm^3 in the control group (average reduction of 70% in tumor volume ($p < 0.05$). No visible sign of toxicity was observed in CuB-treated mice [10]. CuB could suppress human NSCLC cell growth in vitro through its effects on the PI3Kinase and MAPK pathways, which lead to programmed cell death induction, as well as inhibition of cell migration and cell invasion [11]. Additionally, CuB induces cell cycle arrest in A-549 cells and causes DNA double strand breaks. It also produces DNA damage and G2/M phase arrest; this damage could be due to an increase in reactive oxygen species (ROS) formation [12].

The cytotoxic effect of CuB was tested on HeLa and U2OS cells, and the IC_{50} values were 12.2 and 17.07 μM, respectively. The inhibition of tubulin polymerization in vitro was observed with an IC_{50} > 1 mM [13]. CuB from the leaves of Tunisian *E. elaterium* exhibited an anticancer effect and displayed anti-integrin activity in human glioblastoma U87 cells, with no cytotoxicity observed at concentrations up to 500 nM. CuB affected the adhesion and migration of U87 cells to fibronectin with IC_{50} values of 86.2 and 84.6 nM, respectively. Time-lapse video-microscopy showed that CuB significantly reduced U87 cell motility and affected directional persistence. CuB also inhibited cell proliferation with an IC_{50} value of 70.1 nM, as determined using the crystal violet assay. Moreover, CuB inhibited in vitro human microvascular endothelial cell (HMEC) angiogenesis at concentrations up to 10 nM. Interestingly, this work demonstrated for the first time that this effect was specifically mediated by α5β1 integrins. These findings reveal a novel mechanism of action for cucurbitacin B, which displays potential as a specific anti-integrin drug [14].

2.2 23,24-Dihydrocucurbitacin B (DHCB) (2′)

C. tayuya (Cucurbitaceae) is a climbing lignified plant with a large tuber that has long been used in folk medicine as an anti-inflammatory, antitumor, and antirheumatic agent. DHCB (**2′**) was isolated from the roots of *C. tayuya* and assessed in isogenic colon cancer cell lines HCT116 and Hke-3 by the 3-(4,5-dimethylthiazol-2-yl)-2,5-diphenyl tetrazolium bromide (MTT) assay. This compound induced apoptosis in both cell lines with IC_{50} values of 9.8 and 4.7 μM, respectively [15].

DHCB inhibited the viability of human cervical cancer cell lines with an IC_{50} of 40–60 μM, but its cytotoxic effects were less pronounced in normal epithelial fr2 and HerEpiC cells, where the IC_{50} was 125 μM. The underlying mechanisms were studied, and the results showed that DHCB induced apoptosis in HeLa cells and caused ROS-mediated shifts in the $\Delta\Psi m$. Additionally, DHCB caused cell cycle arrest in HeLa cells at the G2/M checkpoint. The phosphoinositide 3 kinase/protein kinase B/mechanistic target of rapamycin (PI3K/AKT/mTOR) cascade may play an important role in cancer tumorigenesis and progression and resistance to chemotherapy. The results indicated that DHCB decreased the expression of important proteins in the PI3K/Akt/mTOR cascade [16].

2.3 23,24-Dihydrocucurbitacin F (DHCF) (3′)

DHCF (**3′**) has been isolated from the roots of *H. amabilis*, an ancient Chinese remedy for bacillary dysentery, gastroenteritis, and cancer. While the toxicity of other cucurbitacins has been explored in several types of cancer, little data exist on the effect of DHCF on human cancers, including prostate cancer (PCa). Human PCa DU145, PC3, and LNCaP cells were treated with graded doses of DHCF in vitro, and the antiproliferative activity of this compound was determined using the MTS assay. DHCF inhibited the proliferation of all three PCa cell lines in a dose-dependent manner. The IC_{50} values of DHCF in DU145, PC3, and LNCaP cells were 15, 7, and 5 μM, respectively [17].

2.4 Cucurbitacin E (4′)

The inhibition of breast cancer metastasis in mouse models by CuE was reported. To evaluate the effect of CuE on the proliferation and apoptosis of inoculated 4T1 and MDA-MB231 cells in vivo, the expression of proliferating cell nuclear antigen (PCNA) and cleaved caspase-3 was tested by immunohistochemical analysis [18]. CuE targets the dissemination of breast cancer cells from the primary tumor but not the outgrowth of established micrometastases in target organs (lung, liver, between others). CuE exerts no significant effect on tumor cell apoptosis or proliferation in vivo [19].

CuE demonstrated cytotoxic activity against human oral squamous cell carcinoma SAS cells with an IC_{50} of 3.69 μM and induced the apoptosis of SAS cells after 24 h of treatment, but not MRC-5 or HS68 cells, which showed a dose-dependent reduction. Microscopic examination showed that following exposure to CuE (2.5 μM) for 6–24 h, the cells displayed a remarkable change in their morphology, and CuE induced the death of cancer cells [20].

The inhibitory effect of CuE on the proliferation of Bcap37 and MDA-MB-231 cells was assessed by the MTT assay. Breast cancer cells were treated with various concentrations (0, 0.1, 1, 10, and 100 μM) of CuE or DMSO as a control for 24, 48, and 72 h. The MTT method was then used to determine the number of viable cells. The data indicated that CuE inhibited cell growth in a concentration- and time-dependent manner (ANOVA, $p < 0.05$). After treatment with 0.1 μM CuE for

24 h, the growth of Bcap37 and MB-231 cells was significantly inhibited. At a CuE concentration of 100 μM, most of the cancer cells detached from the dish [21].

Additionally, CuE was evaluated on the chondrosarcoma SW 1353 cancer cell line, and the IC_{50} values indicated higher toxicity in this cell line than in the previously test lines (MTT assay). The amount of CuE that induced a mortality of 50% was calculated after 6, 12, and 24 h of treatment, and the results were 13.55, 12.65, and 9.16 μM, respectively [22]. The cytotoxic effect of CuE was tested on HeLa and U2OS cells, and the IC_{50} values were 6.43 and 15.07 nM, respectively. The inhibition of tubulin polymerization in vitro had an IC_{50} of 566.91 nM [13].

The effects of CuE from *E. elaterium* fruit on the expression of the BAX, caspase-3, LC3, and VEGF and c-MYC genes in the AGS cell line were investigated. The sub-G1 accumulation of AGS cells treated with CuE was increased compared to that of untreated cells. Moreover, the treatment of AGS cells with CuE-induced cell death. Additionally, the effects of CuE on the mRNA expression levels of the LC3, VEGF, BAX, caspase-3, and c-MYC genes were evaluated using qRT-PCR. LC3 mRNA levels were increased approximately 20-fold after treatment with CuE at a concentration of 0.1 μg/mL for 24 h. However, BAX, caspase-3, and c-MYC mRNA levels at these concentrations were not changed by the treatment [23, 24].

2.5 Cucurbitacin R (5′)

One additional cucurbitacin was discovered in the roots of *C. tayuya* and was identified as cucurbitacin R (CCR) (**5′**). This compound was experimentally assessed in isogenic colon cancer cell lines HCT116 and Hke-3 by the MTT assay and induced the apoptosis of both HCT116 and Hke-3 cells with IC_{50} values 37 and 27 μM, respectively [15].

2.6 Cucurbitacin I (6′)

CuI, also known as elatericin B or JSI 124, has been isolated from different plants, such as *M. balsamina* L. (balsam pear), *C. tayuya* (tayuya), *Cucurbita andreana* (winter squash), and *C. colocynthis* (bitter cucumber). This compound was tested in isogenic colon cancer cell lines HCT116 and Hke-3 and was found to induce apoptosis in both lines, with IC_{50} values of 0.29 and 0.09 μM, respectively [15].

The cytotoxicity IC_{50} values of CuI in SW 1353 cells after 6, 12, and 24 h of treatment were 7.93, 8.31, and 5.06 μM, respectively [22]. The cytotoxic activity of CuI against SW-480 human colon cancer cells was tested. In this case, CuI diminished cell proliferation in a concentration-dependent manner and increased apoptosis, enhancing cycle arrest at the G2/M phase [25].

The cytotoxicity of CuI was tested in HeLa and U2OS cells, and the IC_{50} values were 44.77 and 23.47 nM, respectively. The inhibition of tubulin polymerization in vitro had an $IC_{50} > 1$ mM [13]. The effects of CuI purified from *E. elaterium* fruit on the expression of the BAX, caspase-3, LC3, and VEGF and c-MYC genes in the AGS cell line were investigated. The sub-G1 accumulation of AGS cells treated with CuI was increased compared to that of untreated cells. Moreover, treatment of AGS cells with CuI-induced cell death. Additionally, the effects of CuI on the mRNA expression levels of the LC3, VEGF, BAX, caspase-3, and c-MYC genes were evaluated using qRT-PCR. After treatment, at a concentration of 0.5 μg/mL for 24 h, LC3 mRNA levels were increased approximately 25-fold, and VEGF mRNA levels were increased approximately 4.4-fold. However, BAX, caspase-3, and c-MYC mRNA levels were not considerably changed after treatment with CuI [23, 24].

2.7 Cucurbitacin D (7′)

CuD was evaluated in the chondrosarcoma SW 1353 cancer cell line. Its IC_{50} values against SW 1353 cells after 6, 12, and 24 h of treatment were 16.48, 13.03, and 13.14 μM, respectively [22].

The effects of CuD purified from *E. elaterium* fruit on the expression of the BAX, caspase-3, LC3, VEGF, and c-MYC genes in the AGS cell line were investigated. The sub-G1 accumulation of AGS cells treated with CuD was increased compared to that of untreated cells. Moreover, the treatment of AGS cells with CuD induced cell death. Additionally, the effects of cucurbitacin D on the mRNA expression levels of the LC3, VEGF, BAX, caspase-3, and c-MYC genes were evaluated using qRT-PCR. LC3 mRNA levels were increased approximately 23-fold after treatment with CuD at a concentration of 0.3 μg/mL for 24 h. However, the BAX, caspase-3, and c-MYC mRNA levels were not considerably changed after treatment. Regarding the effects of CuD and CuE on LC3 mRNA expression, CuD's effect was significantly greater than that of CuE [23].

2.8 Cucurbitacin A (8′)

The antiproliferative effects of Cucurbitacin A (CuA) on A-549 cells were determined by using the MTT assay. This compound exhibited a potent cytotoxic effect on A-549 cells. The assay was carried out at different concentrations of CuA (0, 10, 20, 40, 100, 150, and 200 μM) with incubation for 24 and 48 h. CuA showed inhibitory effects on cell proliferation in a dose- and time-dependent manner. However, the effect of the incubation time was more pronounced at higher doses of the compound. CuA also induced morphological changes in these cells, featuring chromatin condensation, cell shrinkage, and apoptotic body formation. G2/M phase cell cycle collapse was also induced by CuA along with inhibition of the expression levels of m-TOR/PI3K/Akt proteins [26].

2.9 2 β,3β,16α,20(*R*),25-Pentahydroxy-22-oxocucurbita-5-en (RPO) (9′)

This compound is a cucurbitacin isolated from *Cayaponia racemosa* Cong. The anticancer activity of RPO was evaluated with in vitro and in vivo models. Cucurbitacin (**9′**) reduced the number of viable HL-60 leukemia cells; however, there was no change in the number of nonviable cells at 5 μg/mL. This compound had no effect on normal proliferating lymphocytes at the concentrations tested (IC_{50} > 25 μg/mL). Morphological analysis of RPO-treated cells showed typical apoptotic features, such as heavy deposition of granules in the cytoplasm (eosinophilia), DNA fragmentation and irregularities in the plasma membrane, and intense vacuolization and disruption of the plasma membrane. Acridine orange/ethidium bromide staining confirmed these findings, revealing an increased number of apoptotic cells. In the sarcoma 180 tumor model, compound (**9′**) showed 52 or 62% antitumor activity when administered alone (25 mg/kg/day) or in association with the chemotherapeutic agent 5-FU (10 + 10 mg/kg/day), respectively. Moreover, treatment with compound (**9′**) either alone or in combination with 5-FU caused an increase in spleen weight and morphological alterations related to immunostimulatory properties [27].

2.10 Cucurbitaglycosides A (10′) and B (11′)

Phytochemical investigation of the fruits of *Cucurbita pepo* cv. dayangua led to the isolation of cucurbitaglycosides A (**10′**) and B (**11′**). This was the first report of

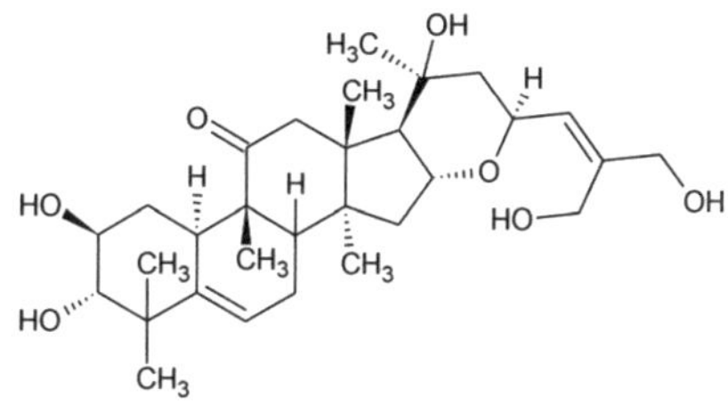

Figure 2.
2β,3β,20(S),26,27-Pentahydroxy-16α,23(S)-epoxycucurbita-5,24-dien-11-one.

cucurbitane triterpenoids with a purine unit. Cucurbitaglycosides A and B showed cytotoxic activity against the human epithelial carcinoma cell line HeLa with IC_{50} values of 17.2 and 28.4 μg/mL, respectively [28].

2.11 Hemslecin A (12′)

Three cucurbitane triterpenoids were isolated from *H. amabilis*, and the main compound was Hemslecin A (HA). This compound showed significant cytotoxic activity against HeLa cells with an IC_{50} value of 0.389 μM. Additionally, 7β-hydroxycucurbitacin F-25-O-acetate (**13′**) and 2β,3β,20(*S*),26,27-pentahydroxy-16α,23(*S*)-epoxycucurbita-5,24-dien-11-one (**14′**) (**Figure 2**) were isolated and showed less cytotoxic activity (IC_{50} values of 12.3 and 387 μM, respectively) than HA [29].

3. Cucurbitane-type triterpene glycosides

Several new cucurbitane-type triterpene glycosides (**Figures 3** and **4**) have been isolated from the fruit pulp of *Momordica charantia* L., and their cytotoxic activity has been evaluated.

Two new cucurbitane-type triterpene glycosides, charantagenins D (**15′**) and E (**16′**), and one new sterol, 7-oxo-stigmasta-5, 25-diene-3-O-β-D-glucopyranoside (**17′**), were isolated from the fruit of *M. charantia* L. together with another six known compounds (**18′–23′**). The cytotoxic activities of the major isolated compounds were evaluated against the lung cancer cell line A549, glioblastoma cell line U87, and hepatoma carcinoma cell line Hep3B using in vitro MTT assays. Two new cucurbitane-type triterpenes, 25-methoxycucurbita-5,23(*E*)-diene-3β,19-diol (**24′**) and 7β-ethoxy-3β-hydroxy-25-methoxycucurbita-5,23(*E*)-dien-19-al (**25′**), together with three known cucurbitane-type triterpenes, 3β,7β,25-trihydroxycucurbita-5,23(*E*)-dien-19-al (**26′**), (23*E*)-3β-hydroxy-7β,25-dimethoxycucurbita-5,23-dien-19-al (**27′**), and 3β-hydroxy-25-methoxycucurbita-6,23(*E*)-dien-19,5β-olide (**28′**), were isolated from the fruit pulp of *M. charantia*. Their cytotoxic activity was evaluated against human hepatoma SK Hep-1 cells with etoposide as a positive control (IC_{50} = 3.7 μM). The results are shown in **Table 1** [19, 30].

3.1 Momordicin VII (29′)

Several new cucurbitane triterpenoids were isolated from the stems and leaves of *M. charantia* and tested against five human cancer cell lines (HL-60, SMMC-7721, A-549, MCF-7, and SW480). Only momordicin VII (**29′**) was slightly active, with IC_{50} values of 16.2, 20.3, 20.5, 16.9, and 14.3 μM, respectively [31].

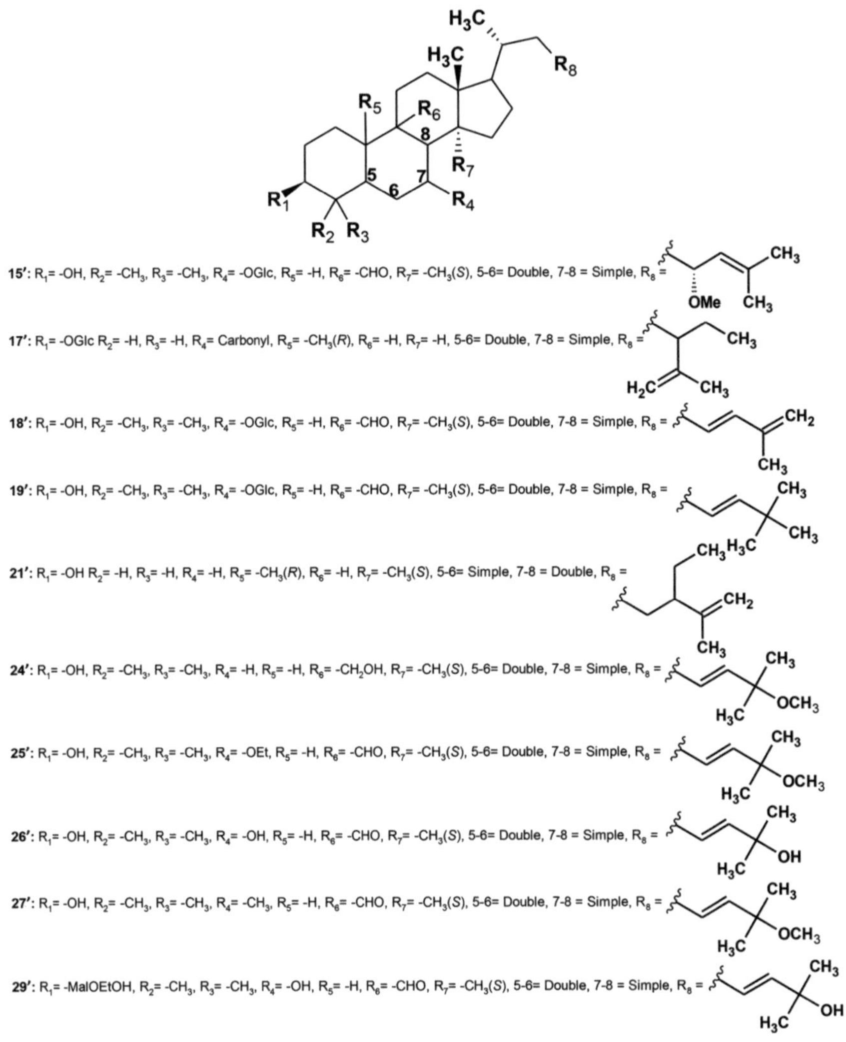

Figure 3.
Structure of cucurbitane-type triterpene glycosides 15′, 17′-19′, 21′, 24′-29′.

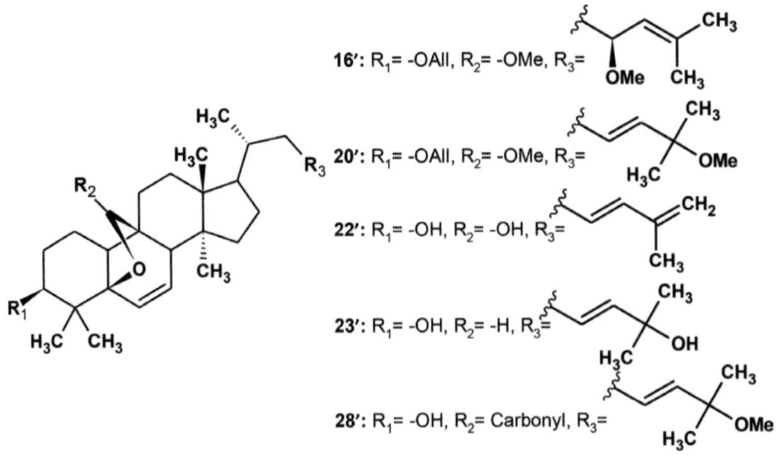

Figure 4.
Structure of cucurbitane-type triterpene glycosides 20′, 22′, 23′, 28′.

Cancer cell line	IC_{50} values (μM)
A549 lung cancer cell line	**15′** = 1.07
	16′ = 3.82
	17′, 22′, 23′ = >100
	18′ = 4.46
	19′ = 4.89
	20′ = 5.32
	21′ = 15.10
U87 glioblastoma cell line	**15′** = 1.08
	16′ = 67.32
	17′,18′,22′,23′ = >100
	19′ = 0.60
	20′ = 0.19
	21′ = 8.65
Hep3B hepatoma carcinoma cell line	**15′** = 14.01
	16′–19′,21′–23′ = >100
	20′ = 19.30
SKHep1 human hepatoma cell line	**24′** = 33.1
	25′ = 24.3
	26′ = >50
	27′ = >13
	28′ = 38.7

Table 1.
Cytotoxic activities of cucurbitane-type triterpene glycosides **15′–28′**.

4. Multiflorane-type triterpenes

Multiflorane-type triterpenes (**Figure 5**), a new class of cucurbitacins, were isolated from seeds of *Cucurbita maxima*, along with three known compounds from *Benincasa hispida* (Thunb.) Cogn., fruits that are widely consumed in China and tropical countries, and these compounds were found to exhibit interesting cytotoxicity activity.

Three new multiflorane-type triterpenes, 7α-methoxymultiflor-8-ene-3α, 29-diol-3-acetate-29-benzoate (**30′**), 7-oxomultiflor-8-ene-3α,29-diol-3-acetate-29-benzoate (**31′**), and multiflora-7,9(11)-diene-3α,29-diol-3-p-hydroxybenzoate-29-benzoate (**32′**), were isolated from seeds of *C. maxima*, along with three known compounds. These compounds exhibited cytotoxicity against HL-60 and P388 cells. Compound (**30′**) did not show significant cytotoxic activity, with an IC_{50} > 100 μM in both lines, but compounds 31 and 32 showed cytotoxic activity against HL-60, with IC_{50} values of 7.1 and 7.1 μM, respectively. The IC_{50} values for P388 were 55.9 and 92.6 μM, respectively [32].

Analysis of *Benincasa hispida* (Thunb.) Cogn. fruits yielded three new triterpenoids, 3α,29-O-di-trans-cinnamoyl-D:C-friedooleana-7,9(11)-diene (**33′**), oleanolic acid 28-O-β-D-xylopyranosyl-[β-D-xylopyranosyl-(1→4)]-(1→3)-α-L-rhamnopyranosyl-(1→2)-α-L-arabinopyranoside (**34′**), and oleanolic acid 28-O-β-D-glucopyranosyl-(1→3)-β-D-xylopyranosyl-[β-D-xylopyranosyl-

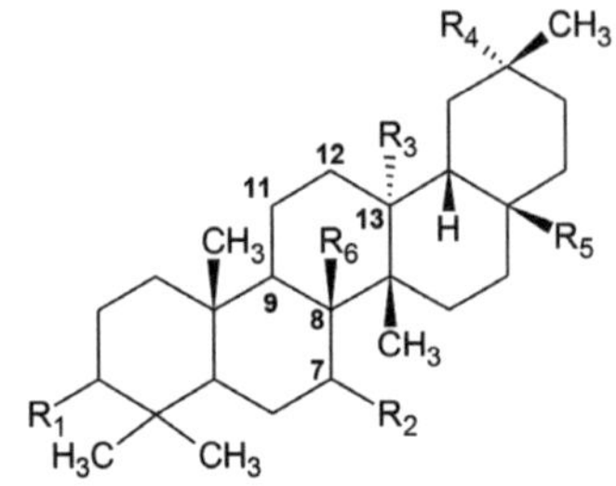

30': R_1= -OAc, R_2= -OCH_3, R_3= -CH_3, R_4= -Benzoate, R_5= -CH_3, R_6= -, 7-8= Simple, 8-9=Double, 9-11= Simple, 11-12= Simple, 12-13= Simple
31': R_1= -OAc, R_2= -Carbonyl, R_3= -CH_3, R_4= -Benzoate, R_5= -CH_3, R_6= -, 7-8= Simple, 8-9=Double, 9-11= Simple, 11-12= Simple, 12-13= Simple
32': R_1= -(*p*-Hydroxy)benzoate, R_2= -H, R_3= -CH_3, R_4= -Benzoate, R_5= -CH_3, R_6= -, 7-8= Double, 8-9= Simple, 9-11= Double, 11-12= Simple, 12-13= Simple
33': R_1= -*trans*-cinnamoyl, R_2= -H, R_3= -CH_3, R_4= --*trans*-cinnamoyl, R_5= -CH_3, R_6= -, 7-8= Double, 8-9= Simple, 9-11= Double, 11-12= Simple, 12-13= Simple
34': R_1= -OH, R_2= -H, R_3= -H, R_4= --CH_3, R_5= -COO-Xyl-[(1→4)-Xyl]-(1→3)-Rha-(1→2)-Ara, R_6= -CH_3, 7-8= Simple, 8-9= Simple, 9-11= Simple, 11-12= Simple, 12-13= Double
35': R_1= -OH, R_2= -H, R_3= -H, R_4= --CH_3, R_5= -COO-Glu-(1→3)-Xyl-[(1→4)-Xyl]-(1→3)-Rha-(1→2)-Ara, R_6= -CH_3, 7-8= Simple, 8-9= Simple, 9-11= Simple, 11-12= Simple, 12-13= Double

Figure 5.
Multiflorane-type triterpenes.

(1→4)]-(1→3)-α-L-rhamnopyranosyl-(1→2)-α-L-arabinopyranoside (**35'**). The cytotoxic activities of compounds (**33'–35'**) were assessed by the MTT assay. These compounds showed no significant cytotoxic activity against HeLa human cervical, HL-60 human hepatoma, and SMMC-7721 human hepatoma cell lines [33].

5. Cyclic bisdesmosides

Cyclic bisdesmosides, new compounds analogous to cucurbitacins, share the tetracyclic triterpenoid core but contain carbohydrates to form a bicycle (**Figure 6**). These compounds were isolated from *Actinostemma lobatum* MAXIM and *Bolbostemma paniculatum* (Maxim) Franquet.

Two new cyclic bisdesmosides elucidated as lobatoside L (**36'**) and lobatoside M (**37'**) and four known cyclic bisdesmosides (**38'–41'**) were isolated from *A. lobatum* Maxim. The inhibitory effects of these six compounds on human cancer cell growth (including the esophageal squamous carcinoma cell line ECA109, lung cancer cell line A549, and gastric cancer cell line MGC-803) were determined using the MTT assay. The six compounds exhibited cytotoxicity against all the cell lines tested, and compounds (**36'**, **38'**, and **40'**) showed significant activity in a dose-dependent manner against all the cell lines. The IC_{50} values for compounds (**36'** and **40'**) against ECA-109 cells were 8.25 and 3.71 μM, respectively. The rest of the results are shown in **Table 2** [34].

Tubeimoside I (**42'**) isolated from *B. paniculatum* (Maxim) Franquet exhibited cytotoxic activity against HepG2 human cancer cells. The IC_{50} values at different times of exposure (24, 48, and 72 h) were 15.5, 11.7, and 9.2 μM, respectively. This compound induced shrinkage, nuclear condensation, fragmentation, and cell cycle arrest in phase G2/M. The inhibition of growth in this case is mediated by a cascade of apoptosis [35].

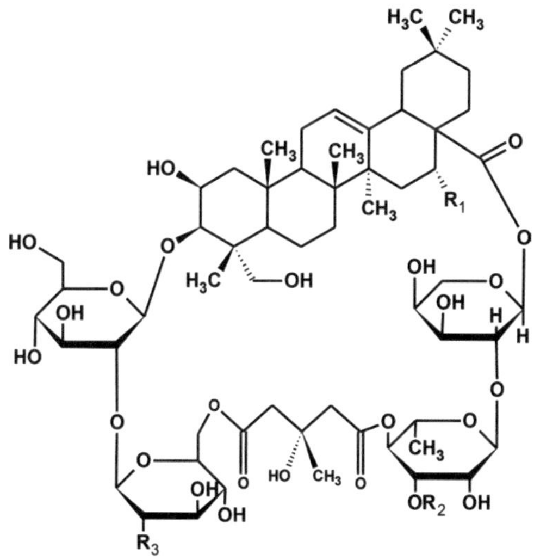

Lobastoside L (36′): R_1= OH, R_2= Glc, R_3= OH
Lobastoside M (37′): R_1= H, R_2= Glc, R_3= OH
38′: R_1= OH, R_2= H, R_3= OH
39′: R_1= H, R_2= H, R_3= OH
40′: R_1= OH, R_2= Xyl, R_3= OH
41′: R_1= H, R_2= Xyl, R_3= OH
Tubeimoside I (42′): R_1= H, R_2= H, R_3= H

Figure 6.
Cyclic bisdesmosides structure.

Cancer cell lines	IC_{50} values (μM)
Esophageal squamous carcinoma cell line ECA-109	**36′** = 8.25
	37′ = 74.14
	38′ = 22.37
	39′ = 71.97
	40′ = 3.71
	41′ = 83.53
Lung cancer cell line A549	**36′** = 26.52
	37′ = 69.28
	38′ = 27.27
	39′ = 77.79
	40′ = 35.12
	41′ = 77.02
Gastric cancer cell line MGC-803	**36′** = 35.33
	37′ = 84.71
	38′ = 36.85
	39′ = 90.49
	40′ = 35.21
	41′ = 96.55

Table 2.
Cytotoxic activities of cyclic bisdesmosides **36′–41'**.

6. Gypenosides

The gypenosides (**Figure 7**) were isolated from *Gynostemma pentaphyllum* and from the aerial parts of *G. pentaphyllum*.

Gypenoside L (**43′**) and gynogenin (**44′**), 20(*S*)-dammar-24-en-2a,3b,12b,20-tetrol, were isolated from *G. pentaphyllum* and tested against A-549 lung carcinoma cells. The IC_{50} values were 34.94 and 12.54 μg/mL, respectively [36]. Some gypenosides were isolated from the aerial parts of *C. pentaphyllum* (**45′–51′**), and their structures were elucidated with spectroscopic and chemical methods. Their cytotoxic activity was determined against different human cancer cell lines, A549, HT-29, MCF-7, and SK-OV-3. All the compounds showed low activity, with IC_{50} values between 62.8 and 19.6 μM [37].

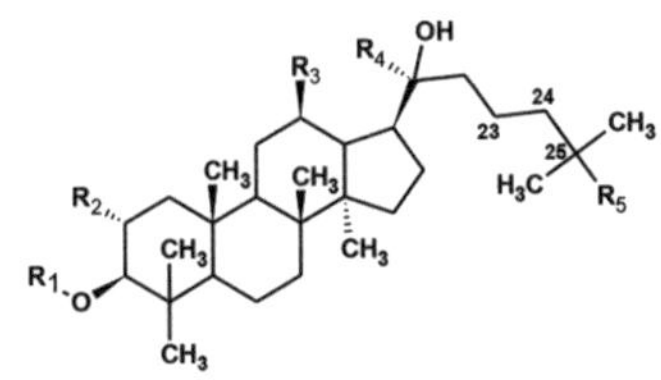

Gypenoside L (43′): R_1= -S^1, R_2= -OH, R_3= -OH, R_4= -CH_3, R_5= -, 23-24= Simple, 24-25= Double

Gynogenin (44′): R_1= -OH, R_2= -OH, R_3= -OH, R_4= -CH_3, R_5= -, 23-24= Simple, 24-25= Double

45′: R_1= -S^2, R_2= -H, R_3= -H, R_4= -S^3, R_5= -, 23-24= Simple, 24-25= Double

46′: R_1= -S^2, R_2= -H, R_3= Carbonyl, R_4= -CH_3, R_5= -, 23-24= Simple, 24-25= Double

47′: R_1= -S^4, R_2= -H, R_3= Carbonyl, R_4= -Glu-1, R_5= -, 23-24= Simple, 24-25= Double

48′: R_1= -S^2, R_2= -H, R_3= Carbonyl, R_4= -Glu-1, R_5= -OH, 23-24= Double, 24-25= Simple

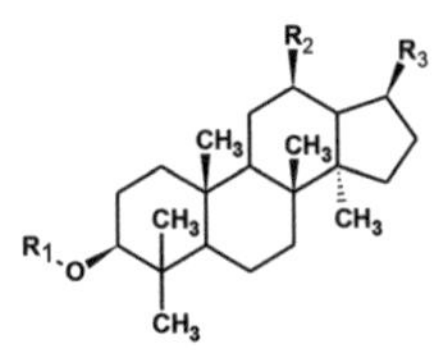

49′: R_1= -S^2, R_2= -OH, R_3= -S^5

50′: R_1= -S^2, R_2= Carbonyl, R_3= -S^5

51′: R_1= -S^2, R_2= -H, R_3= -S^6

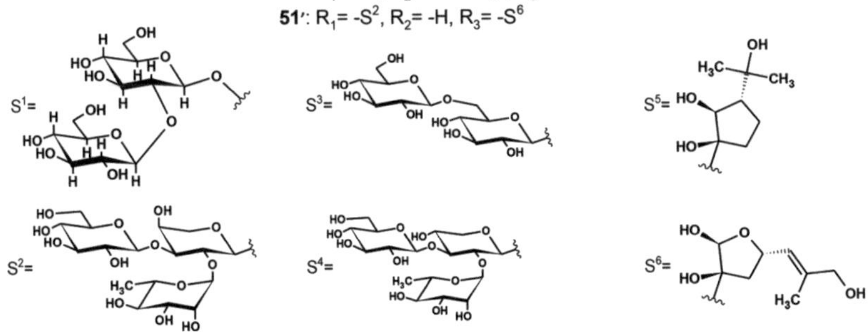

Figure 7.
Gypenosides structure.

7. Other substances of interest

In addition to the cucurbitacins, other substances isolated from the Cucurbitaceae family have been identified, including proteins isolated from the sarcocarp of *Cucurbita moschata* (pumpkin) and from the root of *T. kirilowii* Maxim

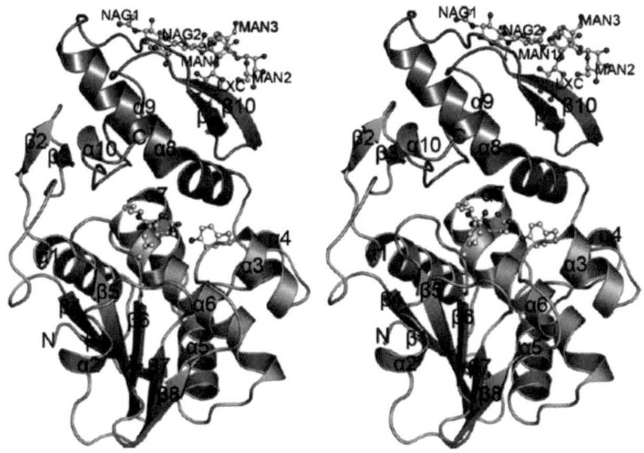

Figure 8.
Overall structure of cucurmosin in stereo view.

(Cucurbitaceae). Additionally, the protein from the root of *T. kirilowii* Maxim has been demonstrated to possess important cytotoxicity activity.

7.1 Cucurmosin

A novel type-1 ribosome-inactivating protein (RIP) designated cucurmosin was isolated from the sarcocarp of *Cucurbita moschata* (pumpkin). Its structure contains two domains: a large N-terminal domain composed of seven α-helices and eight β-strands and a smaller C-terminal domain consisting of three α-helices and two β-strands (**Figure 8**).

Cucurmosin was tested for its cytotoxicity against human leukemia cells (K562), murine melanoma cells (B16), lung adenocarcinoma cancer cells (A549), and peripheral blood lymphocytes using the standard MTT assay. The IC_{50} values of cucurmosin were 88.1, 63.4, and 359.3 nM in human leukemia cells (K562), murine melanoma cells (B16), and lung adenocarcinoma cancer cells (A549), respectively, while its IC_{50} in normal cells (peripheral blood lymphocytes) was higher than 1.4 μM [38].

7.2 Trichosanthin

Trichosanthin was isolated from the roots of *T. kirilowii* Maxim and has been used in traditional Chinese medicine. This compound was tested against HepG-2 and WRL 68 cells, and the IC_{50} values obtained were 10.38 and 15.45 μmol/L, respectively [39].

Tianhua, an extract of *T. kirilowii*, was analyzed to determine its mechanism of action against lung cancer cells (A549) using the MTS assay. This compound induced apoptosis via an anti-telomerase effect but had no effect on stimulating peripheral lymphocytes to produce interferon (IFN)-γ; tianhua inhibited the metastatic ability of cells and inhibited the growth of cancer cells in vivo [40].

8. Conclusion

The aim of this review is to present 51 cucurbitacin compounds and two compounds with different structures isolated from Cucurbitaceae plants, their chemical structures, their biological activities, and the mechanisms by which these compounds reduce the proliferation of cancer cells.

Conflict of interest

The authors declare that there is note conflict of interest.

Author details

Carlos Alberto Méndez-Cuesta, Ana Laura Esquivel Campos, David Salinas Sánchez, Cuauhtemoc Pérez González and Salud Pérez Gutiérrez*
Universidad Autónoma Metropolitana-Xochimilco, Mexico City, Mexico

*Address all correspondence to: msperez@correo.xoc.uam.mx

References

[1] WHO. Cancer, facts and figures about cancer. Available from: http://www.who.int/en/news-room/fact-sheets/detail/cancer [Consulted on: July 18, 2018]

[2] Globocan. Cancer Today 2012: Data visualization tools that present current national estimates of cáncer incidence, mortality and prevalence. Available from: http://gco.iarc.fr/today/home [Consulted on: July 18, 2018]

[3] Takimoto CH, Calvo E. Principles of Oncologic Pharmacotherapy. Cancer Management: A Multidisciplinary Approach. 11th ed. 2008. ISBN-13: 978-1891483622. Available from: http://www.cancernetwork.com/cancermanag?ement-11/

[4] Side effects of cancer treatments. National Cancer Institute. Available from: https://www.cancer.gov/about-cancer/treatment/side-effects [Consulted on: September 4, 2018]

[5] Perez Gutierrez RM. Review of *Cucurbita pepo* (pumpkin) its phytochemistry and pharmacology. Medicinal Chemistry. 2016;**6**(1):12-21. DOI: 10.4172/2161-0444.1000316

[6] Ajuru M, Nmom F. A review on the economic uses of species of cucurbitaceae and their sustainability in Nigeria. American Journal of Plant Biology. 2017;**2**(1):17-24. DOI: 10.11648/j.ajpb.20170201.14

[7] Ahmad Shah SS, Ijaz Hussain M, Kashif Aslam M, Rivera G. Natural products; pharmacological importance of family cucurbitaceae: A brief review. Mini-Reviews in Medicinal Chemistry. 2014;**14**(8):1-11. DOI: 10.2174/13895575 14666140820113055

[8] Soto-Hernández M, Cadena Iñiguez J, Arévalo-Galarza LC, Santiago-Osorio E, Aguiñiga-Sánchez I, Ruíz-Posadas LM. Chapter 12: Lead compounds from cucurbitaceae for the treatment of cancer. In: Rao AV, Rao LG, editors. Phytochemicals: Isolation, Characterization and Role in Human Health. AvE4EvA; Rijeka, Croatia: In Tech; 2015. pp. 289-303. DOI: 10.5772/60048

[9] Duangmano S, Sae-lim P, Suksamrarn A, Domann FE, Patmasiriwat P. Cucurbitacin B inhibits human breast cancer cell proliferation through disruption of microtubule polymerization and nucleophosmin/B23 translocation. BMC Complementary and Alternative Medicine. 2012;**12**:185-197. DOI: 10.1186/1472-6882-12-185

[10] Kausar H, Munagala R, Bansal SS, Aqil F, Vadhanam MV, Gupta RC. Cucurbitacin B potently suppresses non-small-cell lung cancer growth: Identification of intracellular thiols as critical targets. Cancer Letters. 2013;**332**:35-45. DOI: 10.1016/j.canlet.2013.01.008

[11] Silva IT, Geller FC, Persich L, Dudek SE, Lang KL, Balparda Caro MS, et al. Cytotoxic effects of natural and semisynthetic cucurbitacins on lung cancer cell line A549. Investigational New Drugs. 2016;**34**(2):139-148. DOI: 10.1007/s10637-015-0317-4

[12] Guo J, Wu G, Bao J, Hao W, Lu J, Chen X. Cucurbitacin B induced ATM-mediated DNA damage causes G2/M cell cycle arrest in a ROS-dependent manner. PLoS One. 2014;**9**(2):1-12. DOI: 10.1371/journal.pone.0088140

[13] Wang X, Tanaka M, Peixoto HS, Wink M. Cucurbitacins: Elucidation of their interactions with the cytoskeleton. PeerJ. 2017;**5**:e3357:1-18. DOI: 10.7717/peerj.3357

[14] Touihri-Barakati I, Kallech-Ziri O, Ayadi W, Kovacic H, Hanchi B, Hosni

K, et al. Cucurbitacin B purified from *Ecballium elaterium* (L.) A. rich from Tunisia inhibits α5β1 integrin-mediated adhesion, migration, proliferation of human glioblastoma cell line and angiogenesis. European Journal of Pharmacology. 2017;**797**:153-161. DOI: 10.1016/j.ejphar.2017.01.006

[15] Escandell JM, Kaler P, Recio MC, Sasazuki T, Shirasawa S, Augenlicht L, et al. Activated kRas protects colon cancer cells from cucurbitacin-induced apoptosis: The role of p53 and p21. Biochemical Pharmacology. 2008;**76**:198-207. DOI: 10.1016/j.bcp.2008.05.004

[16] Zhang JX, Wei Tan H, Hu CY, Wang WQ, Chu GH, Wei LH, et al. Anticancer activity of 23,24-dihydrocucurbitacin B against the HeLa human cervical cell line is due to apoptosis and G2/M cell cycle arrest. Experimental and Therapeutic Medicine. 2018;**15**(3):2575-2582. DOI: 10.3892/etm.2018.5710

[17] Ren S, Dong-Yun O, Saltis M, Li-Hui X, Qing-Bing Z, Ji-Ye C, et al. Anti-proliferative effect of 23,24-dihydrocucurbitacin F on human prostate cancer cells through induction of actin aggregation and cofilin-actin rod formation. Cancer Chemotherapy and Pharmacology. 2012;**70**:415-424. DOI: 10.1007/s00280-012-1921-z

[18] Zhang T, Li J, Dong Y, Zhai D, Lai L, Dai F, et al. Cucurbitacin E inhibits breast tumor metastasis by suppressing cell migration and invasion. Breast Cancer Research and Treatment. 2012;**135**:445-458. DOI: 10.1007/s10549-012-2175-5

[19] Yun-Wen L, Chiy-Rong C, Jiunn-Jye C, Hui-Chi H, Jue-Liang H, Tzou-Chi H, et al. Cucurbitane triterpenoids from the fruit pulp of *Momordica charantia* and their cytotoxic activity. Journal of the Chinese Chemical Society. 2013;**60**:526-530. DOI: 10.1002/jccs.201200532

[20] Chao-Ming H, Chi-Chang C, Chen-Wei L, Shun-Yao K, Yi-Chiang H. Cucurbitacin E as inducer of cell death and apoptosis in human oral squamous cell carcinoma cell line SAS. International Journal of Molecular Sciences. 2013;**14**:17147-17156. DOI: 10.3390/ijms140817147

[21] Lan T, Wang L, Xu Q, Liu W, Jin H, Mao W, et al. Growth inhibitory effect of cucurbitacin E on breast cancer cells. International Journal of Clinical and Experimental Pathology. 2013;**6**(9):1799-1805. PMID: 24040444

[22] Abbas S, Vincourt JB, Habib L, Netter P, Greige-Gerges H, Magdalou J. The cucurbitacins E, D and I: Investigation of their cytotoxicity toward human chondrosarcoma SW 1353 cell line and their biotransformation in man liver. Toxicology Letters. 2013;**216**:189-199. DOI: 10.1016/j.toxlet.2012.11.014

[23] Jafargholizadeh N, Zargar SJ, Aftabi Y. The cucurbitacins D, E, and I from *Ecballium elaterium* (L.) upregulate the LC3 gene and induce cell-cycle arrest in human gastric cancer cell line AGS. Iranian Journal of Basic Medical Sciences. 2018;**21**(3):253-259. DOI: 10.22038/ijbms.2018.25175.6236

[24] Jafargholizadeh N, Zargar SJ, Yassa N, Tavakoli S. Purification of cucurbitacins D, E, and I from *Ecballium elaterium* (L.) A. rich fruits and study of their cytotoxic effects on the AGS cell line. Asian Pacific Journal of Cancer Prevention. 2016;**17**(10):4631-4635. DOI: 10.22034/APJCP.2016.17.10.4631

[25] Hyeon JK, Jung Han YP, Jin-Kyung K. Cucurbitacin-I, a natural cell-permeable triterpenoid isolated from cucurbitaceae, exerts potent anticancer effect in colon cancer. Chemico-Biological Interactions. 2014;**219**:1-8. DOI: 10.1016/j.cbi.2014.05.005

[26] Wang WD, Liu Y, Su Y, Xiong XZ, Shang D, Xu JJ, et al. Antitumor and apoptotic effects of cucurbitacin a in

A-549 lung carcinoma cells is mediated via G2/M cell cycle arrest and M-TOR/PI3K/Akt signalling pathway. African Journal of Traditional, Complementary, and Alternative Medicines. 2017;**14**(2):75-82. DOI: 10.21010/ajtcam.v14i2.9

[27] Militão G, Dantas I, Pinherio Ferreira PM, Alves AP, Chaves DC, Monte FJ, et al. In vitro and in vivo anticancer properties of cucurbitacin isolated from *Cayaponia racemose*. Pharmaceutical Biology. 2012;**50**(12):1479-1487. DOI: 10.3109/13880209.2012.684691

[28] Da-Cheng W, Xiang H, Li D, Hui-yuan G, Hui C, Li-Jun W, et al. Purine-containing cucurbitane triterpenoids from *Cucurbita pepo* cv dayangua. Phytochemistry. 2008;**69**:1434-1438. DOI: 10.1016/j.phytochem.2008.01.019

[29] Xu-Bing C, Guang-Yong C, Jun-Hua L, Lei M, Yu-Hui M, De-An G, et al. Cytotoxic cucurbitane triterpenoids isolated from the rhizomes of *Hemsleya amabilis*. Fitoterapia. 2014;**94**:88-93. DOI: 10.1016/j.fitote.2014.01.014

[30] Wang X, Sun W, Cao J, Qu H, Bi X, Zhao Y. Structures of new triterpenoids and cytotoxicity activities of the isolated major compounds from the fruit of *Momordica charantia* L. Journal of Agricultural and Food Chemistry. 2012;**60**:3927-3933. DOI: 10.1021/jf204208y

[31] Gao-Ting Z, Jie-Qing L, Yuan-Yuan D, Hai-Zhou L, Jian-Chao C, Zhi-Run Z, et al. Cucurbitane-type triterpenoids from the stems and leaves of *Momordica charantia*. Fitoterapia. 2014;**95**:75-82. DOI: 10.1016/j.fitote.2014.03.005

[32] Kikuchi T, Takebayashi M, Shinto M, Yamada T, Tanaka R. Three new multiflorane-type triterpenes from pumpkin (*Cucurbita maxima*) seeds. Molecules. 2013;**18**:5568-5579. DOI: 10.3390/molecules18055568

[33] Xiao-Na H, Chun-Yu L, Yan-Li L, Qiong-Ming X, Xiao-Ran L, Shi-Lin Y. New triterpenoids and other constituents from the fruits of *Benincasa hispida* (Thunb.) Cogn. Journal of Agricultural and Food Chemistry. 2013;**61**:12692-12699. DOI: 10.1021/jf405384r

[34] Li W, Cao J, Tang Y, Zhang L, Xie Q, Shen H, et al. Cyclic bisdesmosides from *Actinostemma lobatum* MAXIM (Cucurbitaceae) and their in vitro cytotoxicity. Fitoterapia. 2012;**83**:147-152. DOI: 10.1016/j.fitote.2011.10.008

[35] Wang Y, Deng L, Zhong H, Wang Y, Jiang X, Chen J. Natural plant extract Tubeimoside I promotes apoptosis-mediated cell death in cultured human hepatoma (HepG2) cells. Biological & Pharmaceutical Bulletin. 2011;**34**(6):831-838. DOI: 10.1248/bpb.34.831

[36] Dao-Jin C, Hui-Min L, Shao-Fang X, Xiang-Lan P. Cytotoxic activity of gypenosides and gynogenin against non-small cell lung carcinoma A549 cells. Bioorganic & Medicinal Chemistry Letters. 2014;**24**:186-191. DOI: 10.1016/j.bmcl.2013.11.043

[37] Pham Thanh K, Pham Thanh H, Than Kieu M, Pham Tuan A, Phan Van K, Chau Van M, et al. Dammarane-type saponins from *Gynostemma pentaphyllum*. Phytochemistry. 2010;**71**:994-1001. DOI: 10.1016/j.phytochem.2010.03.009

[38] Xiaomin H, Meehan EJ, Xie J, Huang M, Minghuang C, Chen L. Atomic resolution structure of cucurmosin, a novel type 1 ribosome-inactivating protein from the sarcocarp of *Cucurbita moschata*. Journal of Structural Biology. 2008;**164**:81-87. DOI: 10.1016/j.jsb.2008.06.011

[39] Mondal A. A novel extraction of trichosanthin from *Trichosanthes kirilowii* roots using three-phase

partitioning and its in vitro anticancer activity. Pharmaceutical Biology. 2014;**52**(6):677-680. DOI: 10.3109/13880209.2013.864684

[40] Chien-Te L, Ching-Hsiung L, Te-Yu K, Ming-Fang W, Chin-Shui Y, Kun-Tu Y, et al. The mechanisms of action of Tianhua™ on antitumor activity in lung cancer cells. Pharmaceutical Biology. 2010;**48**(11):1302-1309. DOI: 10.3109/13880201003789432

Chapter 11

Natural Polymers as Potential Antiaging Constituents

Pranati Srivastava and Syed Abul Kalam

Abstract

Active pharmaceutical ingredients and pharmaceutical excipients are the core of any pharmaceutical preparation. API's are responsible for the therapeutic activity while excipients are non-pharmacological ingredients which are used in the manufacturing of pharmaceutical preparations. As we know that some polymers have thickening property, also the water based formulations are fluid in nature therefore in order to change the rheology of such formulations various polymers are used. These polymers act by increasing the viscosity of formulations. Starch, guar gum, alginates, pectin, gelatin, agar, carrageenan, cellular derivatives are the examples of natural polymer that are used to increase the viscosity of water based formulations meant for topical application. The present review deals with the use of such natural polymers as constituents of anti-aging formulations. As is well-known that aging is a natural process in which rate of production of new cells reduces while the rate of degradation of old cells increases because the normal physiology of body changes and free radicals produced by mitochondria as a byproduct and are oxygen containing highly reactive molecules. The antiaging preparations basically neutralize the effect of free radicals and protect our cell from premature degradation. On a contrary note, the already in use synthetic polymers have adverse effect on human body as well as on environment. It is well advocated in various researches that natural polymers have no or less side effects in comparison to synthetic polymers, giving them a positive lead for incorporation to various antiaging formulations. The present review gives a deep insight on the nature of polymers used over ages, there applications and incorporation into different cosmeceuticals. It also discusses the process and mechanism of aging and the phenomenon by which cell damage can be overcome. Finally, the authors have concluded with the upcoming scenario of the use of naturally derived polymers in various skin care preparations.

Keywords: polymers, antioxidant, aging, free radicals, antiaging agents

1. Introduction

Polymers are non-pharmacological agents and use as excipients. They possess special properties and are used in site targeting, taste masking and to increase patient compliance [1].

Herman Staudinger, Nobel Prize winner (1953) German scientist coined the term "Macromolecules" in reference to Polymer [2].

The word 'Polymer' is derived from the Greek word and is made up of two words 'Poly' and 'meros'. Poly means 'many' and meros (Mers) mean 'parts or units of high molecular mass'. Polymer molecule consists of a large number of repeated units of monomers by covalent bonds. The monomer is a single structural unit while the polymer is macromolecule.

- Monomer = single structural unit.
- Dimer = two repeated units of monomer.
- Polymer = more than two repeated units of monomers [3].

Polymerization is a chemical process through which two or more than two monomers are attached together and formed a macromolecule (polymers) in which there is repeated units of monomers.

2. Ideal properties of polymers

1. It should be inert and compatible with environment.
2. It should be non-toxic.
3. It should be easily administered.
4. It should be easy and inexpensive to fabricate.
5. It should have good mechanical strength.
6. It must be compatible with body fluids.
7. It should have no pharmacological action [7].

3. Types of polymer

3.1 On the basis of source

1. Natural polymer
2. Semisynthetic polymer
3. Synthetic polymer

Natural polymers: Natural polymers or herbal polymers obtained from nature mean they are obtained from plants and animals. If they are obtained from plant then they are known as "herbal polymers" (**Table 1**).
Example: starch, protein, cellulose.

Semisynthetic polymer: These polymers are prepared by chemical process in which natural polymers are used as raw material.
Example: silicones, cellulose derivatives.

Synthetic polymers: These are pure synthetic material and are prepared by chemical process called polymerization.
Example: polyethylene, synthetic rubbers, nylon, etc.

Sr. no.	Natural polymer	Source	Properties	Reference
1	Starch	Potatoes, maize, rice, wheat, etc.	Act as disintegrant Act as binder	[15–17]
2	Guar gum	Guar beans	Thickening properties Stabilizing properties	[15, 18–22]
3	Alginates	Present in cell wall of brown algae	Thickening properties	[23–27]
4	Pectin	Present in cell wall of terrestrial plants	Thickening properties Stabilizing properties	[28–32]
5	Gelatin	Obtained from animal body parts like bone and skin	Used as a carrier, coating or separating agent	[33–37]
6	Agar	Present in cell wall of Algae *Agarophyte*	Thickener, laxative, appetite suppressant	[15, 38]
7	Carrageenan	Extracted from red edible sea weeds	Thickening properties Stabilizing properties Binding property	[19, 39–41]
8	Tragacanth	Dried gum obtained sap of several species of genus *Astragalus*	Thickening properties Stabilizing properties Binding property	[42]
9	Cellulose	Present in cell wall of green plants, algae and Oomycetes	Thickening properties Stabilizing properties	[8–12, 43–45]
10	Psyllium	Seeds of Plantago	Thickening properties Production of mucilage	[46, 47]

Table 1.
Natural polymers along with their source and properties.

3.2 On the basis of structure

1. Linear polymers
2. Branched polymers
3. Cross linked polymers

Linear polymers: In this, monomers are arranged in a straight-line chain.
Example: PVC.

Branched polymers: In this, there is also a long straight chain, but small monomer chains are attached to this large straight chain.
Example: low density polymers.

Cross-linked polymers: These types of polymers look like a network in which polymeric chains are cross linked with each other [2–6].

4. Advantages of natural polymer over synthetic polymer

1. All synthetic polymers are produced by chemical process so they causes adverse effect on environment as well as human being while natural polymers are produced from natural origin i.e. plants and animals and do not have any adverse effect.

2. The production cost of natural polymer is less than synthetic polymers.

3. Natural polymers are non-toxic and safe for human use as well as for environment while synthetic polymers are pure chemicals they are not as safe as natural polymer.

4. Natural polymers are produced by many countries because of their demand in industries due to their less/no side effect and they are produced in the form of herbs so production is economic [13].

5. Drawbacks of natural polymers

1. The chemical constituent present in natural polymer is affected by various factors like climate or geographical conditions, availability of nutrition, so difference in the chemical constituent in each batch is possible.

2. During production they are directly exposed to environment so risk of microbial contamination is very high.

3. In order to protect herbs from pests various pesticides like DDT are used which is harmful for human being.

4. Herbal polymers are produced by different herb so rate of growth of herb is affected by the environment, altitude, humidity, availability of nutrition, etc.

5. Herbal polymers may adulterated by similar looking herbs so validation is required.

6. The chemical constituent present in herb may be extracted out previously so validation/standardization of herbs is required [13, 14].

6. Applications of polymers in pharmacy

1. Polymers are used to mask the taste and odor of bitter taste of the drug.

2. Enteric coated polymers are useful in the site specific drug delivery.

3. In controlled release drug delivery system, the reservoir containing drug separated from the biological fluids by a water insoluble polymeric film.

4. Sometimes drugs are coated with hydro-swellable polymers for prolonged released.

5. To protect the drug from the acidic environment of the stomach, the water insoluble polymer material is used. Example: ethyl cellulose.

6. Biodegradable polymers are used to make matrix systems in which drug is incorporated in controlled release drug delivery system.

7. Polymers also used as binder (example: ethyl cellulose, HPMC, etc.) and disintegrant (example: PVP, starch, sodium CMC) in tablet manufacturing.

8. Polymers are used as diluents to increase the mass for tablet compression.

9. In order to modifying drug release polymers may be coated with polymeric film. The thickness of film is 10–100 mm.

10. Various hydrophilic polymers are used for enhancing physical stability of pharmaceutical disperse system. Example: alginate, PVP, etc.

11. Drug polymer conjugates are used to alter the pharmacokinetic of drug and ultimately improving bioavailability. This strategy is also used in the treatment of cancer [8–12].

7. Aging process

Aging is a natural process in various changes occurs in normal physiological process and ultimately increases the risk of disease and death of cell, tissue and organ (**Table 1**).

One of the major causes of aging process is the cellular damage that causes the shortening of DNA, leading to the process called apoptosis. Apoptosis is a process in which cell is programmed to be death in given life spam. This process is important when we realized that each cell contain genetic material and mitochondria or power house of cell. As we know that mitochondria serves as an energy generator during normal cell process and free radicals are produced a byproduct and these free radicals damage DNA and creating DNA fragments and triggers cell to apoptosis.

As time passes the more free radicals damages more DNA and fragments increase the process of cell apoptosis and our body cannot generate cells faster enough to maintain or compensate loss, so in older age we have very thin skin in comparison to young age.

In another process, the cellular down-regulation of enzymes such as superoxide dismutase, catalase and glutathione peroxide which are natural oxidative enzymes which making our antioxidant defense lesser efficient with age.

As we grow with age, the process of cellular reproduction increases and body creates non-functional cells along with functional cells, leading to rapid deterioration of the body's function. As we grow with age, the more numbers of useless cells are formed which interfere with normal cellular processes and leading to the aging process.

Free radicals: Free radicals produced by mitochondria as a byproduct and are oxygen containing highly reactive molecules with single electron in the outermost orbital that are very eager to pair up with anything else that has electrons. The life span of free radical is one-millionth of a second. Free radicals attack on cell's DNA and destroy cell prematurely and during young age out antioxidant defense system protect the cell from free radicals but as we grow this system weekend and not be able to work efficiently [48, 49].

7.1 Theories of aging

1. Genetic theory

2. Non-genetic theory

3. Error theory

4. Wear and tear theory

5. Cross linking theory

6. Autoimmune theory

7. Oxidative damage theory

7.1.1 Genetic theory

This theory demonstrates that gene of an animal or human being contains a 'program' of life span. The genetic theory of aging focuses on telomeres which are repeated units deoxyribonucleic acid and are present at the end of chromosome. The number of repeats in a telomere defines the life span of a cell, and multiple repeats are lost when each time a cell divides. When telomere has been reduced to a certain size, the cell reaches at a stage where it is prevented from further dividing, at this stage cell die.

7.1.2 Non-genetic cellular theory

According to this theory accumulation of harmful substance in the cells lead to aging process. Lipofuscin a dark colored insoluble substance that is accumulates day to day. This cellular garbage or cellular waste interferes with the physiology of cells and ultimately lead to death of the cell.

7.1.3 Error theory

Sometime during RNA transmission process a mutant protein or enzyme is produced which is not the exact same copy of original then it is not be able to work well in maintaining life, as a result cell grows and die. As we know that RNA are unstable molecules and formed continuously while DNA are stable molecules and maintained throughout the lifespan of cell and tissue.

7.1.4 Wear and tear theory

Changes in the internal and external environment of the cell cause cell damage and cell will not work their function efficiently. As time passes, changes in the more numbers of the cell functioning lead to change the normal physiology of body and lead to aging and death.

7.1.5 Cross linkage theory

As time passes deoxyribonucleic acid, different molecules and structural molecules develop a cross-linking with each other. These unwanted links/bonding decrease the mobility and elasticity of proteins and other molecules as a result molecule will not work efficiently. This cellular damage stick surround and can cause problems and cross linking appears when weakened immune system is unable to clean up the unwanted glucose in the blood. These sugar molecules react with adjacent neighbor and can cause cross-linking and lead to formation of free radicals.

7.1.6 Immunological theory

Immune system protect our body from different pathogens, disease, etc. they act by producing antibody against antigen and they also act engulfing and digest foreign cell by phagocytosis.

As time passes and we get older out body losses the ability to differentiate between own cells and foreign material and then immune system sometime destroying own cells along with foreign particles.

7.1.7 Oxidative damage theory

Denham Harman proposed free radical theory of aging in 1950s and according to this theory oxygen free radicals formed during normal metabolic process just because of lot of oxidative damage to macromolecules. This theory is further modified and a new theory came in existence that is 'Oxidative Stress Theory of Aging'. According to this theory oxygen species like peroxide and aldehyde are not technically free radicals but they play an important role in oxidative damage to cell. As age passes the imbalance between proxidant and antioxidant leads to an accumulation of oxidative damage in variety of macromolecules and cause failure of normal cellular process and leading to aging [49, 50].

8. Topical anti-aging agent

Antioxidant and cell regulators are the main agents which are used for antiaging action. Antioxidants such as ascorbic acid, polyphenols and flavonoids reduces the collagen degradation by reducing the concentration of free radicals, while cell regulators (retinol, peptide, growth regulators) affect the collagen metabolism and stimulate collagen production.

Ascorbic acid, tocopherol, niacinamide is low molecular weight antioxidant and they have the ability to penetrate skin. L-Ascorbic acid is water soluble photosensitive substance having anti-aging action at the concentration of 5–15% and act by inducing the production of collagen 1 and collagen 3. Several enzymes are also important in the production of collagen.

The combination of vitamin E and vitamin C is more effective in comparison to individual effect of vitamin E and vitamin C.

8.1 Niacinamide (B_3)

Vitamin B_3 regulates the cellular physiology such as metabolism and regeneration and is effective as anti-aging agent at concentration 5%. A result comes from clinical study that elasticity, erythema and pigmentation of study were improved after topical application for 3 months.

8.2 α-Tocopherol (vitamin-E)

Vitamin E is used in the cosmetic cream because of its anti-inflammatory and anti-proliferative activity at the concentration 2–20%. Vitamin E smoothing the skin and act by increasing the cell's ability to maintain humidity and accelerate the process of epithelialization and protect the skin from sunlight but it is not as such effective as combination of vitamin C and vitamin B_3.

Some botanicals such as isoflavones from soya and topical application of green tea polyphenols decreases the number of langerhans cells and reduces deoxyribonucleic acid damage in skin.

Cell regulators such as retinol derivatives (retinaldehyde and tretinoin), polypeptides and botanicals act by affective collagen metabolism and increase the production of collagen and elastic fibers.

Retinol and its derivative such as retinaldehyde and tretinoin are antioxidant and have anti-aging action. They stimulate the synthesis of collagen and reduce the expression of matrixmetaloproteinase-1. Retinol is most commonly used topical cosmetic preparation in comparison to tretinoin because it causes less irritation.

Tretinoin is the nonaromatic retinoid of the first generation and is approved by United States for topical application as an anti-aging treatment at the concentration of 0.05%. It is used for the treatment of wrinkles, ultra violet induced skin aging, pigmentation and loss of skin elasticity.

Polypeptides also have a capacity to stimulate collagen synthesis and activate dermal metabolism [51–53].

9. Types of antioxidant

Three types of anti-oxidant found in nature i.e. phytochemicals, vitamins and enzymes. Potent anti-oxidants are found in plants because plants are exposed to ultra violet light throughout of the day. Plants generate high quantity of free radicals but they do not cause cellular damage, because they are protected by naturally occurring anti-oxidant defense system.

9.1 Anti-oxidant enzymes

These enzymes are basically antioxidant and are synthesized in human body when eat proteins and minerals as our daily diet. The examples of these enzymes are superoxide dismutase, glutathione peroxide, glutathione reductase and catalases. They require co-factors such as iron, copper, selenium, magnesium and zinc for anti-oxidant activity.

9.2 Anti-oxidant vitamins

Human body is not able to synthesize or produce these anti-oxidant vitamins naturally but they require for maintaining normal physiology and health, so we take these vitamin in our daily diet. Retinol, L-ascorbic acid, α-tocopherol, folic acid and beta-carotene are the examples of anti-oxidant vitamins.

Retinol is important in tissue repair, for eye health, for improving immune system as well as for improving cholesterol level. L-Ascorbic acid protects our skin from ultra violet light damage and it stimulates immune system by providing resistance from infection and helps in regulating cholesterol level.

α-Tocopherol play an important role in maintaining health of blood vessels and it also improve the skin condition by protect the cell's membrane. Folic acid is useful in the process of erythropoiesis.

Various phytochemicals such as carotenoid provide protection against singlet oxygen and free radicals. These carotenoids are found in orange-colored vegetables like carrot as well as in dark green vegetables like kale, etc.

9.3 Anti-oxidant phytochemicals

Phytochemicals are natural anti-oxidant and they are found in plants and used by plants in order to protect themselves from free radicals. Phytochemicals are naturally fount in whole foods like whole grains, fruits and vegetables. Phytochemicals may be dividing into following category.

1. Carotenoids

2. Flavonoids

3. Polyphenols

4. Allyl sulfides [54]

10. Natural anti-oxidant in human body

As we know that free radicals attack on DNA and interferes with normal physiology of cell and to protect DNA from these attacks a series of defense mechanism is developed by body. Anti-oxidant act at different levels and by different mechanism in the defense system such as preventive mechanism, radical scavenging and repair and adaptation (**Table 2**).

1. First line of defense

2. Second line of defense

3. Third line of defense

4. Fourth line of defense

10.1 First line of defense

Preventive oxidants are the first line of defense and they act by suppressing the formation of free radicals. Catalase (CAT), glutathione peroxide (GPx) and superoxide dismutase (SOD) are the examples of enzymatic oxidants.

10.2 Second line of defense

In second line of defense include retinol, α-tocopherol, uric acid, bilirubin, albumin and thiols. This anti-oxidant scavenges the active radicals and breaks the chain propagation reaction and suppresses chain initiation.

10.3 Third line of defense

Third line of defense includes proteolytic enzymes, proteinases and peptidases present in the cytosols and in the mitochondria of mammalian cells, etc. they act by repair deoxyribonucleic acid.

10.4 Fourth line of defense

Fourth line of defense include adaptation, in this signals for the production and reaction of free radicals induce the formation of antioxidant and they also transport the suitable antioxidant to the right place.

Various types of natural antioxidant fount in nature and they are differ in their specifications, mechanism of action and their composition, etc. [55–59]

11. Enzymes

These enzymes act as antioxidant and act by converting reactive oxygen species and reactive nitrogen species into stable compound and is important in the repairing of damaged DNA, Proteins and oxidized peroxides.

11.1 Superoxide dismutase (SOD)

Superoxide dismutase catalyzes the breakdown of superoxide anion into hydrogen peroxide and oxygen. These enzymes are present in aerobic cells as well as in extra cellular fluids. In plants, superoxide dismutase are present in chloroplast, peroxisomes and apoplast in cytosol, while in human body superoxide dismutase-1 present in cytoplasm and superoxide dismutase-2 in mitochondria and superoxide dismutase-3 in extracellular [59–64].

11.2 Catalase

Catalase is an enzyme and present in almost all living organism which are exposed to oxygen and its function is to catalyze the decomposition of hydrogen peroxide into water and oxygen. As we know that hydrogen peroxide is harmful substance and produced by various metabolic processes and to prevent damage from hydrogen peroxide, catalase converts the hydrogen peroxide into water and oxygen [65].

11.3 Glutathione

Glutathione is a cysteine containing peptide found naturally in aerobic organism and it is not required in daily diet because it is synthesized in cells from amino acids [66]. Thiol group in its cysteine moiety of glutathione is responsible for antioxidant activity. Glutathione is one of the most important cellular antioxidant enzymes which present in high concentration and play an important role in maintain redox state of cell [67].

11.4 High molecular weight compounds

Metal catalyzed free radicals production is restricted by few high molecular weight compounds like albumin, transferrin, ceruplasmin, etc. [68]

11.5 Low molecular weight compound

Low molecular weight compounds like Tocopherol, quinines, bilirubin are lipid soluble antioxidant while ascorbic acid, uric acid are water soluble antioxidants [69].

11.6 Minerals

Selenium, copper, manganese, zinc are mineral antioxidants. Copper shows antioxidant activity through SOD while zinc is necessary for normal growth and reproduction of body [70].

11.7 Vitamins

Vitamins re organic molecules and essential for normal growth of body and helpful in maintain normal physiology of body. Retinol, ascorbic acid and tocopherol are popular antioxidant agent [71, 72].

11.8 Ascorbic acid

L-Ascorbic acid or vitamin-C is a monosaccharide antioxidant found in animals as well as in plants e.g., citrus fruits. Human body is not able to synthesize vitamin-C, so it is taken in food as regular diet. Inside the cell, it is maintained in its reduced form by reacting with glutathione, which further catalyzed by protein disulfide, glutaredoxins and isomerase [73].

Actually vitamin-C is a reducing agent and can reduce, thereby neutralize reactive oxygen species, such as hydrogen peroxide [74].

11.9 Tocopherol and tocotrienols

Vitamin E is fat soluble vitamin with antioxidant properties, and a collective set of eight related tocopherol and tocotrienols [75]. α-Tocopherol is one of the most important lipid soluble antioxidant and it protect the cell membrane from oxidant by reacting with lipid radicals which are formed in lipid peroxide chain reaction [76]. These free radical intermediates are then removed and prevents the propagation reaction from continuing. In this reaction oxidized α-tocopherol radicals are formed which recycled back to the active reduced form through reduction reaction by other antioxidants such as vitamin-A, etc. [77]

11.10 Melatonin

Melatonin is produced by the pineal gland and have bleaching action on skin pigment i.e. melanin. Melatonin is used as a protective agent against various processes and agents which damage the tissue via free radicals. Melatonin is found in all living organism. As we know that melatonin is a naturally occurring hormone and chemically is N-acetyl-5-methoxytryptamine [78] and found in animals and in algae [79].

Melatonin is highly lipophilic in nature and having an ability to cross various barriers like cell membrane as well as highly selective barriers like BBB [80]. Melatonin also known as 'suicidal anti-oxidant' because it cannot be recycled when it reduced to its former state [81].

11.11 External anti-oxidant

As we know that our body is programmed to generate own antioxidants to protect life but body is also designed to fight inflammation, disease and toxins naturally. In order to support these internal antioxidant systems we also take some external antioxidant in our diet as regular meal. External antioxidant include vitamins and some specific food products, etc.

Peoples who eats fresh fruits and vegetables regularly have lower risk of health loss. Some heart disease is also prevented by taking tocopherol as nutritional supplement [82].

Nutritional supplement include specific antioxidant chemicals like polyphenol, resveratrol and some other minerals and vitamins. Spices like turmeric, coriander, cumin, fennel also have medicinal properties. Food and part of foods which provide medicinal benefit known as "Nutraceuticals". These nutraceuticals also helpful in maintaining normal physiology of body [83] (**Table 2**).

Sr. no.	Antiaging agent	Source	Mechanism of action	Reference
1	Retinol	Eggs, dairy products, cod liver oil, cheese, liver, butter, etc.	Act by inducing the production of collagen-1 and collagen-2	[71]
2	Tocopherols	Olive oil, almond oil, sunflower oil, peanut oil, oats, goat's milk, almonds, poppy seed oil, carrots and asparagus, etc.	It act by smooth the skin and increase the ability of stratum corneum to hold humidity and increase the process of epithelial cell formation	[76]
3	Ascorbic acid	Orange, lemon, strawberry, apple, carrot, pear, grape fruits, pine apple, banana and avocado, etc.	It act by neutralizing reactive oxygen species such as hydrogen peroxide	[74]
4	Hydroxy acid	Pine apple, lemons, grape fruits, papaya, tomato and plain yogurt, etc.	It act by removing old dead skin and promote formation of new skin	[84]
5	Co-enzyme (ubiquinone)	Red meat, soybean oils, rapaseed oils, sesame oils, oily fish like tuna and salmon, etc.	Act by neutralizing free radicals and increase the production of collagen	[85]
6	Tea extract	Leaves of green and black tea e.g. *Camellia sinensis*	Polyphenols present in tea act by reduce the formation of free radicals	[86]
7	Grape seed extract	Seeds of grapes	Grape seeds contain phytochemicals like gallic acid, catechin, and epicatechin and these phytochemicals are useful in the production of antioxidative supplements	[87]
8	Niacinamide	Sword fish, tuna fish, white meat, corn, green vegetables, grains, yeast, etc.	Maintain moisture content in skin as well as regulate cell regeneration	[88]
9	N-acetyl glucosamine	Shells of crabs, shitake mushroom, shark cartilage, dumontiaceae (red Japanese algae)	Act by improving skin moisturization	[89]
10	Peptides	Milk, eggs, grain, soybean etc.	It act by increasing collagen production and inhibit the breakdown of collagen	[90]

Table 2.
Antiaging agents, natural source along with their mechanism of action.

12. Role of polymers in anti-aging preparations

1. As thickeners

2. As structuring agent

3. In hair products

4. As delivery system

12.1 As thickeners

As we know that some polymers have thickening property and water based formulations are fluid in nature and in order to change the rheology of these formulations these polymers are used. These polymers are used to increase the viscosity of these formulations.

12.1.1 Natural thickeners

Starch, guar gum, alginates, pectin, gelatin, agar, carrageenan, cellular derivatives are the examples of natural polymer that are used to increase the viscosity of water based formulations.

12.1.2 Synthetic thickeners

Polyacrylate derivatives, polyacrylamide are most commonly used synthetic polymers in cosmetic industry.

12.1.3 Role of natural polymers as thickening agent in antiaging preparations

Thickening agent or thickener is a substance which are used to increase the viscosity of fluid.

12.1.4 Xanthan gum

Xanthan is a polymer and consist of a repeating units of pentasaccharides (two D-glucopyranosyl unit, two D-mannopyranosyl unit and one D-glucopyranosyluronic unit). It is a free flowing powder and gives a viscous solution in hot as well as in cold water even at low concentration. It is widely used in cosmetic, toothpaste as well as in antiaging preparations.

12.1.5 Pectin

Pectin is obtained from various citrus peels like orange peel and other peels of various family but citrus peels have highest concentration i.e. 20–30%. In pharmaceutical industry pectin is used as binding agent in tablets as well as used to increasing the viscosity of fluids.

12.1.6 Carrageenan

It is obtained from the various species of red seaweed of class Rhodophyceae like *Chondrus crispus*, *Eucheuma cottonii*.

Carrageenan is used in the manufacturing of shells of soft and hard gel capsules as substitution of gelatin. Carrageenan is also used to increase the viscosity of formulations which are liquid in nature.

12.1.7 Guar gum

The botanical source of guar gum is *Cyamopsis tetragonoloba*. The composition of guar gum is sugar galactose and mannose. It is used as stabilizer, thickening agent in liquid formulation and as a binder and disintegrant in solid dosage form i.e. tablet [1].

12.2 Structuring agent

In order to add rigidity natural and synthetic waxes, lanolin, long-chain fatty alcohols and triglycerides are used. Poly α olefin is used in the preparation of lip products. Glycol stearates is used as opacifier, which gives a pearlizing affect.

12.3 In hair products

Cationic polymers are used in hair products since hair is negatively charged.

12.3.1 Natural polymers in hair product

Polysaccharides (starch and cellular derivatives), natural gums and hydrolyzed proteins are used as natural polymer in hair product.

12.3.2 Synthetic polymers in hair product

Silicones, polyurethanes, poly vinyl amides, poly vinyl pyrrolidone and acetate polyurethanes are the examples of synthetic polymers.

12.4 Delivery system

Sometime polymers are used as a carrier to deliver active pharmaceutical agent i.e. antioxidant. Natural antioxidant include ascorbic acid, tocopherols, grape seed extract along with synthetic extract like butylated hydroxyl anisole/butyl hydroxyl toluene. E.g. polyanhydride ester is used as a carrier to deliver salicylic acid (anti-acne agent) [91, 92] (**Table 3**).

13. Conclusion

The attitude and lifestyle of society changes from last decades and they are more conscious for their health and appearance due to this change various new antiaging formulations are introduced in market. Antiaging formulations generally contain antioxidants and vitamins like vitamin-E (tocopherol), ascorbic acid, etc. The cosmetic industry is one the growing industries in the India, not even in India but throughout the world. Various new formulations like creams, face washes, face pack, emulsions are introduced day by day. As we know that synthetic chemicals show various side effects on human body, due to this peoples prefer polyherbal

Sr. no.	Work done	Formulation	Polymer used	Author	Year	Reference
1	Formulation and evaluation of natural antioxidants creams comprising methanolic peel extract of *Dimocarpus longan*	Cream	Stearic acid	Alifah Ilyana et al.	2016	[93]
2	Formulation and characterization of herbal face wash/scrubber	Face wash	Carbopol 940	D.K. Sanghi et al.	2016	[94]
3	Formulation and evaluation of herbal vanishing cream	Cream	Stearic acid	Dr. Satyanarayan et al.	2016	[95]
4	Formulation and evaluation of polyherbal face wash gel	Face wash	Carbopol	X. Fatima grace et al	2015	[96]
5	Preparation and evaluation of turmeric herbal formulation	Cream	Stearic acid	Ramya Kuber et al.	2015	[97]
6	Formulation and in-vitro evaluation of the topical antiaging preparation of the fruit *Benincasa hispida*	Cream	Methyl Cellulose	Vidya Sabale et al.	2015	[98]
7	Antiaging activities of polysaccharides from *Athyrium multidentatum* (Doll.) Ching	Paste	Protein	Dongmei Liu et al.	2015	[99]
8	A novel *Cassia fistula* (L.)-based emulsion elicits skin anti-aging benefits in human	Cream	Stearic acid	Barkat Ali Khan et al.	2015	[100]
9	Development and evaluation of antimicrobial herbal cosmetic preparation	Cream	Stearic acid	Sonika Pandey et al.	2014	[101]
10	Formulation and evaluation of polyherbal cosmetic cream	Cream	Stearic acid	X. Fatima grace et al	2014	[102]
11	Promotion and computation of inhibitory effect on tyrosinase activity of herbal cream by incorporating indigenous medicinal plant	Cream	Stearic acid	Amit Roy et al.	2014	[103]

Sr. no.	Work done	Formulation	Polymer used	Author	Year	Reference
12	Formulation and evaluation of herbal antioxidant face cream of nordostachys collected from Indian Himalayas region	Face cream	Stearic acid	Priyanka Tiwari et al.	2014	[104]
13	Formulation and development and compositions comprising arbutin, tretinoin and triamcinolone	Cream	Stearic acid	V. Muruganantham et al.	2014	[105]
14	Formulation and evaluation of antiaging poly herbal cream	Cream	Methyl cellulose, microcrystalline cellulose, sodium alginate	Santhosh Aruna et al.	2014	[106]
15	Formulation and evaluation of antiwrinkle activity of cream and nano emulsion of *Moringa oleifera* seed oil	Cream and nanoemulsion	Stearic acid	Asma Shaheda et al.	2014	[107]
16	Development of antiaging cream from chicken feather	Cream	Keratin	Kausar et al.	2014	[108]
17	Preparation of antiaging collagen face mask	Face mask	Soluble starch, sodium carboxy methyl cellulose	Zibin Shu et al.	2014	[107]
18	Preparation and evaluation of polyherbal cosmetic cream	Cream	Stearic acid	Ashish Aswal et al.	2013	[109]
19	Formulation and development of whitening polyherbal cream	Cream	Stearic acid	Sahu R.K. et al.	2012	[110]
20	Formulation and development of face cream containing natural products.	Cream	Stearic acid	Sahu R.K. et al.	2012	[111]
21	Formulation and evaluation of herbal cream containing *Curcuma longa*	Cream	Stearic acid	Sujith S. Nair et al.	2012	[112]
22	Formulation and evaluation of curcuminoid based herbal face cream	Cream	Saric acid	Sahu Alakh N. et al.	2011	[113]
23	Formulation and evaluation of *Cyperus rotundus* and *Cucumis sativus* based herbal face cream	Cream	Stearic acid	Shailini Sharma et al.	2011	[114]

DOI: http://dx.doi.org/10.5772/intechopen.80808

Sr. no.	Work done	Formulation	Polymer used	Author	Year	Reference
24	Formulation and evaluation of herbal cosmetic preparation using safed musli	Cream	Stearic acid	V.V. Painthankar et al.	2010	[115]
25	Formulation and evaluation of cream of *Azadirachta indica* leaves extract on skin renewal rate	Cream	Stearic acid	Kamlesh J. et al.	2009	[131]

Table 3.
Natural antiaging agent reported till date.

formulations which contain antioxidant along with natural polymers. Polymer in antiaging formulations serve as a thickening agent like guar gum, pectin etc. and as a structuring agents.

Polymers non-pharmacological agents and used as an ingredient in various formulations. Natural and synthetic both polymers are used in pharmaceutical industry but because of the side effects of synthetic polymers, the attitude of the people changed and they prefer natural polymers containing antiaging formulations. The demand of natural polymer containing antiaging agents increases day by day, this change causes change in manufacturer to use herbal polymers instead of synthetic polymers.

Author details

Pranati Srivastava* and Syed Abul Kalam
Amity Institute of Pharmacy, Amity University Uttar Pradesh, Lucknow, UP, India

*Address all correspondence to: psrivastava6@lko.amity.edu

References

[1] Kaushik K, Sharma RB, Agarwal S. Natural polymers and their applications. International Journal of Pharmaceutical Sciences Review and Research. 2016;**2**:30-31

[2] https://www.acs.org/content/acs/en/education/whatischemistry/landmarks/staudingerpolymerscience.html [Accessed: 10/09/2017]

[3] Gowariker VR, Viswanathan NV, Shreedhar J. Polymer Science. New Delhi: New Age International; 2005. pp. 1-15

[4] Pandey R, Khuller GK. Polymer based drug delivery systems for mycobacterial infections. Current Drug Delivery. 2004;**1**:195-201

[5] Chamarthy SP, Pinal R. Plasticizer concentration and the performance of a diffusion-controlled polymeric drug delivery system. Colloids and Surfaces, A: Physiochemical and Engineering Aspects. 2008;**331**:25-30

[6] Alonso-Sande M, Teijeiro D, Remuñán-López C, Alonso MJ. Glucomannan a promising polysaccharide for biopharmaceutical purposes. European Journal of Pharmaceutics and Biopharmaceutics. 2009;**72**(Suppl 2):453-462

[7] Patrick, Sinko J. Physical Chemical and Biopharmaceutical Principles in the Pharmaceutical Sciences. 6th ed. China: Lippincott Williams & Wilkins; 2011. pp. 492-515

[8] Chambin DC, Debray C, Rochat-Gonthier MH, Le MM, Pourcelot M. Effects of different cellulose derivatives on drug release mechanism studied at a pre-formulation stage. Journal of Controlled Release. 2004;**95**(1):101-108

[9] Obae HI, Imada K. Morphological effect of microcrystalline cellulose particles on tablet tensile strength. International Journal of Pharmaceutics. 1999;**182**:155-164

[10] Westermark S, Juppo AM, Kervinen L, Yliruusi J. Microcrystalline cellulose and its microstructure in pharmaceutical processing. European Journal of Pharmaceutics and Biopharmaceutics. 1999;**48**: 199-206

[11] Orawan S, Uracha R, Pitt S. Electrospun cellulose acetate fiber mats containing asiaticoside or *Centella asiatica* crude extract and the release characteristics of asiaticoside. Polymer. 2008;**49**(19):4239-4247

[12] Abdelrahman T, Newton H. Wound dressings: Principles and practice. Surgery. 2011;**29**(2011):491-495

[13] Jani GK, Shah DP, Prajapati VD, Jain VC. Gums and mucilages: Versatile excipients for pharmaceutical formulations. Asian Journal of Pharmaceutical Sciences. 2009;**4** (Suppl 5):309-332

[14] Shirwaikar A, Prabu SL, Kumar GA. Herbal excipients in novel drug delivery systems. Indian Journal of Pharmaceutical Sciences. 2008;**70**:415-422

[15] Kokate CK, Purohit AP, Gokhale SB. Pharmacognosy. 22nd ed. India: Nirali Prakashan; 2003. pp. 133-166

[16] Te-Wierik GH, Eissens AC, Bergsma J, Arends-Scholte AW, Bolhuis GK, A new generation starch product as excipient in pharmaceutical tablets, III: Parameters affecting controlled drug release from tablets based on high surface area retrograded pregelatinized potato starch, International Journal of Pharmaceutics. 1997 157, 181-187

[17] Kaushik K, Sharma RB, Agarwal S. Natural polymers and their applications. International Journal of Pharmaceutical Sciences Review and Research. 2016;**2**:30-37

[18] Doyle JP, Lyons G, Morris ER. New proposals on hyperentanglement of galactomannans: Solution viscosity of fenugreek gum under neutral and alkaline conditions. Food Hydrocolloids. 2008;**23**:1501-1510

[19] Coviello T, Alhaique F, Dorigo A, Matricardi P, Grassi M. Two galactomannans and scleroglucan as matrices for drug delivery: Preparation and release studies. European Journal of Pharmaceutics and Biopharmaceutics. 2007;**66**:200-209

[20] Sharma RL. Synthesis and characterization of graft copolymers of N-vinyl-2-pyrrolidone onto guar gum for sorption of Fe2+ and Cr6+ions. Carbohydrate Polymers. 2011;**83**:1929-1936

[21] Murthy S, Hiremath S, Paranjothy K. Evaluation of carboxymethyl guar films for the formulation of transdermal therapeutic systems. International Journal of Pharmaceutics. 2004;**272**:11-18

[22] Dürig T, Fassihi R. Guar-based monolithic matrix systems: Effect of ionizable and nonionizable substances and excipients on gel dynamics and release kinetics. Journal of Controlled Release. 2002;**80**:45-56

[23] Haug A, Larsen B, Smidsrod O. Studies on the sequence of uronic acid residues in alginic acid. Acta Chemica Scandinavica. 1967;**21**: 691-704

[24] Haug A, Larsen B. Quantitative determination of the uronic acid composition of alginates. Acta Chemica Scandinavica. 1962;**16**:1908-1918

[25] Tuğcu-Demiröz F, Acartürk F, Takka S, Konuş-Boyunağa O. Evaluation of alginate based mesalazine tablets for intestinal drug delivery. European Journal of Pharmaceutics and Biopharmaceutics. 2007;**67**:491-497

[26] Moebus K, Siepmann J, Bodmeier R. Alginate–poloxamer microparticles for controlled drug delivery to mucosal tissue. European Journal of Pharmaceutics and Biopharmaceutics. 2009;**72**:42-53

[27] Davidovich-Pinhas M, Harari O, Bianco-Peled H. Evaluating the mucoadhesive properties of drug delivery systems based on hydrated thiolated alginate. Journal of Controlled Release. 2009;**136**:38-40

[28] Mohnen D. Pectin structure and biosynthesis. Current Opinion in Plant Biology. 2008;**11**:266-277

[29] Fry SC. Primary cell wall metabolism, tracking the careers of wall polymers in living plant cells. The New Phytologist. 2004;**161**:641-675

[30] Sriamornsak P, Thirawong N, Weerapol Y, Nunthanid J, Sungthongjeen S. Swelling and erosion of pectin matrix tablets and their impact on drug release behavior. European Journal of Pharmaceutics and Biopharmaceutics. 2007;**67**:211-219

[31] Cárdenas A, Goycoolea FM, Rinaudo M. On the gelling behaviour of 'nopal' (Opuntia ficus indica) low metholoxyl pectin. Carbohydrate Polymers. 2008;**73**:212-222

[32] Vervoort L, Kinget R. In vitro degradation by colonic bacteria of inulinhp incorporated in Eudragit RS films. International Journal of Pharmaceutics. 1996;**129**:185-190

[33] Vervoort L, Van den Mooter G, Augustijns P, Kinget R. Inulin hydrogels I. Dynamic and equilibrium swelling

properties. International Journal of Pharmaceutics. 1998;**172**:127-135

[34] Sudhakar Y, Kuotsu K, Bandyopadhyay AK. Buccal bioadhesive drug delivery—A promising option for orally less efficient drugs. Journal of Controlled Release. 2006;**114**:15-40

[35] Sarmento B, Ribeiro A, Veiga F, Sampaio P, Neufeld R, Ferreira D. Alginate/chitosan nanoparticles are effective for oral insulin delivery. Pharmaceutical Research. 2007;**24**:2198-2206

[36] Ching AL, Liew CV, Heng PWS, Chan LW. Impact of cross-linker on alginate matrix integrity and drug release. International Journal of Pharmaceutics. 2008;**355**:259-268

[37] Nerurkar J, Jun HW, Price JC, Park MO. Controlledrelease matrix tablets of ibuprofen using cellulose ethers and carrageenans: Effect of formulation factors on dissolution rates. European Journal of Pharmaceutics and Biopharmaceutics. 2005;**61**:56-68

[38] Trease GE, Evans WC. Text Book of Pharmacognosy. 15th ed. London: Balliere, Tindall; 2002. pp. 200-201

[39] Mohamadnia Z, Zohuriaan-Mehr MJ, Kabiri K, Jamshidi A, Mobedi H. Ionically cross-linked carrageenan-alginate hydrogel beads. Journal of Biomaterials Science, Polymer Edition. 2008;**19**:47-59

[40] Varshosaz J, Tavakoli N, Eram SA. Use of natural gums and cellulose derivatives in production of sustained release Metoprolol tablets. Drug Delivery. 2006;**13**:113-119

[41] Mythri G. Novel mucoadhesive polymers—A review. Journal of Applied Pharmaceutical Science. 2011;**01**(08):37-42

[42] Ghayempour S, Montazer M, Mahmoudi RM. Tragacanth gum as a natural polymeric wall for producing antimicrobial nanocapsules loaded with plant extract. International Journal of Biological Macromolecules. 2015;**81**:514-520. DOI: 10.1016/j.ijbiomac.2015.08.041 Epub 2015 Aug 24

[43] Nishiyama Y, Langan P, Chanzy H. Crystal structure and hydrogen-bonding system in cellulose Iβ from synchrotron X-ray and neutron fiber diffraction. Journal of the American Chemical Society. 2002;**124**(Suppl 31): 9074-9082

[44] Scheller HV, Jensen JK, Sørensen SO, Harholt J, Geshi N. Biosynthesis of pectin. Physiologia Plantarum. 2007;**129**:283-295

[45] Hon DN-S. Cellulose and its derivatives: Structures, reactions and medical uses. In: Dumitriu S, editor. Polysaccharides in Medicinal Applications. New York, NY, USA: Marcel Dekker, Inc; 1996. pp. 87-106

[46] Kulkarni GT, Gowthamrajan K, Rao BG, Suresh B. Evaluation of binding properties of plantago ovata and Trigonella foenum graecum mucilages. Indian Drugs. 2002;**38**:422-468

[47] Chavanpatil MD, Jain P, Chaudhari S, Shear R, Vavia PR. Novel sustained release, swellable and bioadhesive gastroretentive drug delivery system for ofloxacin. International Journal of Pharmaceutics. 2006;**316**:86-92

[48] https://www.nuskin.com/en_ZA/corporate/company/science/skin_care_science/the_process_of_aging.html

[49] Prakash L. Natural ingredients nurture skin health from theinside and out. Nutracos. 2008;**4**:6-9

[50] https://www.afar.org/docs/migrated/111121_infoaging_guide_theories_of_agingfr.pdf

[51] Bissett DL, Miyamoto K, Sun P, Li J, Berge CA. Topical niacinamide reduces yellowing, wrinkling, red blotchiness, and hyperpigmented spots in aging facial skin. International Journal of Cosmetic Science. 2004;**26**: 231-238; PMID:18492135. DOI: 10.1111/j.1467-2494.2004.00228.x

[52] Haftek M, Mac-Mary S, Le Bitoux MA, Creidi P, Seité S, Rougier A, et al. Clinical, biometric and structural evaluation of the long-term effects of a topical treatment with ascorbic acid and madecassoside in photoaged human skin. Experimental Dermatology. 2008;**17**:946-952. DOI: 10.1111/j.1600-0625.2008.00732.x

[53] Nusgens BV, Humbert P, Rougier A, Colige AC, Haftek M, Lambert CA, et al. Topically applied vitamin C enhances the mrna level of collagens I and III, their processing enzymes and tissue inhibitor of matrix metalloproteinase 1 in the human dermis. The Journal of Investigative Dermatology. 2001;**116**:853-859. DOI: 10.1046/j.0022-202x.2001.01362.x

[54] http://www.nutrex-hawaii.com/types-of-antioxidants [Accessed: 1/10/2017]

[55] Cadenas E. Basic mechanisms of antioxidant activity. BioFactors. 1997;**6**:391-397

[56] Niki E. Antioxidant defences in eukaryotic cells. In: Poli G, Albano E, Dianzani MU, editors. Free Radicals: From Basic Science to Medicine. Basel, Switzerland: Birkhauser, Verlag; 1993. pp. 365-373

[57] Sies H. Oxidative stress: Oxidants and antioxidants. Experimental Physiology. 1997;**82**:291-295

[58] Prior RL, Cao G, Martin A, Sofic E, Mcewen J, O'Brien C, et al. Antioxidant capacity as influenced by total phenolic and anthocyanin content, maturity and variety of vaccinium species. Journal of Agricultural and Food Chemistry. 1998;**46**(7):2686-2693

[59] Zelko I, Mariani T, Foln R. Superoxide dismutase multigene family: A comparison of the Cuzn–SOD (SOD1), Mn-SOD (SOD2) and EC-SOD (SOD3) gene structures, evolution, and expression. Free Radical Biology & Medicine. 2002;**33**: 337-349

[60] Banniste J, Bannister W, Ratilio G. Aspects of the structure, function and application of superoxide dismutase CRC. Critical Reviews in Biochemistry. 1987;**22**:111-180

[61] Johnson F, Giulin C. Superoxide dismutases and their impact upon human health. Molecular Aspects of Medicine. 2005;**26**:340-352

[62] Wuereges J, Lee JW, Yim YI, Yim HS, Kang SO, Djinovic Carugo K. Crystal structure of nickel containing superoxide dismutase reveals another type of active site. Proceedings of the National Academy of Sciences. 2004;**101**:8569-8574

[63] Corpas FJ, Barroso JB, del Rio LA. Peroxisomes as a source of reactive oxygen species and nitric oxides signal molecules in plant cells. Trends in Plant Science. 2001;**6**:145-150

[64] Corpas FJ, Fernandez–Ocana A, Carreras A, Valderrama R, Luque F, Esteban FJ, et al. The expression of different superoxide dismutase forms in cell type dependant in olive (*Olea europaea* L.) Leaves. Plant & Cell Physiology. 2006;**47**:984-994

[65] Chelikani P, Fita I, Loewen PC. Diversity of structures and

properties among catalases. Cellular and Molecular Life Sciences. 2004;**61**:192-208

[66] Meister A, Anderson A. Glutathione. Annual Review of Biochemistry. 1983;**52**:711-716

[67] Matill HA. Antioxidants. Annual Review of Biochemistry. 1947;**16**:177-192

[68] Khanam S, Shivprasad HN, Devi K. Invitro antioxidant screening models: A review. Indian Journal of Pharmaceutical Education and Research. 2004;**38**(4):180-183

[69] Blosis MS. Antioxidant determinations by the use of a stable free radical. Nature. 1958;**181**:1199-1200

[70] Shirwairkar A, Rajendran K, Kumar CD. In vitro antioxidant studies of *Annona squamosa* Linn. leaves. Indian Journal of Experimental Biology. 2004;**42**:80

[71] Fogliano V, Verde V, Randazzo G, Ritieni A. Method for measuring antioxidant activity and its application to monitoring the antioxidant capacity of wines. Journal of Agricultural and Food Chemistry. 1999;**47**:1035-1040

[72] Mantena SK, Jagdish Badduri SR, Siripurapu KB, Unikrishnan MK. In vitro evaluation of antioxidant properties of *Cocos nucifera* Linn. water. Nahrung Food. 2003;**2**:12-131

[73] Meister A. Glutathione-ascorbic acid antioxidant system in animals. The Journal of Biological Chemistry. 1994;**269**:9397-9400

[74] Padayatty S, Katz A, Wang Y, Eck P, Kwon O, Lee J, et al. Vitamin C as an antioxidant: Evaluation of its role in disease prevention. Journal of the American College of Nutrition. 2003;**22**:18-35

[75] Herrera E, Barbas C. Vitamin E: Action, metabolism and perspectives. Journal of Physiology and Biochemistry. 2001;**57**:43-56

[76] Traber MG, Atkinson J. Vitamin E, antioxidant and nothing more. Free Radical Biology & Medicine. 2007;**43**:4-15

[77] Wang X, Quinn P. Vitamin E and its function in membranes. Progress in Lipid Research. 1999;**38**:309-336

[78] Nassar E, Mulligan C, Taylor L, Kerksick C, Galbreath M, Greenwood M, et al. Effects of a single dose of N-acetyl-5-methoxytryptamus (Melatonin) and resistance exercise on the growth harmone/IGF—1 axis in young males and females. Journal of the International Society of Sports Nutrition. 2007;**4**:14

[79] Caniato R, Filippini R, Piovan A, Puricelli L, Borsarini A, Cappeletti E. Melatonin in plants. Advances in Experimental Medicine and Biology. 2003;**527**:593-597

[80] Reiter RJ, Carneiro RC, Oh CS. Melatonin in relation to cellular antioxidative defence mechanisms. Hormone and Metabolic Research. 1997;**29**:363-372

[81] Tan DX, Manchestor LC, Reiter RJ, Qi WB, Karbownik M, Calvo JR. Significance of melatonin in antioxidative defence system: Reactions and products. Biological Signals and Receptors. 2000;**9**:137-159

[82] Stanner SA, Hughes J, Kellyc N, Buttriss J. A review of the epidemiological evidence for the antioxidant hypothesis. Public Health Nutrition. 2004;**7**(3):407-422. DOI: 10.1079/PHN2003543

[83] Defelice SL. Nutraceuticals: Oppurtunities in an emerging market. Scrip Magazine. 1992;**9**:14-15

[84] http://www.stylecraze.com/articles/amazing-benefits-of-alpha-hydroxy-acid-for-your-skin/#gref

[85] https://www.drugs.com/npc/ubiquinone.html

[86] https://skincareclub.wordpress.com/2011/03/20/skin-benefits-green-tea-extract/

[87] https://nccih.nih.gov/health/grapeseed/ataglance.htm

[88] WHO Model Formulary 2008 (PDF). World Health Organization. 2009. pp. 496, 500. ISBN: 978-924-154765-9 [Retrieved December 8, 2016]

[89] Wertz PW, van der Bergh B. The physical, chemical and functional properties of lipid in the skin and other biological barrier. Chemistry and Physics of Lipids. 1998;**91**:85-96

[90] Kadajji VG, Betageri GV. Water soluble polymers for pharmaceutical applications. Polymer. 2011;**3**: 1972-2009. DOI: 10.3390/polym3041972

[91] https://www.polymersolutions.com/blog/polymers-and-cosmetics/

[92] Ravindran M, Alifah I, Fithriyaani N'A, Najihah NA, Asyiqin N, Sekar M. Formulation and evaluation of natural antioxidant cream comprising methanolic peel extract of *Dimocarpus longan*. International Journal of Pharmaceutical and Clinical Research. 2016;**8**(9):1305-1309

[93] Sanghi DK, Tiwle R. Formulation and characterization of herbal face wash/scruber. ejpmr. 2016;**3**(11): 274-278

[94] Nirmala kumari D, Satyanarayana DT, Sai Kumar CH, Moulabi SK, Pullarao B, Gavamma A, et al. Formulation and evaluation of herbal vanishing cream containing *Punica granatum*. Indo American Journal of Pharmaceutical Research. 2016;**6**(03):1-3

[95] Sowmya KV, Darsika C, Fatima Grace X, Shanmuganathan S. Formulation and evaluation of a polyherbal face wash gel. World Journal of Pharmacy and Pharmaceutical. 2016;**4**(06):585-588

[96] Ramya Kuber B, Hema Latha D, Chetash CH, Lakshmi M. Preparation and evaluation of turmeric herbal formulations. Journal of Scientific and Innovative Research. 2015;**4**(3): 286-295

[97] Vidya S, Harish K, Prafulla S. Formulation and in vitro evaluation of the topical antiageing preparation of the fruit of *Benincasa hispida*. Journal of Ayurveda and Integrative Medicine. 2015;**2**(3):1-4

[98] Liu D, Sheng J, Qi H, Zhang W. Anti-aging activities of polysaccharides from *Athyrium multidentatum* (Doll.) Ching. Journal of Chemical and Pharmaceutical Research. 2015;7(1):386-389

[99] Khana BA, Akhtar N, Menaa A, Menaa F. Novel *Cassia fistula* (L.)-based emulsion elicits skin anti-aging benefits in humans. Cosmetics. 2015;**2**:368-383

[100] Pandey S, Seth A, Tiwari R, Singh S, Behl HM, Singh S. Development and evaluation of antimicrobial herbal cosmetic preparation. African Journal of Pharmacy and Pharmacology. 2014;**8**(20):514-528, 529

[101] Fatima Grace X, Joan Vijetha R, Shanmuganathan S, Chamundeeswari D. Formulation and evaluation of polyherbal cosmetic cream. 2014;**3**:14-17

[102] Ram KS, Amit R, Jaya D, Amit KJ. Promotion and computation of inhibitory effect on tyrosinase activity of herbal cream by incorporating indigenous medicinal plant. Pakistan

Journal of Biological Sciences: PJBS. 2014;**17**(1):1-5

[103] Mishra AP, Saklani S, Milella L, Tiwari P. Formulation and evaluation of herbal antioxidant face cream of Nardostachys jatamansi collected from Indian Himalayan region. Asian Pacific Journal of Tropical Biomedicine. 2014:1-4

[104] Muruganantham V, Sreedharan NKK, Jaykar B, Palanisamy P. formulation development and evaluation of topical compositions comprising Arbutin. Tretinoin and Triamcinolone Acetonide Cream. 2014;**8**(10):1480-1490

[105] Surya PM, Santhosh A, Mamidi G, Raghavamma STV, Rama Rao N. Formulation and evaluation of anti aging poly herbal cream. International Journal of Pharmaceutical Sciences Review and Research. 2014;**24**(2):133-136

[106] Duraivel S, Shaheda A, Rabbani Basha S, Eesaf Pasha S, Jilani S. Formulation and evaluation of antiwrinkle activity of cream and nano emulsion of *Moringa oleifera* seed oil. IOSR Journal of Pharm acy and Biological Sciences (IOSR-JPBS). 2014;**9**(4):58-73

[107] Aswal A, Kalra M, Rout A. Preparation and evaluation of polyherbal cosmetic cream. Der Pharmacia Lettre. 2013;**5**(1): 83-88

[108] Shu Z, Zou S, Yang H. Preparation of anti-aging collagen face mask. Journal of Chemical and Pharmaceutical Research. 2014;**6**(8):97-101

[109] Sahu RK, Roy A, Kushwah P, Khare M, Mudotiya R. Formulation and development of whitening polyherbal face cream. Research Journal of Topical and Cosmetic Science. 2012;**3**(1): 23-27

[110] Sahu RK, Roy A, Kushwah P, Khare M, Mudotiya R. Formulation and development of whitening polyherbal face cream. Research Journal of Topical and Cosmetic Science. 2012;**3**(1):22-28

[111] Nair SS, Mathew M, Sreena K. Formulation and evaluation of herbal cream containing *Curcuma longa*. International Journal of Pharmaceutical and Chemical Sciences. 2012;**1**(4):1-4

[112] Sahu AN, And JS, Dubey SD. Formulation & evaluation of curcuminoid based herbal face cream. Indo-Global Journal of Pharmaceutical Sciences. 2011;**1**(1):77-84

[113] Rajvanshi A, Sharma S, Khokra SL, Sahu RK, Jangde R. Formulation and evaluation of *Cyperus rotudus* and *cucumis sativus* based herbal face cream. Pharmacologyonline. 2011;**2-8**:1238-1244

[114] Paithankar VV. Formulation and evaluation of herbal cosmetic preparation using Safed musli. International Journal of PharmTech Research. 2010;**2**(4):2261-2264

[115] Wadher KJ, Lakhotia CL, Umekar MJ. Formulation and evaluation of cream of *Azadirachta indica* leaves extracts on skin renewal rate. International Journal of ChemTech Research. 2009;**1**(1):88-95

Section 4

Pharmacology

Chapter 12

Pharmacology Evaluation of Bioactive Compounds that Regulate Cervical Cancer Cells

Mauricio Salinas-Santander, Patricia Alvarez-Ortiz, Juan Alberto-Ascacio Valdes, Raul Rodriguez-Herrera, Alejandro Zugasti-Cruz, Ricardo Rangel-Zertuche, Victor de Jesus Suarez Valencia and Antonio Morlett-Chavez

Abstract

Cancer has been a public health problem that has gained a lot of death. However, in spite of the advances in the diagnosis and treatment of cervical cancer, women follow the struggle versus this disease. Also, those patients suffer from limited efficacy and specificity, undesirable effects, drug resistance, and a high cost of treatments. Currently, several studies have demonstrated the efficiency of natural products, called bioactive compounds, against cervical cancer cell lines. Bioactive compounds, including polyphenols and phenolic acids or flavonoids, etc., have antioxidant and pro-oxidant properties. These compounds are efficacy and show high specificity because probably they act as anti-oxidant and pro-oxidant. The pro-oxidant activity obstructs growth factors related to different signalling pathways that trigger cancer. Although, usually this kind of compounds helps for dispatching the apoptosis in cervical cancer cell. The aim of this chapter is reviewing how bioactive compounds affect the signalling pathways.

Keywords: HeLa, cervical cancer, bioactive compounds, signalling pathway, polyphenols

1. Introduction

Cancer is a term for diseases in which abnormal cells divide without control and can invade nearby tissues. Typically, cells in healthy tissues only share if they receive growth stimulatory signals known as growth factors, those that together with the cytokines regulate the progression of the cell cycle [1]. The progressive transformation of normal cells into malignant derivatives implies the accumulation of some genetic changes, which can be carried in the germ line, by the development of somatic mutation throughout the life of the individual, or by the incorporation of viruses, which eventually produce alterations in the cell cycle and DNA repair mechanisms [2, 3]. That triggers several oncogenic signalling pathways, leading to a series of drastic phenotypic and biochemical changes in the cell. These alterations refer to various areas, such as growth factor signalling, cell-cell adhesion, gene expression, motility or cell shape [4].

IntechOpen

Cancer rates continue to rise, particularly in the developed world, becoming one of the leading public health problems in many countries [5]. Many cancers are associated with longevity, and the possibility of their appearance increases as the life expectancy of individuals lengthens [6]. On the other hand, cancers of high prevalence are related to environmental factors and lifestyles, which involve a series of modifiable risk factors for their development such as smoking, drinking, diet, sun exposure and others [7]. Currently, many anticancer agents are available, including alkylating agents, antimetabolites, antitumor antibiotics, natural products and hormones [8]. However, treatments available for cervical cancer show low efficacy and specificity, undesirable effects, a high cost of treatment, relapsed among patients who had improved, drug resistance and a decreased quality of life [9–11].

The bioactive compounds present in plants, fruits and vegetables, are antioxidant or stopping different signalling pathways including apoptosis and Wnt (Wingless/Integrates) [9–12]. Also, this kind of biocompounds has a selective cytotoxic effect, attacking only to the cancer cells [9, 10]. But, before its use, it is necessary to evaluate the activity of these therapies through in vitro antiproliferation assays, using cultures containing both tumour and non-tumour cells and different cell models [7]. Also, only few of these compounds have the potential to be therapeutic against cancer. This work describes the advance rise regarding the capacity of biocompounds to trigger or re-establish the antioxidant capacity or blocking oncogenes that participate in HeLa cancer cells.

2. Cervical cancer generalities

Cervical cancer (CC) is a principal cause of death in women in the whole world [9, 11, 13]. Prior reports indicated this cancer contributed with approximately 500,000 new cases and produced between 270,000 and 300,000 deaths in 2015 [9, 11, 13–15]. However, is clear that Hispanic women have a high incidence of cervical cancer and a significant death rate than other women in the world [16, 17]. The described above probably is due to the interaction between genetic factors of the population, geographic locations and environment exposures [18, 19]. In general, the susceptibility to the pathogens as human papillomaviruses (HPV), lifestyle and cultural factors and inadequate medical system contribute to the development of cervical cancer [17–19].

2.1 Cancer cervical and human papilloma virus (HPV)

Current information noticed that almost 100 serotypes of HPV exist. But, 2 of these, 16 and 18 serotypes, are related to the development of cervical cancer in Latin women [14, 17]. During cervical carcinogenesis, a viral protein E6 sequesters to p53 protein. Also, another viral protein called E7 participates in the same process, sequestering Rb protein. In consequence, the arrest of both proteins p53 and Rb induces deregulation in the cell cycle. However, possibly the HPV is not an exclusive aetiology agent that produces this disease. Further information noticed that sex steroid hormone participates in the early stages of cervical carcinogenesis [14]. Previous report evidenced the possible relationship between E7 viral and E_2 (17β, also spelled oestradiol), but this is poorly understood [14]. Perhaps, our knowledge about the risk factors that derive from the developed cancer will be increasing but also is necessary to improve our awareness of the prevention and treatment of disease.

2.2 Current therapies against cervical cancer

In this context, in Mexico 15% of women are detected with precancerous lesions of cervical cancer, and they could be potentially prevented. Currently, chemotherapy, radiotherapy, hormonal therapy, biological therapy and surgery are the treatments majority employed in the early stages of CC [10, 20, 21]. But, the treatments above mentioned often are associated with certain disadvantages, such as toxicity of chemical agent or drug resistance [22]. For example, *cisplatin* in combination with *bevacizumab* can increase the expectations of survival, but they are scarce to the population. In another case, *paclitaxel* is a chemotherapeutic agent used against ovarian carcinoma, but there is evidence of the resistance for this agent [11]. Also, the use of chemotherapy represents other drawbacks, the undesirable effects, the high cost of treatment and recurrence among patients who had improved [10, 20]. All of these adverse effects are due to the lack of a specific target cancer cell, because chemotherapeutics do not have a cancer-specific receptor, protein or DNA [20]. Another limit, in Mexico, there is one radiotherapy machine available for 2 million Mexican. But, reducing the doses of the chemical agent or employing natural compounds can overcome this significant barrier that exists to eliminate CC [11]. Natural or bioactive compounds are used against multiple illnesses including rheumatic, anthelmintic, diuretic, hypoglycaemia and cancer [23].

2.3 Relationship between ROS and cervical cancer

The diseases above mentioned, including CC, could produce free radicals that induce damage to the cells, tissues and organs [12]. However, the proper function of cells depends on the mitochondria's ability to regulate metabolic processes and produce molecules, including free radicals as reactive oxygen species (ROS) [11, 24, 25]. ROS controls both physiological and pathological process related to cell proliferation, invasion cell, and tumour hypoxia and drug resistance [11, 12, 26, 27]. Also, in the cell, a defence system against ROS includes several enzymes such as superoxide dismutase, catalase, glutathione peroxidase, glutathione reductase and glutathione S-transferase [28]. However, when the cellular antioxidant systems are damaged, antioxidants are insufficient to neutralise ROS, and then oxidative stress occurs [27, 29]. Moreover, in a pathological process, ROS are responsible for damaging proteins, lipids and nucleic acids [29, 30]. Nonetheless, bioactive compounds are strongly linked to the radical scavenging capacity and protect the cell against oxidative DNA damage [12, 25, 31].

2.4 Alternative therapy among cervical cancer

The plants, fruits and vegetable contain large amounts of bioactive compounds that act as antioxidant, and they can be used with therapeutic purpose [27, 32, 33]. Among antioxidants, different subclasses are described, (a) flavonoids, (b) phenolic acids and polyphenols, (c) stilbenoids, (d) catechins and (e) tannins, and they are abundant and available in natural products previously mentioned [20, 31, 34]. Other compounds related with their oxidant capacity and ROS productions are listed in **Table 1**. The antioxidants that are most well-known, curcumin, resveratrol and gallic acid, have activity against cancer cell line in vitro [15, 24, 28, 35]. For example, galangin is a flavonoid with various biological effects in different cancer cells [25]. Also, the green tea has cancer-preventive effects due to containing catechins known as EGCG (−)-epicatechin-3-gallate, (−)-epigallocatechin and (−)-epicatechin. Also, CTS extract possesses chlorogenic acid, (+)-catechin, caffeic acid, phloretic acid, veratric acid, hesperidin, quercetin and naringenin. Additionally, fucoidan is a major bioactive

Compound	Anti-carcinogenic effects
Terpenes and steroids	Inhibit cancer cell proliferation and metastasis; cell cycle arrest, apoptosis, anti-angiogenesis, anti multidrug resistance
Alkaloids	Target DNA replication or protein synthesis, resulting in apoptosis of the neoplastic cells
Phenolic compounds	
Chalcones	Anticancer, anti-inflammatory, antioxidant; cytotoxic activities through multiple mechanisms which include cell cycle disruption, angiogenesis inhibition, tubulin polymerization inhibition, apoptosis induction and blockade of nuclear factor-kappa B (NF-B) signalling pathway
Coumarins	Antioxidants and anti-inflammatory; anti-proliferative activity may be due to inhibition of CDK2 activity
Flavonoids	Antioxidant and cytotoxic effect, cell growth and proliferation inhibition; modulate the metabolism of carcinogen, inhibition of multidrug resistance, anti-angiogenesis effect, induce apoptosis and cell cycle arrest
Hydroxybenzoic acids	Antioxidant capacity; inhibit cell proliferation and cell cycle progression; metalloproteinase inhibition
Hydroxycinammic acids	Anti-proliferative effect; suppressive effects of signalling pathways that are related to NF-κB, ERK, protein kinase C, calcium signalling, phosphatidylinositol 3-kinase (PI3K) and nuclear transcription activity
Lignins	Antioxidant and cytotoxic effect
Lignans	Cytotoxic potential; angiogenesis and metastasis inhibition induces apoptosis
Stilbenes	Antioxidant activity; inhibition of cancer cell proliferation, induces apoptosis and reduces angiogenesis
Xanthones	Antioxidant and pro-apoptotic effect; anti-proliferative, cell-cycle arrest

Antioxidant properties can be risen with phenolic compounds described here. However, possible signalling pathways, apoptotic or inflammation, can be affected by this kind of compounds.

Table 1.
List of phenolic compounds. Antioxidant properties can be risen with phenolic compounds described here. However, possible signalling pathways, apoptotic or inflammation, can be affected by this kind of compounds.

compound in *Sargassum polycystum* and demonstrated anti-proliferation, antitumor and anticancer properties [13]. Moreover, pterostilbene can be found in berries and grapes and showed therapeutic effects in a variety of cancer types [36]. Other biocompounds such as triptolide, celastrol and tripchlorolide were isolated from *Tripterygium wilfordii*; these compounds are immunosuppressive and anticancer [37]. Gallic acid is a natural phenolic compound with the potential to act against different cancers or viruses [38]. Further information, extracts from *Annona muricata* leaves were shown to have the capacity to induce apoptosis in HeLa cells, suggesting that the extracts have the potential to be used as a treatment against virus-induced cancer cells [39]. Also, this compound can be used in combination with a chemotherapeutic agent to increase the efficiency of chemotherapy [11].

Also, the genus *Annona* has been shown to have promising compounds, called Annonaceous acetogenins (AGEs), that can be utilised in the treatment of cancer because they induce cell cytotoxicity by inhibiting the mitochondrial complex I, and their capacity of acetogenins to inhibit NADH oxidase was also shown to be important for their antitumour function [40, 41]. However, the biological activities of the compounds obtained from *Annona* species are diverse. For example, the crude extract of *A. crassiflora* significantly alters cell viability of cervical cancer cell lines as well as proliferation and migration and induces cell death [42]. Many studies have described, or continuous screening the anticancer bioactive compounds, and explained the potential of plants against illness [25]. Though, the success of the prevention or treatment depends on the quality and quantity of bioactive compounds. But, the biological effects and mechanisms of action of flavonoids, phenolic acids, stilbenoids and tannins have been studied lightly.

2.5 Antioxidant and ROS cancer prevention

Antioxidant capacities describe the biological mechanism of bioactive compounds and how consequence prevents the oxidative stress in normal cell [11, 31, 35, 43]. But these compounds also can act as pro-oxidant agent and increase the ROS production in cancer cell [11, 31, 35, 43]. However, Gu et al. mentioned that those compounds are antioxidants in lower concentration and can be a pro-oxidant at a high level [31]. Also, the intake of polyphenols and phenolic compounds has multiple protective functions against inflammation and tumorigenesis. However, the success of the prevention and treatment also depends on the quality and quantity of bioactive compounds. But, more critical is the fact that the consumption and bioavailability of polyphenols are insufficiently studied to determine the efficacy for disease prevention or disease treatment [15, 35]. From this, derive the relationship among bioactive compounds and the induction of apoptosis, anti-proliferation, antimetastasis and anti-angiogenesis [12]. Further information notices the interaction of the phenolic compound is involved with receptor or enzymes in signal transduction [31]. This interaction may downregulate or upregulate essential proteins in signalling pathways that control the biological process [35].

2.6 Signalling pathways blocked by polyphenols

In addition to the antioxidant effects above mentioned, these bioactive compounds can induce two phases during ROS activation. Phase I starts when polyphenols inhibit cytochrome P450 (CYPs) including CYP1A1 and CYP1B1, and the increase and excretion of polar metabolites and prevention of the formation of DNA adducts remark phase II [35, 44]. But, pro-oxidant activities mediated by polyphenols and phenolic compounds increase the ROS production. Lin et al. reported that resveratrol induced apoptosis in HeLa cell line [15]. The extract of *Cudrania tricuspidata* stem (CTS) on cell viability was investigated in HPV-positive cervical cancer cells. CTS induced apoptosis by downregulating the E6 and E7 viral oncogenes. Also, the mRNA expression levels of extrinsic pathway molecules such as Fas, death receptor 5 (DR5) and TNF-related apoptosis-inducing ligand (TRAIL) were increased by CTS. CTS induced apoptosis by activating the extrinsic pathway in SiHa cervical cancer cells. Chlorogenic acid has been reported to have anticancer, antioxidant and antidiabetic effects. Also, galangin increased ROS, which induced the activation of cell death via various mechanisms including apoptosis or arrest of cell cycle [15, 20, 25]. Bruges reported that pyrogallol induced mitochondrial apoptotic response. Mitochondrial pathway probably begins with the activation of BH3-only proteins. This protein causes the production of BAK1 and BAX, which promote a membrane permeabilisation. Last, in cytoplasm increasing cytochrome C level, this allows apoptosome formation and caspase-9 activations. In extrinsic apoptosis pathway, binding of the cell death ligands and cell death receptors activates caspase-8 and caspase-3 (**Figure 1**) [35, 45]. Similarly, *Terminalia sericea* enabled caspases-7 and -8 and poly (ADP-ribose) polymerase (PARP) in HeLa cancer cell line [31]. Also, pyrogallol induces superoxide anion, and this generates activation of caspase-3 and phosphatidylserine [45]. Silva et al. mentioned that the hexane partition derived from the crude extract presented cytotoxic effect in SiHa cells and initiates cell responses, such as DNA damage (H2AX activity), apoptosis via intrinsic pathway (cleavage of caspase-9, caspase-3, poly (ADP-ribose) polymerase (PARP) and mitochondrial

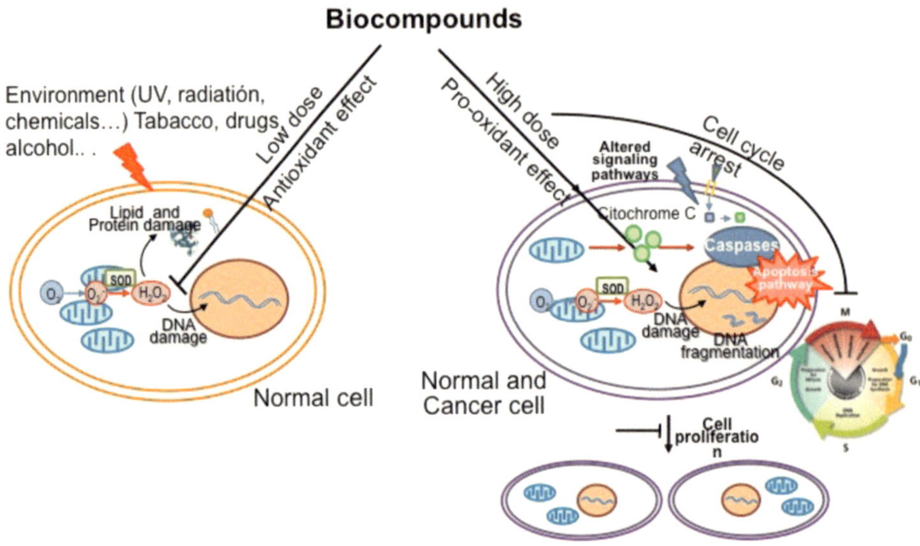

Figure 1.
Effect of biocompounds in cellular processes. In the figure, it is observed that at low concentrations, biocompounds (left) can exert an antioxidant effect, whereby it acts by reducing reactive oxygen species. However, at high concentrations (right), biocompounds have pro-oxidant effects, which can affect both normal and carcinogenic cells and result in alteration of key pathways for homeostasis of the cell, causing cell cycle arrest and stop cell proliferation, damage to DNA and apoptosis, among others, cellular process.

membrane depolarization) and decreased p21 expression by ubiquitin proteasome pathway [42]. Fusi et al. reported that the antioxidant activity of resveratrol, catechin, curcumin, etc. increases sirtuin 1 (SIRT1) expression and monophosphate-activated protein kinase (AMPK) activation in HeLa cell line [27, 44]. Prior reports indicated AMPK is an enzyme that inhibits anabolic process and increases catabolic activity. Perhaps, the relationship between SIRT1 and AMPK may protect against oxidative stress [27, 44]. On the other hand, pro-oxidant activities induced by polyphenols generate ROS and produce [1] cell cycle arrest, and [2] induction of apoptosis and DNA fragmentation. In HeLa cells, autophagy-signalling pathways are modulated by polyphenols, i.e. resveratrol, curcumin and genistein, and act on epidermal growth factor kinase B (EFGR)/AMPK, and this inhibits the mammalian target of rapamycin (mTORC1) via TSC1/2. Also, these three polyphenols inhibit nuclear factor kappa-light-enhancer of activated B cells (NF-κB), and these compounds plus quercetin stop phosphatidilinositide 3-kinases/protein kinase B (PI3K/Akt), and last, rottlerin breaks PKC5 [35, 44]. Last, safflower polysaccharide (SPS) is a major active component of *Carthamus tinctorius*. SPS inhibited proliferation and increased apoptosis of HeLa cells through downregulation of the phosphatidylinositol-3-kinase/AKT pathway [46].

3. Conclusions

The potential disadvantage that represents the strategies against cervical cancer or other cancers is the resistance, high cost, secondary effects and disposal of pharmaceuticals. However, extracts of plants, including phenolic acid and polyphenolic, flavonoids, etc., have gained remarkable interest such as new treatment or strategies versus cervical cancer. The antioxidant properties of plants were demonstrated with multiple investigations, some of which are pointed out in this chapter, especially for its antioxidant properties, influence on cellular apoptosis, ROS increase, etc.

DOI: http://dx.doi.org/10.5772/intechopen.82258

Currently the efforts to discover new anticancer agents continue, and it is possible that plants containing compounds still unknown and that compounds could modulate the pathways that government cancer. Also, the signalling pathways regulated by these compounds have been superficially studied. Unfortunately, these foods are not always available to all people, and in the case of those who have them within reach, they do not consume them. Also, it is important that people change their hygienic dietary habits and improve the quality of their immune system and the level of cellular oxidative stress does not increase the risk for development of cancer.

Acknowledgements

JM acknowledges to each one of the authors that contributed to the writing, reading and editing of this MS. Also, the authors want to thank CGEPI-UADEC and IMSS who facilitate the edition of this work.

Conflict of interest

Authors declare no conflict of interest.

Author details

Mauricio Salinas-Santander[1], Patricia Alvarez-Ortiz[4],
Juan Alberto-Ascacio Valdes[2,3], Raul Rodriguez-Herrera[2], Alejandro Zugasti-Cruz[3],
Ricardo Rangel-Zertuche[6], Victor de Jesus Suarez Valencia[1]
and Antonio Morlett-Chavez[2,4,5]*

1 Research Department, Medicine School at Saltillo, Autonomous University of Coahuila, Saltillo, Coahuila, Mexico

2 Molecular Biology, Autonomous University of Coahuila, Saltillo, Mexico

3 Toxicology Laboratory, Food Research Department, Autonomous University of Coahuila, Saltillo, Mexico

4 Clinical Analysis and Molecular Diagnosis Laboratory, Autonomous University of Coahuila, Saltillo, Coahuila, Mexico

5 Clinical Laboratory Department, General Hospital No. 2, Mexican Institute of Social Security, Saltillo, Coahuila, Mexico

6 Health Research Department, Mexican Institute of Social Security, Saltillo, Coahuila, Mexico

*Address all correspondence to: antoniomorlett@uadec.edu.mx

References

[1] Stull MA, Rowzee AM, Loladze AV, Wood TL. Growth factor regulation of cell cycle progression in mammary epithelial cells. Journal of Mammary Gland Biology and Neoplasia. 2004;**9**(1):11

[2] Witsch E, Sela M, Yarden Y. Roles for growth factors in cancer progression. Physiology (Bethesda, Md.). 2010;**25**(2):85-101

[3] Biswal BN, Das SN, Das BK, Rath R. Alteration of cellular metabolism in cancer cells and its therapeutic prospects. Journal of Oral and Maxillofacial Pathology. 2017;**21**(2):244-251

[4] Efferth T, Leber MF. Molecular principles of cancer invasion and metastasis (review). International Journal of Oncology. 2009;**34**(4):14

[5] Mahshid Ghoncheh HS. Inequality in the incidence and mortality of all cancers in the world. Iranian Journal of Public Health. 2016;**45**(12):2

[6] White MC, Holman DM, Boehm JE, Peipins LA, Grossman M, Henley SJ. Age and cancer risk: A potentially modifiable relationship. American Journal of Preventive Medicine. 2014;**46**(3 Suppl 1):S7-S15

[7] Han HW, Qiu HY, Hu C, Sun WX, Yang RW, Qi JL, et al. Design, synthesis and anti-cancer activity evaluation of podophyllotoxin-norcantharidin hybrid drugs. Bioorganic & Medicinal Chemistry Letters. 2016;**26**(14):3237-3242

[8] Masood I, Kiani MH, Ahmad M, Masood MI, Sadaquat H. Major contributions towards finding a cure for cancer through chemotherapy: A historical review. Tumori. 2016;**102**(1):6-17

[9] Tan BL, Norhaizan ME, Chan LC. ROS-mediated mitochondrial pathway is required for *Manilkara Zapota* (L.) P. Royen leaf methanol extract inducing apoptosis in the modulation of caspase activation and EGFR/NF-kappaB activities of HeLa human cervical cancer cells. Evidence-based Complementary and Alternative Medicine. 2018;**2018**:6578648

[10] Susianti S, Yanwirasti Y, Darwin E, Jamsari J. The cytotoxic effects of purple nutsedge (*Cyperus Rotundus* L.) tuber essential oil on the HeLa cervical cancer cell line. Pakistan Journal of Biotechnology. 2018;**15**(1):5

[11] Sanchez-Carranza JN, Diaz JF, Redondo-Horcajo M, Barasoain I, Alvarez L, Lastres P, et al. Gallic acid sensitizes paclitaxel-resistant human ovarian carcinoma cells through an increase in reactive oxygen species and subsequent downregulation of ERK activation. Oncology Reports. 2018;**39**(6):3007-3014

[12] Rached W, Zeghada FZ, Bennaceur M, Barros L, Calhelha RC, Heleno S, et al. Phytochemical analysis and assessment of antioxidant, antimicrobial, anti-inflammatory and cytotoxic properties of *Tetraclinis articulata* (Vahl) masters leaves. Industrial Crops and Products. 2018;**112**:460-466

[13] Firdaus M, Setijawati D, Islam I, Nursyam H, Kartikaningsih H, Yufidasari HS, et al. The reducibility of HeLa cell viability by *Sargassum polycystum* extracts. IOP Conference Series: Earth and Environmental Science. 2018;**137**:1-4

[14] Munguia-Moreno JA, Diaz-Chavez J, Garcia-Villa E, Albino-Sanchez ME, Mendoza-Villanueva D, Ocadiz-Delgado R, et al. Early synergistic interactions between the HPV16E7 oncoprotein and 17beta-oestradiol for repressing the expression of

Granzyme B in a cervical cancer model. International Journal of Oncology. 2018;**53**(2):579-591

[15] Li L, Qiu RL, Lin Y, Cai Y, Bian Y, Fan Y, et al. Resveratrol suppresses human cervical carcinoma cell proliferation and elevates apoptosis via the mitochondrial and p53 signaling pathways. Oncology Letters. 2018;**15**(6):9845-9851

[16] Ager BJ, Gallardo-Rincon D, de Leon DC, Chavez-Blanco A, Chuang L, Duenas-Gonzalez A, et al. Advancing clinical research globally: Cervical cancer research network from Mexico. Gynecologic Oncology Reports. 2018;**25**:90-93

[17] Morales-Campos DY, Snipes SA, Villarreal EK, Crocker LC, Guerrero A, Fernandez ME. Cervical cancer, human papillomavirus (HPV), and HPV vaccination: Exploring gendered perspectives, knowledge, attitudes, and cultural taboos among Mexican American adults. Ethnicity & Health. 2018;**1**:1-19

[18] Castle PE, Wheeler CM, Campos NG, Sy S, Burger EA, Kim JJ, et al. Inefficiencies of over-screening and under-screening for cervical cancer prevention in the U.S. Preventive Medicine. 2018;**111**:177-179

[19] Pinheiro PS, Callahan KE, Stern MC, de Vries E. Migration from Mexico to the United States: A high-speed cancer transition. International Journal of Cancer. 2018;**142**(3):477-488

[20] Parida PK, Mahata B, Santra A, Chakraborty S, Ghosh Z, Raha S, et al. Inhibition of cancer progression by a novel trans-stilbene derivative through disruption of microtubule dynamics, driving G2/M arrest, and p53-dependent apoptosis. Cell Death & Disease. 2018;**9**(5):448

[21] Ordikhani F, Erdem Arslan M, Marcelo R, Sahin I, Grigsby P, Schwarz JK, et al. Drug delivery approaches for the treatment of cervical cancer. Pharmaceutics. 2016;**8**(3):23

[22] Dandawate PR, Subramaniam D, Jensen RA, Anant S. Targeting cancer stem cells and signaling pathways by phytochemicals: Novel approach for breast cancer therapy. Seminars in Cancer Biology. 2016;**40-41**:192-208

[23] Pereira JM, Peixoto V, Teixeira A, Sousa D, Barros L, Ferreira I, et al. *Achillea millefolium* L. hydroethanolic extract inhibits growth of human tumor cell lines by interfering with cell cycle and inducing apoptosis. Food and Chemical Toxicology. 2018;**118**:635-644

[24] Wedel S, Manola M, Cavinato M, Trougakos IP, Jansen-Durr P. Targeting protein quality control mechanisms by natural products to promote healthy ageing. Molecules. 2018;**23**(5):1219-1244

[25] Kumar R, Tiku AB. Galangin induces cell death by modulating the expression of glyoxalase-1 and Nrf-2 in HeLa cells. Chemico-Biological Interactions. 2018;**279**:1-9

[26] Hou L, Klug G, Evguenieva-Hackenberg E. Archaeal DnaG contains a conserved N-terminal RNA-binding domain and enables tailing of rRNA by the exosome. Nucleic Acids Research. 2014;**42**(20):12691-12706

[27] Fusi J, Bianchi S, Daniele S, Pellegrini S, Martini C, Galetta F, et al. An in vitro comparative study of the antioxidant activity and SIRT1 modulation of natural compounds. Biomedicine & Pharmacotherapy. 2018;**101**:805-819

[28] Hejazi II, Khanam R, Mehdi SH, Bhat AR, Rizvi MMA, Thakur SC, et al. Antioxidative and anti-proliferative potential of *Curculigo orchioides* Gaertn in oxidative stress induced cytotoxicity: In vitro, ex vivo and in silico studies.

Food and Chemical Toxicology. 2018;**115**:244-259

[29] Kouka P, Chatzieffraimidi G-A, Raftis G, Stagos D, Angelis A, Stathopoulos P, et al. Antioxidant effects of an olive oil total polyphenolic fraction from a Greek Olea europaea variety in different cell cultures. Phytomedicine. 2018;**47**:135-142

[30] Joshi KB, Mandavia MK, Golakiya AB. Growth inhibition and induction of apoptosis in different carcinoma cell lines by *Euphorbia tirucalli* stem extracts. International Journal of Current Microbiology and Applied Sciences. 2018;**7**(04):1439-1447

[31] Gu B, Shalom JE, Cock I. Anti-proliferative properties of *Terminalia sericea* Burch. Ex dc leaf extracts against $CaCo_2$ and HeLa cancer cell lines. Pharmacognosy Journal. 2018;**10**(3):408-415

[32] Joghatai M, Barari L, Mousavie Anijdan SH, Elmi MM. The evaluation of radio-sensitivity of mung bean proteins aqueous extract on MCF-7, HeLa and fibroblast cell line. International Journal of Radiation Biology. 2018;**94**(5):478-487

[33] Losada-Echeberria M, Herranz-Lopez M, Micol V, Barrajon-Catalan E. Polyphenols as promising drugs against main breast cancer signatures. Antioxidants (Basel). 2017;**6**(4):88-112

[34] Rajagopal C, Lankadasari MB, Aranjani JM, Harikumar KB. Targeting oncogenic transcription factors by polyphenols: A novel approach for cancer therapy. Pharmacological Research. 2018;**130**:273-291

[35] Amawi H, Ashby CR, Samuel T, Peraman R, Tiwari AK. Polyphenolic nutrients in cancer chemoprevention and metastasis: Role of the epithelial-to-mesenchymal (EMT) pathway. Nutrients. 2017;**9**(8):911-934

[36] Mak KK, Wu AT, Lee WH, Chang TC, Chiou JF, Wang LS, et al. Pterostilbene, a bioactive component of blueberries, suppresses the generation of breast cancer stem cells within tumor microenvironment and metastasis via modulating NF-κB/microRNA 448 circuit. Molecular Nutrition & Food Research. 2013;**57**(7):1123-1134

[37] Wong KF, Yuan Y, Luk JM. Tripterygium wilfordii bioactive compounds as anticancer and anti-inflammatory agents. Clinical and Experimental Pharmacology & Physiology. 2012;**39**(3):311-320

[38] Govea-Salas M, Rivas-Estilla AM, Rodriguez-Herrera R, Lozano-Sepulveda SA, Aguilar-Gonzalez CN, Zugasti-Cruz A, et al. Gallic acid decreases hepatitis C virus expression through its antioxidant capacity. Experimental and Therapeutic Medicine. 2016;**11**(2):619-624

[39] Astirin OP, Artanti AN, Fitria MS, Perwitasari EA, Prayitno A. *Annonaa muricata* Linn leaf induce apoptosis in cancer cause virus. Journal of Cancer Therapy. 2013;**04**(07):1244-1250

[40] Yajid AI, Ab Rahman HS, Wong MPK, Wan Zain WZ. Potential benefits of *Annona muricata* in combating cancer: A review. Malaysian Journal of Medical Sciences. 2018;**25**(1):5-15

[41] Gavamukulya Y, Abou-Elella F, Wamunyokoli F, Ael-Shemy H. Phytochemical screening, antioxidant activity and in vitro anticancer potential of ethanolic and water leaves extracts of *Annona muricata* (Graviola). Asian Pacific Journal of Tropical Medicine. 2014;**7**:S355-SS63

[42] Silva VAO, Alves ALV, Rosa MN, LRV S, Melendez ME, Cury FP, et al. Hexane partition from *Annona crassiflora* Mart. promotes cytotoxity and apoptosis on human cervical cancer cell lines. Investigational New Drugs. 2018;**1**;1-14

[43] Jaradat N, Al-lahham S, Abualhasan MN, Bakri A, Zaide H, Hammad J, et al. Chemical constituents, antioxidant, cyclooxygenase inhibitor, and cytotoxic activities of *Teucrium pruinosum* Boiss. essential oil. BioMed Research International. 2018;**2018**:1-9

[44] Abdal Dayem A, Choi HY, Yang GM, Kim K, Saha SK, Cho SG. The anti-cancer effect of polyphenols against breast cancer and cancer stem cells: Molecular mechanisms. Nutrients. 2016;**8**(9)

[45] Bruges G, Venturini W, Crespo G, Lopez-Zambrano M. Pyrogallol induces apoptosis in human platelets. Folia Biologica. 2018;**64**:8

[46] Yang J, Wang R, Feng Q, Wang YX, Zhang YY, Wu WH, et al. Safflower polysaccharide induces cervical cancer cell apoptosis via inhibition of the PI3K/Akt pathway. South African Journal of Botany. 2018;**118**:209-215

Chapter 13

Pharmacognostic Study of a Plant Seed Extract

Maxwell Osaronowen Egua

Abstract

Most research work on plant source for medicines end up without the researcher reaching a conclusive indication of the implicated chemical name/structure for the cure claimed. A large majority stop at just authenticating the claimed folkloric use of the crude extract of the said plant. A thorough authentication experimental process from plant identification, literature, and methodology to bioassay-guided pursuance of the active compound is carefully penned down. In addition, a vivid descriptive literature of the separation process, difficulty encountered, financial implication of the process, and joy in achievement of results is discussed in a friendly read. Furthermore, a close of the chapter with a plea to researches to endeavor to provide answers in their quest, rather than unending questions.

Keywords: *Corchorus olitorius*, crude extract, separation, liquid-liquid partitioning, fractionation, column chromatography

1. Introduction

Most research work on plant source for medicines end up without the researcher reaching a conclusive indication of the implicated chemical name/structure for the cure claimed. A large majority stops at just authenticating the claimed folkloric use of the crude extract of the said plant. Another group of researchers search for the bioactivity even when there is not a history or folkloric evidence giving lead to their quest. In the hunger of researchers' quest and bid not to "perish" and the unavailability of fund, we are satisfied with the mere authentication of crude plant extract. This is seen in the richness of the literature that abounds on the Internet with multiple claims of almost every disease cure and plant use. The "publish or perish" syndrome which is not matched with the provision of research funds or available research grants and the stiff promotion requirements seem to be counterproductive in terms of paucity of robust quality research especially in the developing world.

The researcher, in most times is like a child who wants to know the reason for everything around him. The child does not just stop at the first answer but persist to the exact utmost reason for his curiosity. The difficulties encountered in a conclusive end of a research quest are numerous though. That notwithstanding there should be some effort at our very best. In so doing, our goal would be met with genuine success and mind-blowing inventions. There could be some difficulty in the knowledge of how to go about the research work, and such the available becomes the only option. And being that the majority seen in the source (internet) is inconclusive, we satisfy our minds at the ease of a publishable authentication of the crude extract. This chapter is met to follow up from the identification of a choice of plant part particularly seed, through to the process of isolation of the active ingredient and structural characterization.

Our ancient fathers knew the natural source of medicines which was once the only option known to man. They used this source to cure every disease that came their way. Over the centuries several options of drug source and discovery were uncovered. The era of synthetic substances (synthesized drugs) relegated our once popular natural gift of nature. The history of drug discovery has cited several drugs from natural sources with plant source earning a reasonable portion [1]. The notion that is still held high about natural products is its likelihood of being accepted by the body than synthetic substances [2]. Herbs due to their high chemical diversity and broad biological functionality have consistently been considered the leading source of pharmaceuticals, employed in the treatment of various human diseases [3]. An important drug used in treatment of diabetes, metformin, is a derivative of plant-derived compound guanidine from *Galega officinalis* [4]. It is now commonplace to include herbal or botanical extracts as a part of medical treatment (as an adjunct to hypoglycemia agents) [5]. It is obvious there still lay in nature's bank a lot of uncovered chemicals useful for the treatment of the numerous diseases that inflict man. These await researchers dogged enough to uncover them. They may remain hidden (researches) if we satisfy ourselves with just the authentication of herbal use. There is need therefore to conduct pharmacognostic and pharmacological studies conclusively, to ascertain chemicals with therapeutic values.

In the bid to guide researchers through a thorough authentication experimental process from plant identification, literature, methodology to bioassay-guided pursuance of the active compound, a bias toward diabetes and a seed plant part research would be described with some effort at generalizing the process.

2. Research study justification

In Africa, hundreds of plants are used traditionally for the management of diabetes mellitus; however, only a few of these African medicinal plants have received scientific scrutiny, even though the World Health Organization has recommended medical and scientific examinations of these plants that are undertaken [6]. Diabetes mellitus, a serious endocrine syndrome, is a group of multiple disorders with different etiologies and characterized by derangement of carbohydrate, protein, and fat metabolism caused by a complete or relative insufficiency in insulin secretion and/or insulin action [7]. Approximately 140 million people worldwide are estimated to suffer from diabetes mellitus [8]. The side effects of taking insulin and oral hypoglycemic agents have brought about a growing interest among patients for using natural products having antidiabetic activity [9]. Pharmacology and toxicological evaluations of medicinal plants are essential for drug discovery, and not to forget, there lay in nature's bank a lot of uncovered chemicals useful for the treatment of numerous diseases that inflict man.

In the guide of the above paragraph, and with a lead to its use, such as a traditional medicine practitioner use whose patient was patronizing an orthodox medical practitioner that was noticed a once poorly controlled diabetic patient having an almost normal control by laboratory test, the choice of the plant seed was drawn from the concoction implicated. Several lead modest stories abound literatures for numerous plants as with the choice of a seed plant part, *Corchorus olitorius* explored for antidiabetic property [10]. Worldwide, a number of plants with acclaimed antidiabetic properties are being studied, among these are *Treculia africana* and *Bryophyllum pinnatum* [11], *Gynostemma pentaphyllum* tea [12], *Ganoderma lucidum*

[13] ginger and garlic [14], *Phyllanthus niruri* [15] *Ficus religiosa* [16], *Boerhaavia diffusa* and *Ocimum sanctum* [17], and *Fumaria parviflora* [18]. Other plants reported study the world over, of hypoglycemic effect are *Fructus Mume* formula [19], Diabetan tablet (a blend of *Salvia officinalis, Trigonella foenum*, and *ginseng)* [20], flower heads of *Artemisia maritima* [21], *Eriobotrya japonica* seeds [22], and fenugreek (*Trigonella-foenum graecum*) seed [23] to mention few.

After this lead choice of the plant (seed), the plant identity is sort, with the help of a botanist, following purchase from traders of seeds of farm produce. The plant and part (seed) of the plant of interest are deposited in the researchers' institution with a herbarium voucher specimen number obtained. The ecology of the choice plant is a necessary literature to be included in the researcher's write-up. *Corchorus olitorius* plant grows in grassland and does well on abandoned fields, often close to marshes, rivers, and lakes, ranging from warm temperate through tropical desert to wet forest life zones, at up to 1250(−1750) m altitude [24]. It thrives best under hot and humid conditions [24]. The geographical origin of *Corchorus olitorius* is often disputed; it is rather pantropical in distribution [24]. In the savanna and Sahel zone, it grows best during the hot rainy season [24]. It is cultivated where annual rainfall averages 600–2000 mm [24]. The optimal temperature is 25–32°C, and growth stops below 15°C [24]. *Corchorus olitorius* is a short-day species. In Nigeria a day length of 12.5 hours caused a much stronger vegetative growth expressed in weight of roots, stems, and leaves than a day length of 11.5 hours, but the fruit and seed production was higher at a photoperiod of 11.5 hours [24]. The plant grows best in sandy loam soils rich in organic matter and grows poorly on heavy clay [24]. It is a leading leaf vegetable in Côte d'Ivoire, Benin, Nigeria, Cameroon, Sudan, Kenya, Uganda, and Zimbabwe [24]. It is also cultivated as a leaf vegetable in the Caribbean, Brazil, India, Bangladesh, China, Japan, Egypt, and the Middle East [24]. *Corchorus* is genus of about 40–100 species of flowering plants in the family *Malvaceae* [24]. The specie of interest is *Corchorus olitorius*, others are *Corchorus capsularis*, *Corchorus tridens*, *Corchorus walcottii*, etc. [24].

The following description of the process of seed preparation, extraction, fractionation, and bioassay is guided by works of Egua et al. [10, 25–27]. Care is taken here at the generalization of the procedure for all seeds and plant parts and advice for an educated modification in choice of solvents for intending users.

3. Preparation of seed extract

The dried seeds are grinded to powder using a blending machine. Soxhlet extractor is used for extraction of the dried powdered seed using ethanol as the solvent. A 10 g of the powdered seed extract is placed inside the thimble made from thick filter paper, which is loaded into the main chamber of the Soxhlet extractor. The Soxhlet extractor allows for several cycles to repeat many times, over hours and days with the desired compound dissolved in the warm ethanol solvent. During each cycle, a portion of the nonvolatile compound (powdered extract) dissolved in the solvent. After many cycles the desired compound is concentrated in the distillation flask. The advantage of this system is that instead of many portions of warm solvent passing through the sample, just one batch of solvent is recycled. After extraction, the solvent is removed by means of a rotary evaporator, yielding the extracted compound (which is weighed). The non-soluble portion of the extract remains in the thimble and is weighed also before it is discarded. These values would help in the calculation of the yield of crude extract from the seed.

The crude extract is first tested for the acclaimed bioactivity before the fractionation procedure is carried out. At this stage, the entire model met for sufficient scientific authentication of the disease is used as it is documented later. And the crude extract is also tested for its phytochemical properties.

4. Extraction and fractionation procedure

Extraction and fractionation were according to Gandhi et al. [28] and Leila et al. [29] with some modification in the choice of primary solvent (water) and partitioning solvents (hexane, chloroform, ethyl acetate, and butanol) [26]. The solvents are chosen in order of polarity. The advantage is to allow for different chemical compounds in the plant part (seed) to selectively dissolve in solvents they are accommodated in (as with the chemical axiom "like dissolves like"). The extracted compound is collected from the rotary evaporator under vacuum at 45°C and is ready for use.

The ethanol extract residue obtained is dissolved in 100% water (500 ml) and exhaustively extracted by consecutive liquid/liquid partition with hexane (500 ml), chloroform (500 ml), ethyl acetate (500 ml), and saturated butanol (500 ml) using a separating funnel (1000 ml). That is, on your initial fill of the separating funnel with primary solvent (500 ml water) and the extracted compound, shake vigorously to make a solution before adding the next solvent. The content is again shaken vigorously following the addition of the next solvent, before it is left to stand till the obvious separation of both solvents. The separated solvent is let out into a container and labeled the solvent (say hexane) extract. The next solvent (500 ml) of choice (chloroform) is again added to the remaining water extract solution left in the separation funnel and again shaken vigorously. The higher the number of solvent used is, the better the expected result and further ease at subsequent separation. The experiment takes advantages of the immiscibility of the solvents with water (the primary solvent used to dissolve the extracted compound).

The hexane, chloroform, ethyl acetate, saturated butanol, and last remaining aqueous fractions are evaporated to obtain fractions [26]. It should be borne in mind that each of the fractions contains a portion of some of the chemical constituent in the primary water-extract mixture in the initial fill of the funnel. The fractions obtained (hexane, chloroform, ethyl acetate, saturated butanol, and last remaining aqueous) are bioassayed for bioactivity. At this stage, the entire model met for sufficient scientific authentication of the disease (investigated) is used as with the case of the crude extract [25]. That is tested for antidiabetic and phytochemical properties in the case of this writer/researcher.

5. Further fractionation in column chromatography

The most potent fraction is selected and subjected to fractionation in column chromatography using silica gel. The column fractions are eluted using hexane, hexane ethyl acetate, ethyl acetate, ethyl acetate methanol, and methanol (in order of polarity) as mobile phase. The obtained pure compounds are isolated and identified through thin layer chromatography (TLC) and functional group analysis by nuclear magnetic resonance (NMR) spectroscopy [26, 27].

A glass chromatography column is set up. A piece of wool is placed in the bottom of the column and tamped down with a glass rod. The column is attached to a clamp stand and securely fastened in a vertical position. The column is then filled with hexane. Some (about 20) grams (20 g) of silica gel (60 mesh) is poured into a flask containing hexane; the slurry (mixture of hexane and silica gel) is then packed into the column while tapping the glass. After packing, the excess solvent is drained (using the tap at the bottom of the column) until it just reached the top level of the silica gel. A thin layer of cotton (adsorbent) is placed on top of the column to prevent it from being disturbed when fresh solvent is added. The setup is ready for loading of the choice fraction with the best bioactivity. In the case of this research, the chloroform fraction was chosen. A quantity (say 2 g) of the chosen (chloroform) most bioactive fraction is mixed with little quantity (2 g) of silica gel and left to air dry.

The chloroform fraction and silica gel is loaded dried to the top of the column. A small amount of the eluting solvent (hexane) with which the setup was loaded is added and allowed to drain in until the mixture was a little way into the adsorbent (cotton), and then the column was filled to the top with eluting solvent (hexane). The solvent system, starting with 100% hexane and 0% ethyl acetate, with subsequent increase in the polarity by 1%, is added. The eluent (fluid/solvent mixture) is collected in numbered test tubes of 15 ml each from the tap below. The column fractions are further eluted using hexane ethyl acetate (i.e., 99–1%...1–99%), ethyl acetate, (in order of polarity) as mobile phase. This was done by increasing the polarity by 1% alteration in eluent solvents' ratio (i.e., ethyl acetate 100%; ethyl acetate 99%/methanol 1%; till methanol 100%) [27]. The process is guided by thin layer chromatography (TLC) monitoring, for an effective separation in the eluent (solution containing "pure compound"). The procedure was stopped on eluent of the last pure compound. The solvent level is never allowed to drop below the top of the adsorbent. The eluent with the same bands of compounds are pooled. It should be said that the researcher could at this stage harvest pure compounds, seen in the TLC as single band. The process is discontinued when the compound(s) desired are off the column. The eluents collected in pools are put in the rotary evaporator and run to harvest the compound (pure or in two or three).

6. Separation with preparative TLC plate

Finally the compounds in two or three bands are separated using a preparative TLC plate after collecting compound in the rotary evaporator. There are different types of preparative plates. The difference lies in the capacity of how much compound it can separate and whether it has a concentration zone or not. Though expensive, the relaying researcher advices for the preparative TLC plate with concentration zone and avoidance of locally made ones that may input impurities with poor separation quality. The quantity (concentration) of the compound to be loaded onto the preparative plate at the concentration zone is dependent of the type purchased. It should be stated here that the loading of the compound is the crucial skill for a successful separation. So if the type purchased can only separate 50 mg at a go, make sure you load say 48 mg for a successful uniform separation.

In preparation one would have first found out the solvent system that would best separate the compound through thin layer chromatography (TLC) testing. This solvent system is what is poured into the preparative TLC chamber (made of thick glass) that can accommodate a 20 by 20 cm preparative TLC plate with concentration zone. The procedure starts with first weighing out 50 mg of the compound to be separated and making into a fine dissolved solution ready to be loaded onto the plate at the concentration zone. The loading is done with a pipette such that it is diligently spread uniformly onto the plate from one end of the concentration zone to the other, just avoiding the very edges (right and left). Allow the plate to dry after the loading. Prepare the developing chamber (thick glass preparative TLC chamber) by making sure it's clean and dry before pouring in your solvent system of choice for the separation. The solvent level in the developing chamber should not be higher than the level of the concentration zone (or the point of load of the compound). It should be just below the loading point when the preparative plate is dropped gently into the developing chamber and allowed to separate for an hour tops. The time is guided by a virtualized capillary movement of the solvent seen on the preparative plate. The plate is removed from the chamber after completion of the capillary movement to almost the tip of the plate and dried at very low temperature say 40°C. The separated compounds are located in the plate by using an ultraviolent light source, and the positions are marked. Since the compound would have traveled the same distance on the plate, it is easy to mark the region and scrape out the position on the plate into a clean beaker. A solvent is then poured into the beaker to dissolve the separated pure compound. The content of the beaker is then filtered to collect the solution (solvent and dissolved separated pure compound) which is allowed to evaporate by low temperature heat of 40°C.

The described procedures are repeated until the researcher has the desired quantity (mg) for both bioassay and structural elucidation. It is advised that one should have secured a research grant because several repeat processes are expected before a reasonable quantity can be gotten that would warrant for a successful bioassay.

7. Bioassay

At this point of the bioassay with the most active pure compound, the methodology chosen should be definitive and not the whole array of test for the particular disease of interest.

7.1. The experimental model of a disease

The experimental model of a disease aids not only the understanding of the pathophysiology of the disease but also the development of drugs for its treatment [30]. In the bias of the relaying researcher, the several animal models existing for studying diabetes mellitus (DM) are treated below. And with this knowledge, the reader can deduct relevant idea to use in her/his field of interest. It should be noted that certain disease state may have more than one model for scientific study. And the choice of test may be the use of more than one model which would be sufficient to satisfy the general entity of the pathophysiology of the disease state.

7.1.1 Normoglycemic animal model

Normal healthy animals are used for testing potential oral hypoglycemic agents. This method allows for the effect of the drug to be tested in the animal with an intact pancreatic activity [30]. This is a valid screening method often used in addition to diabetic animal models [31]. This means that using this model alone would not be sufficient for the study of this disease of interest.

7.1.2 Oral glucose loading animal model

In this method the animals are fasted overnight, then an oral glucose load (1.0–2.5 g/kg body weight) is given, and blood glucose level is monitored. This method is often referred to as physiological induction of DM because there is no damage to the pancreas even with raised blood glucose level. And in the clinical setting, it is referred to as oral glucose tolerance test (OGTT), used for diagnosis of borderline DM [30].

7.1.3 Chemical induction of DM

The most frequently used drugs are streptozotocin and alloxan. Both drugs exert their diabetogenic action on parenteral administration (intravenously, intraperitoneally, or subcutaneously) [30]. The dose required for DM induction depends on the animal species, route of administration, and nutritional status of the animal [32].

7.1.3.1 Alloxan model of DM

Alloxan is a well-known diabetogenic agent widely used to induce type 2 DM in animals [33]. The animals are administered with a single dose of alloxan 140–180 mg/kg (usually 150 mg/kg) as a 5% w/v in distilled water after overnight fast intraperitoneally in the case of rats and mice. Alloxan causes selective necrosis of pancreatic islet β cells producing different grades of the severity of DM by varying dose used. These may be classified by measuring the animals' fasting blood sugar (FBS) level. Moderate DM is defined as FBS level of 180–250 mg/dl and severe DM as FBS level above 250 mg/dl in rabbits [34]. The simplistic argument made against the use of alloxan to induce type 2 DM is that alloxan produces β cell damage, thus leading to type 1 rather than type 2 DM. But studies showed that there are no differential responses to hypoglycemic agents by alloxan and glucose loading hyperglycemic (with intact pancreatic cells) rats [30]. The best known drug-induced DM is the alloxan-induced DM, capable of inducing both type 1 and type 2 DM with proper dosage selection [30].

7.1.3.2 Streptozotocin model of DM

Streptozotocin prevents DNA synthesis in mammalian cells (and bacteria cells) resulting in mammalian cell death. The induction of DM with streptozotocin takes some time. Diabetes develops gradually and may be assessed after a few days, usually 4 days in mice and 7 days in rats. Single dose of streptozotocin in sterile citrate buffer may be used: rats 80 mg/kg; mice 150 mg/kg administered intraperitoneally. This may produce a serum glucose level of about 180–500 mg/dl as DM induction. Although it is the most commonly used model, problems involved in its use include spontaneous recovery from high blood glucose levels by development of functioning insulinoma [35] and high incidence of kidney and liver tumors, due to the oncogenic action of streptozotocin [36].

7.1.3.3 Other chemical methods

Other chemical methods are ferric nitrilotriacetate, ditizona, and anti-insulin serum [30].

7.1.4 Surgical model of DM

This model employs more recently partial pancreatectomy with large resection (over 80% of the pancreas in rats) required to obtain mild to moderate hyperglycemia. Another technique is complete removal of the pancreas (total pancreatectomy). Few researchers have employed this model due to the limitations of the technique which include high technical expertise and adequate surgical room environment, major surgery and high risk of animal infection, adequate postoperative analgesia and antibiotic administration, supplementation, and loss of pancreatic counter regulatory response to hyperglycemia [30].

7.1.5. Genetic model of DM

7.1.5.1. Two types exist

7.1.5.1.1. Spontaneously developed diabetic rats

An example is the diabetic Gato-Kakizaki rat which is a genetic lean model of type 2 diabetes originating from selective breeding over many generations of glucose-intolerant nondiabetic wistar rats [37]. One great advantage of these models is that they can be employed as model of atherosclerosis which represents the long-term complication of diabetes mellitus and tested against several natural products and is without the interference of side effects induced by chemical drugs [38]. Mutant strains obese diabetic mice are available such as the C57BL/Ksj-db/db. With this model it is possible to test for effects of plant extracts on blood sugar, body weight, insulin production, and insulin resistance [38].

7.1.6. Genetically engineered diabetic mice

In this case, rodents may be produced to over- (transgenic) or under (knockout)-expressed proteins thought to play a key part in glucose metabolism [39]. Certainly, the high cost restricts their study in sophisticated protocols which explore mechanism of potential therapeutic agents that stimulate pancreatic β-cell death [40]. Insulin-dependent diabetes mellitus (IDDM) can be developed by inserting into the unique viral protein of mice which is then expressed as a self-antigen in the pancreatic islets of Langerhans. Another is lymphocytic choriomeningitis virus (LCMV)-induced IDDM mice [41]. This procedure is relatively new and rarely used because of the sophisticated techniques, cost, and equipment required.

It suffices here to know that in the choice of assessing a compound, not all the available methods are chosen. Like in the case of the relaying researcher, the following were used to screen for an active compound especially at the stage of crude extract and the liquid-liquid partitioning fractions: normoglycemic animal model, oral glucose loading animal model, and alloxan model of DM. The choice for these three models was influenced by fund, availability, technical skill, and satisfaction of study requirement. At the stage of bioassaying (testing) the pure compound, the only model used was the definitive alloxan-induced DM [27].

After a successful bioassay of the pure compounds, that (pure compound) with the best activity is sent for structural elucidation through functional group analysis by nuclear magnetic resonance (NMR) spectroscopy and confirmed with gas chromatography and mass spectroscopy (GC MS) [27]. The readings are then read out by an experienced chemist. At this point the researcher would be fulfilled for such hard work to be graced by a chemical structure implicated for the bioactivity claimed.

It suffices here to note that there are some quests undertaken by the relaying researcher, not earlier mentioned in this chapter, such as lethal dose estimation (LD50) test of the extract; subacute toxicity; chronic toxicity study [10]; phytochemical analysis [25]; and peroxidatation test of the extract, that were necessary for a successful, question answering research (by providing parameters that aided the meaning/answers of the whole research quest).

8. Conclusion

The best research tends to answer and satisfy the questions asked before the quest, in such a manner that little or no questions are being asked by the research work itself. Though it is impossible for a research work not to leave some unsolved curiosity, after its conclusion, we should have solved or answered to a point that subsequent questions/quests would be too minute to matter. I therefore indulge every intending researcher to engage in research with such resort to have a conclusive end that would be truly conclusive. A thorough authentication experimental process from plant identification, literature, methodology to bioassay guided pursue of the active compound and chemical structural identification of the implicated active compound.

Acknowledgements

The following people are acknowledged for their support and supervision rendered to me during my study period:

Professor Emmanuel Udo Etuk (Department of Pharmacology, Usmanu Danfodio University, Sokoto, Nigeria); Professor Shaibu Oricha Bello (Department of Pharmacology, Usmanu Danfodio University, Sokoto, Nigeria); and Professor Sanusi Wara Hassan (Department of Biochemistry, Usmanu Danfodio University, Sokoto, Nigeria).

Conflict of interest

There is no conflict of interest, as I here declare.

Author details

Maxwell Osaronowen Egua
Department of Pharmacology and Therapeutics, Faculty of Basic Medical Sciences, College of Health Sciences, University of Abuja, Abuja, Nigeria

*Address all correspondence to: limax3m@yahoo.com

References

[1] Evans WC. Plants in medicine: The origins of pharmacognosy. In: Trease and Evans Pharmacognosy. 16th ed.; 2009

[2] Paulo RD, Ana MC, Anderson JM. Reprodutive evaluation on aqueous crude extract of *Achillea millefolium L.* (Asteracceace) in wistar rats. Journal of Pharmaceutical Sciences. (FUNPAR); 2003. 25. 420

[3] Ahmad M, Khan M, Arshad M, Zafar M. Ethnophytotherapical Approaches for the Treatment of Diabetes by the Local Inhabitants of District Attock (Pakistan). Southen Illinois University; 2004. Private ed. Available online at: http://www.sui.edu/ebl/leaflets/phyto.htm

[4] Bailey CJ, Day C. Short report metformin: Its botanical background. Practical Diabetes International. 2004;**21**(3):115-117

[5] Osemene KP, Elujoba AA, Ilori MO. A comparative assessment of herbal and orthodox medicine in Nigeria. Research Journal of Medicinal Sciences. 2011;**5**(5):280-285. DOI: 10.3923/rjmsci.280-285

[6] World Health Organization. WHO Study Group Report on Prevention of Diabetes Mellitus. WHO technical report series No. 844. Geneva: WHO; 1994. pp. 181.1

[7] Edwards CRW, Band JD, Frier BM, Shephend JADT. Endocine and metabolic diseases, including diabetes mellitus, (Chapter 12). In: Davisons Principles and Practices of Medicine. 17th ed.; 1995. ELBS Low Priced Books

[8] World Health Organization. Diabetes mellitus. Facts sheet numbers 138 and 236. Geneva; 1999

[9] Holman RR, Turner RC. Oral agent and insulin in the treatment of NIDDM. In: Pickup J, Williams G, editors. Textbook of Diabetes. Oxford: Blackwell Publication; 1991. pp. 467-469

[10] Egua MO, Etuk EU, Belloc SO, Hassan SW. Toxicological evaluations of ethanolic crude seed extract of *Corchorus olitorius*. African Journal of Pharmacy and Pharmacology. 2014;**8**(9):259-276. DOI: 10.5897/AJPP2013.3892. ISSN 1996-0816 Copyright©2014 http://www.academicjournals.org/AJPP

[11] Ogbonnia SO, Odimegwu JI, Enwuru VN. Evaluation of hypoglycaemic and hypolipidaemic effects of aqueous ethanolic extracts of *Treculia africana Decne* and *Bryophyllum pinnatum Lam*. and their mixture on streptozotocin (STZ)-induced diabetic rats. African Journal of Biotechnology. 2008;**7**(15):2535-2539

[12] Huyen VTT, Phan DV, Thang P, Hoa NK, Östenson CG. Clinical study *Gynostemma pentaphyllum* tea improves insulin sensitivity in type 2 patients. Hindawi Publishing Corporation. Journal of Nutrition and Metabolism. 2013. Article ID 765383:1-7. DOI: 10.1155/2013/765383

[13] Mohammed A, Adelaiye AB, Abubakar MS, Abdurahman EM. Effects of aqueous extract of *Ganoderma lucidum* on blood glucose levels of normoglycemic and Alloxan-induced diabetic Wistar rats. Journal of Medicinal Plant Research: Planta Medica. 2007;**1**(2):34-37

[14] Shahidul IM, Haymie C. Comparative effects of dietary ginger (*Zingiber officinale*) and garlic (*Allium sativum*) investigated in type 2 diabetes model of rats. Journal of Medicinal Food. 2008;**11**:152-159

[15] Nwanjo HU. Studies on the effect of aqueous extract of *Phyllanthus Niruri*

leaf on plasma glucose level and some hepatospecific markers in diabetic wistar rats. The Internet Journal of Laboratory Medicine. 2006;**2**(2):1-6

[16] Rucha P, Ashish P, Arti J. Antidiabetic effect of *Ficus religiosa* extract in streptozotocin-induced diabetic rats. Journal of Ethnopharmacology. 2010;**2**:32

[17] Dwividendra KN, Pratap S, Rakesh C, Bhaumic G, Narendra K, Rakesh KD. Clinical evaluation of anti-hyperglycemic activity of *Boerhaavia diffusa* and *Ocimum sanctum* extracts in streptozocin induced T2DM rat models. International Journal of Pharma and Bio Sciences. 2013;**4**(1):30-34. ISSN No: 0976-5263

[18] Fatemeh F, Sanaz H, Mohamad KK, Arash K. Hypoglycemic activity of *Fumaria parviflora* in streptozotocin-induced diabetic rats. Advanced Pharmaceutical Bulletin. 2013;**3**(1):207-210

[19] Xiang T, Chun Guang X, Fei Wang Q, Zhi Huang Z, Qiong Z, Xing Shuan W, et al. Fructus mume formula in the treatment of type 2 diabetes mellitus: A randomized controlled pilot trial. Hindawi Publishing Corporation. Evidence-Based Complementary and Alternative Medicine. 2013:8. DOI: 10.1155/2013/787459. Article ID 787459

[20] Behradmanesh MS, Ahmadi MA, Rafieian-kopaei M. Effect of diabetan on blood glucose, glycosylated hemoglobin, lipid profile, liver and kidney function tests of diabetic patients: A clinical, double blind, randomized trial. African Journal of Pharmacy and Pharmacology. 2013;**7**(2):50-53. Available Online at: http://www.academicjournals.org/AJPP

[21] Hayat M, Poonam W, Varinderpal S. Hypoglycaemic activity of flower heads of *Artemisia maritima* in normal and alloxan - induced diabetic rats. Journal of Natural Remedies. 2013;**13**(1):9-14. ISSN: 2320-3358. www. jnronline.com

[22] Kazunari T, Shoko N, Nozomi MT, Osamu T, Ikuo I. Hypoglycemic activity of *Eriobotrya japonica* seeds in Type 2 diabetic rats and mice. Bioscience, Biotechnology, and Biochemistry. 2008;**72**(3):686-693

[23] Soeren O, Martin K, Shusmita K, Shamim HT, Hans H. Traditional medicinal plants used for the treatment of diabetes in rural and urban areas of Dhaka, Bangladesh–An ethnobotanical survey. Journal of Ethnobiology and Ethnomedicine. 2013;**9**:43

[24] Fondio L, Grubben GJH. *Corchorus olitorius* L. In: Grubben GJH, Denton OA, editors. PROTA 2: Vegetables/Légumes. Netherlands: PROTA Foundations/Backhuys Publishers/CTA Wageningen; 2004. pp 217-221

[25] Egua MO, Etuk EU, Belloc SO, Hassan SW. Anti diabetic activity of ethanolic seed extract of *Corchorus olitorius*. International Journal of Sciences: Basic and Applied Research (IJSBAR). 2013;**12**(1):8-21

[26] Egua MO, Etuk EU, Belloc SO, Hassan SW. Antidiabetic potential of liquid-liquid partition fractions of ethanolic seed extract of *Corchorus olitorious*. Journal of Pharmacognosy and Phytotherapy. 2014;**6**(1):4-9. DOI: 10.5897/JPP2013.0294. ISSN 2141-2502 ©2014 http://www.academicjournals.org/JPP

[27] Egua MO, Etuk EU, Belloc SO, Hassan SW. Isolation and structural characterization of the most active antidiabetic fraction of *Corchorus olitorius* seed extract. Journal of Advances in Medical and Pharmaceutical Sciences. 2015;**2**(3):75-88. Article no.JAMPS.2015.011 Sciencedomain International.www.sciencedomain.org

[28] Gandhi AP, Joshi KC, Jha K, Parihar VS, Srivastav DC, Raghunadh P, et al. Studies on alternative solvents for the extraction of oil-I soybean. International Journal of Food Science and Technology. 2003;**38**(3):369-375

[29] Leila z, Eliandra d S, Luisa HC, Anildo CJ, Moacir GP, Bruno S, et al. Effect of crude extract and fractions from *Vitex megapotamica* leaves on hyperglycemia in alloxan-diabetic rats. Journal of Ethnopharmacology. 2007;**109**:151-155

[30] Etuk EU. Animals models for studying diabetes mellitus. Agriculture and Biology Journal of North America. 2010. ISSN Print; 21517517, ISSN Online; 2151-7525

[31] Williamson EM, Okpoko DT, Evans FJ. Pharmacological Methods in Phytotherapy Research. Third Avenue, New York, USA: John Wiley and sons, Inc; 1996. pp. 155-167. ISBN0471 942162

[32] Federiuk IF, Casey HM, Quinn MJ, Wood MD, Ward WK. Induction of type 1 diabetes mellitus in laboratory rats by use of alloxan; route of administration, pitfalls, and insulin treatment. Comprehensive Medicine. 2004;**54**:252-257

[33] Viana GS, Medeiros AC, Lacerda AM, Leal LK, Vale TG, Matos FJ. Hypoglycemic and anti-lipemic effects of the aqueous extract from *Cissus sicyoides*. BMC Pharmacology and Toxicology. 2004;**8**:4-9

[34] Huralikuppi JC. Antidiabetic effect of *Nelumbo nucifera* extract: Part 2. Phytotherapy Research. 1991;**5**:217-223

[35] Iwase M, Nnunoi K, Wakisaka M, Kikuchi M, Maki Y, Sadoshima S, et al. Spontaneous recovery from non insulin-dependent diabetes mellitus induced by neonatal streptozotocin treatment in spontaneously hypertensive rats. Metabolism. 1991;**40**:10-14

[36] Kazumi T, Yoshino G, Fuji S, Baba S. Tumonigenic action of streptozotocin on the pancreas and kidney in male wister rats. Cancer Research. 1978;**38**:2144-2147

[37] Chen D, Wang MW. Development and application of rodent models for type 2 diabetis. Diabetis, Obesity and Metabolism. 2005;**7**:307-317

[38] Wu KK, Huan Y. Diabetic atherosclerosis mouse models. Atherosclerosis. 2007;**191**:241-249

[39] Masiello P. Animal model of type 11 diabetes with reduce pancreatic β-cell mass. The International Journal of Biochemistry and Cell Biology. 2006;**38**:873-893

[40] Meiton P. Reversal of type 1 diabetes in mice. The New England Journal of Medicine. 2006;**355**:89-90

[41] Oldstone MBA, Nerenberg M, Southern P, Price J, Lewicki H. Virus infection triggers insulin-dependent diabetes mellitus in a transgenic model: Role of anti-self (virus) immune response. Cell. 1991;**65**:319-331

Chapter 14

Natural Products in Drug Discovery

Akshada Amit Koparde, Rajendra Chandrashekar Doijad and Chandrakant Shripal Magdum

Abstract

Drug discovery using natural products is a challenging task for designing new leads. It describe the bioactive compounds derived from natural resources, its phytochemical analysis, characterization and pharmacological investigation. It focuses on the success of these resources in the process of finding and discovering new and effective drug compounds that can be useful for human resources. From many years, natural products have been acting as a source of therapeutic agents and have shown beneficial uses. Only natural product drug discovery plays an important role to develop the scientific evidence of these natural resources. Research in drug discovery needs to develop robust and viable lead molecules, which step forward from a screening hit to a drug candidate through structural elucidation and structure identification through GC–MS, NMR, IR, HPLC, and HPTLC. The development of new technologies has revolutionized the screening of natural products in discovering new drugs. Utilizing these technologies gives us an opportunity to perform research in screening new molecules using a software and database to establish natural products as a major source for drug discovery. It finally leads to lead structure discovery. Powerful new technologies are revolutionizing natural herbal drug discovery.

Keywords: natural products, herbal, drug discovery, phytochemicals, bioactive

1. Introduction

Natural products and traditional medicines are of great importance. Natural products and their derivatives have been recognized for many years as a source of therapeutic agents and structural diversity. Natural products have a wide range of diversity of multidimensional chemical structures; in the meantime, the utility of natural products as biological function modifiers has also won considerable attention [1].

Drug discovery is leading to be a challenging scientific task to find robust and viable lead candidates, which is nothing but the process flow from a screening of natural product to a new isolate that requires expertise and experience. However, in addition to their chemical structure diversity and their biodiversity, the development of new technologies has revolutionized the screening of natural products in discovering new drugs [2]. Applying these technologies offers a unique opportunity to reestablish natural products as a major source for drug discovery. The present article attempts to describe the process of isolation, characterization, and utilization of bioactive compounds derived from natural products as drug candidates called as lead, which focus on the success of pharmacological activity in the process of finding new and effective drug compounds; this process is commonly referred to as "natural product in drug discovery."

Natural products played a vital role on this earth, so man's existence has been made possible. The outstanding phenomenon of nature always stands as golden mark for achieving the herbal drug discovery [3].

From earlier decades medicinal plants existed on earth. Thus, medicinal herbs are of global and paramount importance. The world is decorated with medicinal herbs, which is a rich wealth of endurance. Every plant is identified by its own different therapeutic properties due to active bioactive molecule. In the modern system of medicine, natural drug substances are reported to be vital and have appreciable roles. Their therapeutic role was justified by the presence of their bioactive molecules. Due to disease-inhibiting capabilities, they are extremely useful as natural drugs, provide basic bioactive compounds that are less toxic and more effective, and bring biological and chemical means of modification and extraction of natural products into potent drug.

The raw materials for Ayurvedic medicines were mostly obtained from plant sources in the form of crude drugs such as dried herbal powders or their extracts or mixture of products. Apart from these systems, there has been a rich heritage of ethnobotanical usage of herbs by various colorful tribal communities in the country [4].

It has been estimated that nearly 75,000 species of higher plants exist on the earth, and only 10% have been used in traditional medicine. Only 1 to 5% have been studied scientifically and are known to have therapeutic value [5].

Around the globe, herbal medicine is based on traditional medicine. As per the oral survey made in many regions of the world, it has been said that traditional medicines have their own importance and basic philosophy. So exploration of the chemical constituents of the plants and their pharmacological screening may provide us the basis for developing a lead molecule through herbal drug discovery. The very important life-saving drugs have been provided by herbs in modern medicine. But among the estimated 4-lakh plant species, only 6% have been studied for their activity and very less not more than of 20% have been investigated phytochemically [6]. Thus, there is a need of investigating the various bioactive fractions and the phytoanalysis and phytopharmacological evaluation of herbal drugs for achieving the dreams of herbal drug discovery.

Working role of every green herbal drugs from plant source and synthesis of bioactive products in their own way as God's gift and preserve them within which are extractable and used raw material as and when required through various scientific process for various scientific investigations and study of herbal drug discovery. Many pharmaceutical compounds contain secondary metabolites of plants that are of vital importance in drug designing. However, in order to have a good supply of the source material, some factors like environmental changes, diverse geographical distribution, labor cost, and selection of the superior plant should be taken care of by green plant developers so that good plants will be beneficial to pharmaceutical industry to develop good-quality herbal drugs [7].

Natural products have played, and will continue to play, a key role in drug discovery and are therefore traditionally claimed as the cornerstones of drug discovery and development. Many drugs that are available in market today were discovered from natural sources [8]. An important example is the analgesic activity of aspirin [22], which is so far the world's best known and most universally used medicinal agent. Its origin is from the plant genera *Salix* spp. and *Populus* spp. and it is related to salicin. A good example is serendipitous discovery of the antibiotic penicillin [22] in the laboratory from the fungus *Penicillium notatum.*

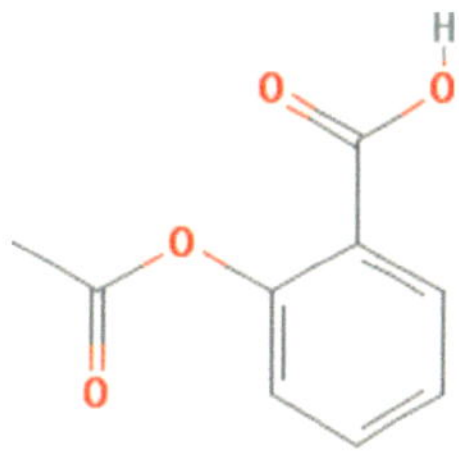

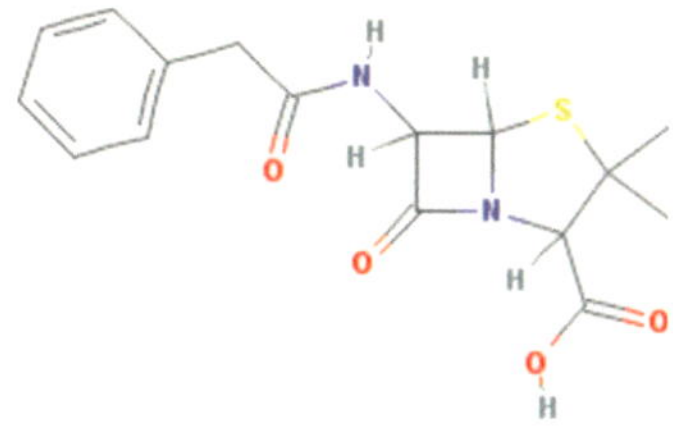

Aspirin [22] Penicillin [22]

Many other examples show the value and importance of natural products from plants and microorganisms in modern days. Paclitaxel (Taxol [22]), which was first isolated from the bark of the Pacific yew tree *Taxus brevifolia* (Taxaceae), is the most recent example of an important natural product that has made an impact in medicine. Activity against a variety of retroviruses, including HIV, two compounds isolated from *Hypericum perforatum* (Guttiferae) are hypericin and pseudohypericin. They are of paramount importance due to inhibition of release of reverse transcriptase by stabilizing the structure of the HIV capsid and thus preventing the uncoating process [9, 10].

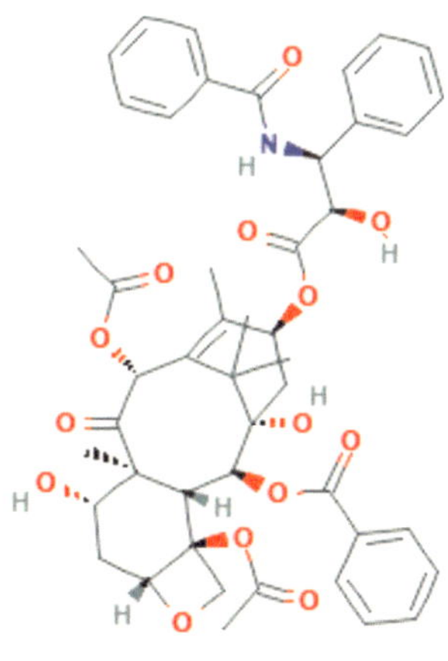

Taxol [22]

In four different ways, medicinal plants having good therapeutic properties are valuable for modern system of herbal and natural drug discovery.

1. They are used as direct sources of therapeutic and bioactive agents.

2. Bioactive fractions serve as raw material base for the elaboration and development of herbal-based more complex semisynthetic chemical compounds.

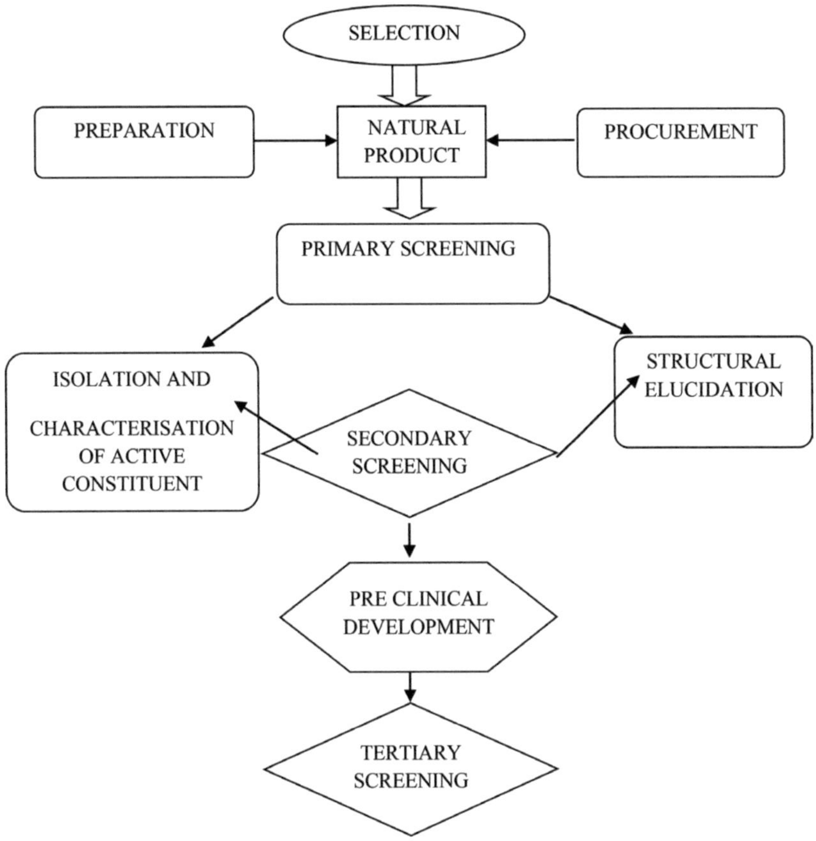

Figure 1.
Various strategies for the discovery of drugs from natural resources.

3. The isolated structures derived from herbal plant species can be used as lead for new drug discovery in developing herbal compounds.

4. Lastly, plants can be used as bioactive markers for the spectroscopic and chromatographic analysis along with the discovery of new compounds.

Various strategies for the discovery of drugs from natural resources can be seen in **Figure 1**.

2. Important steps for successful completion of natural drug discovery

Phytochemistry or phytoanalysis of natural product in chemistry research is the backbone and pillar of herbal pharmaceutical as well as food industry. To achieve success in natural drug discovery and use of herbals in modern medicine, the steps to be followed are listed below [11]:

1. Extraction, isolation with chromatographic separation, purification, and characterization of new phytoconstituents having good bioactivity

2. Use of newly isolated phytoconstituents as "lead" compound for designing of new analogues with either improved therapeutic activity or reduced toxicity

3. Conversation of lead phytoconstituents into medicinally important drugs by herbal drug discovery and herbal drugs used by common people showing socioeconomic benefit

3. Practical outlook of herbal drug discovery

The following facets represent outlook of the stages involved in the development of bioactive molecule as pure drug from a plant source [12].

1. Collection and identification of the plant, authentication, and deposition of sample in herbarium like the botanical survey of India

2. Literature survey and analysis on the plant species along with the activity present in the selected plants for studies

3. Extraction of nonpolar to polar solvent and preparation of extracts for phytochemical analysis and their biological testing [13]

4. Evaluation of plant extracts by judging of different biological test methods

5. Chromatographic analysis by activity-guided fractionation of the extract, monitoring each chromatographic fraction, its isolation calculating Rf values,area as per the computer based software's and comparison with available bioactive markers which leads to the investigation

6. Structure elucidation using spectroscopic techniques of bioactive isolates using chemical methods

7. Testing of each bioactive compound in all in vitro and in vivo phytopharmacological test methods, in order to determine potency and selectivity of the herbal extract or isolates for the discovery of herbal drugs

8. Performing molecular modeling studies and preparing derivatives of the active compound of interest

9. When total synthesis is not practical, carrying out large-scale reisolation of interesting active compounds for toxicological and pharmacological studies

10. Clinical trials (phase I–III).

First of all, in order to study medicinal plants, selection of plant and which type of pharmacological activity is to be studied should be clear to the researcher. Five principles of selection of plants are very important to know which are the random, the taxonomic, the phytochemical, the ethno-medical and the information-managed approach (**Figure 2**) [14].

- In the random selection, collection of all available plants in the area, which is to be studied, is collected based only on visualization and observation without having knowledge and experience about the selected plants.

- In the taxonomic approach, prior knowledge about the plants of interest with their specific genus or family and their different locations should be known.

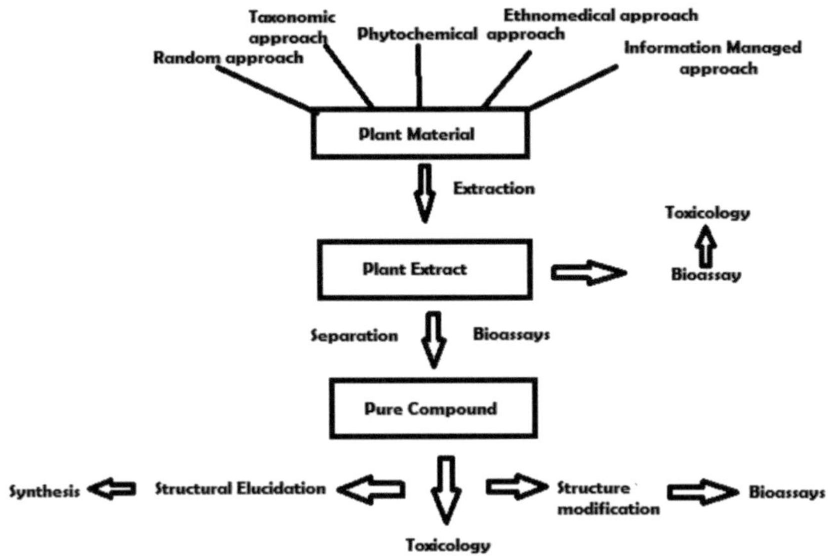

Figure 2.
General procedure for obtaining active principles from plants.

- The phytochemical (chemotaxonomic) approach is based on the knowledge of bioactive chemical type for treating particular disease of interest should be known and are collected. Taxonomic and the phytochemical approaches are interrelated.

- In the ethnomedical approach, selection is totally based on the information of the medicinal use of that particular plant in various areas.

- Lastly, information managed approach is basically collection of plants based on survey and use of plants from their local area that gives prior idea about their usage and activity and then their evaluation scientifically.

4. Position of herbal drugs

In the current era, new and newer diseases are causing threat to common people around the world. Thus, disease percentage differs in every part of the world, but diseases are not new; due to global warming, they are detected newly. Prevention is better than cure, so WHO had taken the vouch of providing "Health for all" by 2000 AD.

Multidisciplinary research on plants has led to many new drugs, as well as prototype active molecules and biological tools; for examples, see [14].

5. Natural drugs available in market: anti-inflammatory

5.1 Himalaya *Boswellia*

Himalaya herbals are developed herbal product from Boswellia, which are a pure herb extract. The bioactive molecule constituent in the gum resin of Shallaki or *Boswellia serrata* was boswellic acid. Pyrazoline as a lead molecule is present in boswellic acid. It acts through the mechanism of supporting the body's natural immune response and preventing inflammation and providing healthy joints and muscle. *Boswellia* is a natural and safe herb for joint health, as it gently cares for it. *Boswellia* is a good promoter of healthy cholesterol and triglyceride levels and provides broad health and immune-modulating benefits. *Boswellia* has been used extensively in Ayurveda for arthritis and to provide an overall sense of well-being.

5.2 Ginger

From long years ago, herbal medicine has paid hats off to ginger due to its ability to boost the immune system. It is believed that ginger is used in day-to-day life because it plays an important role in warming the body. It can help to clean our body from accumulated toxins by its break down in your body. It's also known to cleanse the lymphatic system, our body's sewage system. Ginger prevents the accumulation of toxins and a person's body is highly safe guarded from viral, fungal, and bacterial infections. Medicinal plant ginger also shows many health benefits. It is specially used as natural remedy for nausea and pain alleviation and for its anti-inflammatory properties and inhibiting diabetes.

5.3 Licorice root

Licorice is becoming evident and lighten up in various researches for treatment and prevention of diseases like hepatitis C, HIV, and influenza. From a study, it confirms the antiviral activity of licorice root due to its triterpenoid content. It notes that licorice's antioxidant, free radical-scavenging and immuno-stimulating effects. Licorice root benefits also include pain relief.

5.4 Olive leaf

The olive leaf has antiviral properties, giving it the ability to treat the common cold and dangerous viruses.

5.5 Oregano

Oregano oil benefits are lightening up to be more superior to some antibiotics, with no harmful side effects on health, and can be used in day-to-day life. Carvacrol and thymol are the bioactive molecules isolated and studied and reported to have powerful properties and uses. They act upon viral infections, as well as allergies, tumors, parasites and disease-causing inflammation.

6. Future avenues in herbal drug discovery

In the current era, in many developed countries, priorities has been given to scientific research on medicinal plants is growing need of an hour in various research institutes, universities and pharmaceutical laboratories as well as in the clinics thereof. This research is put forward in mainly two directions: first, bioactive molecule of plants that have long been known and used for their healing properties based on the prior knowledge of the survey and literature. The second phase of basic research has led to the discovery of new medicinal plants with new bioactive molecules, new bioactivity, and new drugs from the more remote regions of the world [15].

Drugs of Ayurveda, Unani, and Siddha need scientific investigation of each and every traditional medicine, which should be put forward for testing and validation. Many government and private companies like CSIR, New Delhi, are already involved in this filed and have validated about thousands of formulations for different activities. This is a welcome trend and it plays a vital role to correlate the traditional practice with modern knowledge for the betterment of health. WHO has emphasized the need to ensure the quality control of herbs and herbal formulations by using modern techniques. Almost many countries have their own herbal pharmacopeias and make time to time amendments for new monographs and procedures to maintain their quality of herbal products that are benefited by common man. Example Ayurvedic pharmacopeia of India includes many basic quality parameters, isolation techniques, separation, and spectroscopic identification for more than hundred common herbal drugs.

6.1 Analytical methodologies

It plays an eminent role in herbal natural drug discovery, and without analytical methodologies, it is hardly impossible. Spectroscopic characterization is the backbone and pillar of herbal drug discovery. The knowledge of this plays an important role in developing the new lead, which can be used for designing new molecules with short modification. The important steps are the extraction, isolation, and characterization of active ingredients from herbal plants [16]. Different techniques of extraction are well known as extraction is the most important step toward the analysis of bioactive constituents. Microwave-assisted extraction and conventional extraction should be studied specifically, which give the ideas about the yield obtained. Further, it highlights the isolation of active molecules by chromatographic techniques like TLC, column chromatography. The most important step toward analysis of bioactive compounds present in the plant extracts is characterization, which includes phytochemical screening assays that give ideas about the presence of secondary metabolites used to cure the health problems. Highly sophisticated techniques for structure identification of lead molecule bioactive fraction are high-performance liquid chromatography (HPLC), high-performance thin-layer chromatography (HPTLC), Fourier-transform infrared spectroscopy (FTIR), nuclear magnetic resonance (NMR), and gas chromatography–mass spectrometry (GC–MS). These techniques are the heart and key challenges in research of natural drug discovery giving rise to natural products in drug discovery.

6.2 Isolation, identification, and characterization of phytochemicals

The combination of various types of bioactive compound or phytochemicals is usually present in different plant extracts. The different bioactive compounds have different polarities. Separation, identification, and characterization of bioactive compounds are a big challenging job in the herbal drug development process.

6.3 Phytochemical screening assay

Phytochemical screening assay is a simple, quick, and inexpensive procedure that tells about various types of phytochemicals in a mixture and an important tool in bioactive compound analyses. Phytochemical examinations are carried out for all extracts as per the standard methods [15].

6.3.1 Tests for carbohydrates

Preparation of test solution: the test extract was prepared by dissolving with water. Add 1 volume of 2 N HCl so that it gets hydrolyzed and is further subjected to the following chemical tests:

- Molisch's test (general test): take 2 ml of extract, add two drops of α-naphthol solution in the alcohol and shake, and then add five drops of concentrated H_2SO_4 to the sides of the test tube to observe violet ring at the junction of two liquids.

- Fehling's test: in a test tube, add 1 ml Fehling's A and 1 ml Fehling's B solutions and mix and boil for 1 min. Add equal volume (2 ml) of test solution. Heat in boiling water bath for 5 min. Observe for yellow and then brick red precipitate.

- Benedict's test: add 1 ml of Benedict's reagent and 1 ml of test solution in a test tube and then mix well. Heat in boiling water bath for 5 min. The solution may appear green, yellow, or red depending on the amount of reducing sugar present in test solution.

- Barfoed's test: add 1 ml of Barfoed's reagent and 1 ml of test solution in the test tube. Heat for 1–2 min, in boiling water bath, and cool. Observe for red precipitate.

6.3.2 Tests for proteins

- Biuret test (general test): for a 2 ml test solution, add two drops of 4% NaOH and two drops of 1% $CuSO_4$ solution, and observe for violet or pink color.

- Millon's test (for proteins): add 2 ml of TS and mix with 4 ml of Millon's reagent; observe for white precipitate. Precipitate if warm, turns brick red or precipitate dissolves giving red color.

- Xanthoproteic test (for protein containing tyrosine or tryptophan): mix 2 ml TS with 0.5 ml concentrated H_2SO_4, and observe for white precipitate.

6.3.3 Tests for amino acids

- Ninhydrin test (general test): add 2 ml TS and two drops of 5% ninhydrin solution, and heat in boiling water bath for 5 min. Observe for purple or bluish color.

- Test for tyrosine: add 2 ml TS and two drops of Millon's reagent. Heat the solution and observe for dark red color.

- Test for tryptophan: add 2 ml of TS and 2 drops of glyoxylic acid and concentrated H_2SO_4 and observe for reddish violet ring at the junction of the two layers.

- Test for cysteine: add 2 ml of TS and few drops of 40% sodium hydroxide and 10% lead acetate solution. Boil. Black ppt. of lead sulfate is formed.

6.3.4 Tests for steroid and triterpenoid

- Salkowski reaction: add 3 ml of extract, 3 ml of chloroform, and 3 ml of concentrated H_2SO_4 in a test tube; shake well; and observe whether chloroform layer appeared red and acid layer showed greenish yellow fluorescence.

- Liebermann-Burchard reaction: add 2 ml extract with 2 ml of chloroform and add 1–2 ml acetic anhydride and 2 drops of concentration H_2SO_4 from the side of test tube. Observe for first red, then blue, and finally green color.

- Liebermann's reaction: add 3 ml of extract with 3 ml acetic anhydride. Heat and cool. Add few drops of concentrated H_2SO_4 and observe for blue color.

6.3.5 Tests for glycosides

Preparation of test solution: the test solution was prepared by dissolving extract in the alcohol or hydro-alcoholic solution.

a. Tests for cardiac glycosides:

- Baljet's test: add a test solution with 1 ml of sodium picrate and observe for yellow to orange color.
- Legal's test (for cardenolides): to 1 ml of test solution, add 1 ml pyridine and 1 ml sodium nitroprusside. Observe for pink to red color.
- Test for deoxysugars (Keller-Kiliani test): to 2 ml extract, add 0.5 ml glacial acetic acid, one drop of 5% $FeCl_3$, and concentrated H_2SO_4. Observe for reddish brown color at the junction of the two liquid and upper layers bluish green.
- Liebermann's test (for bufadienolides): add 2 ml extract to 2 ml acetic anhydride. Heat and cool. Add few drops of concentrated H_2SO_4 and observe for blue color.

b. Tests for saponin glycosides:

- Foam test: the extract was mixed with water and shaken vigorously. Persistent foam was observed.
- Hemolytic test: add test solution to one drop of blood placed on the glass slide. Hemolytic zone appears.

c. Tests for anthraquinone glycosides:

- Borntrager's test: to 3 ml extract, add dil. H2SO4. Boil and filter. To cold filtrate, add equal volume benzene or chloroform. Shake well. Separate the organic solvent. Add ammonia. Ammoniacal layer turns pink or red.
- Modified Borntrager's test: to 3 ml extract, add 3 ml 5% FeCl3 and 3 ml dil. HCl. Heat for 5 min in boiling water bath. Cool and add benzene, shake well, and separate organic layer. Add equal volume dil. ammonia in organic layer. Ammoniacal layer shows pinkish red color.

6.3.6 Tests for flavonoids

Flavonoids are present in hydrolyzed plant extracts. Its presence is maximum in parts of the leaves and they are highly soluble in methanol. The flavonoids are all derived structurally from the important substance called flavone. The flavonoids occur in the free form as well as bound to sugars as glycosides. Flavonoids are found maximum in herbal plants and have good phytopharmacological activities.

Preparation of test solution:

i. To 1 ml of extract, equal volume of 2 M HCl was added and heated in a test tube for 30 to 40 min. at 100°C.

ii. The cooled extract was filtered, and extracted with ethyl acetate.

iii. The ethyl acetate extract was concentrated to dryness and used to test for flavonoids.

- Shinoda test: to 2 ml of extract, add 5 ml of 95% ethanol, 5 drops of concentrated HCl, and 0.5 g magnesium turnings. Pink color was observed. To small quantity of residue, acetate solution was added and observed for yellow colored precipitate. Addition of sodium hydroxide to the residue showed yellow coloration, which was decolorized after addition of dilute hydrochloric acid.

- Ferric chloride test: to 2 ml of test solution, add few drops of ferric chloride solution, which shows intense green color.

- Alkaline reagent test: 2 ml of test solution was treated with 2 ml of sodium hydroxide solution, which showed intense yellow color that became colorless on addition of few drops of dilute hydrochloric acid.

- Lead acetate solution test: 2 ml of test solution with few drops of lead acetate solution (10%) gives yellow precipitates.

6.3.7 Tests for alkaloids

- Mayer's test: test solution treated with Mayer's reagent (potassium mercuric iodide); cream colored precipitate was not obtained.

- Wagner's reagent: the test solution treated with Wagner's reagent (iodine in potassium iodide); brown precipitate was not obtained.

- Hager's test: the test solution treated with Hager's reagent (saturated picric acid solution); gives yellow precipitate.

- Dragendorff's test: the test solution treated with Dragendorff's reagent (potassium bismuth iodide); reddish brown precipitate was not obtained.

6.3.8 Tests for tannins and phenolic compounds

To 2–3 ml of extract, add few drops of the following reagents:
5% $FeCl_3$ solution shows deep blue-black coloration.
Addition of lead acetate solution shows white precipitate.
Addition of gelatin solution shows white precipitate.
Addition of bromine water shows decoloration of bromine water.
Addition of acetic acid solution shows red colored solution.
Addition of dilute iodine solution shows transient red color.
Addition of dilute HNO_3 shows reddish to yellow color.
Addition of dilute $KMnO_4$ shows disappearance of Pink color.

7. Chromatography techniques

Chromatography is a technique where the molecules are separated based on their shape, size, and charge. In any extract, there are hundreds of unknown components and many of them are in very low amount. During chromatography, analyte in solvent and move through solid phase that acts as a sieving material. As molecule proceeds further through molecular sieve, it gets separated. Moreover, there usually exists variability within the same herbal materials. Hence, it is very important to obtain reliable chromatographic fingerprints that represent pharmacologically active and chemically characteristic components of the herbal medicine. Thin layer chromatography is a chromatographic technique that readily provides qualitative information and through which it becomes possible to obtain quantitative data [17].

7.1 Thin layer chromatography (TLC)

Stahl gave the first practical application of thin layer chromatography. TLC is a most versatile technique and it shows its separation with good speed. Advantage of TLC is its sensitivity. TLC works on the principle of an adsorption chromatography in which samples were separated. Separation is based on the interaction between a thin layer of adsorbent attached on the plate and solvent system. The technique is mostly used for the separation of low molecular weight compounds. Many different adsorbents are used in TLC like silica gel, aluminum, cellulose powder, starch, etc. and can be used to separate various compounds like amino acids, alkaloids, phenols, steroids, vitamins, etc.

It is being implemented extensively due to the following reasons:

1. It carries out good speedy separation and rapid analysis of herbal extracts.

2. It shows with minimum sample clean-up requirement.

3. It has the ability for calculating qualitative and semiquantitative information of the separated compounds with Rf values.

4. It enables the quantification of chemical constituents (**Table 1**).

7.2 High performance thin layer chromatography (HPTLC)

HPTLC is a more powerful separation tool for quantitative analysis and it uses the technique in a more optimized way. High performance thin layer chromatography (HPTLC) is based on the principle of planar chromatography where separation of sample components is achieved on high performance layers with detection and data evaluation. These high performance layers on TLC plates are precoated with an adsorbent of 6 micron particle size and a 160 microns layer thickness. The lesser the thickness of layer and particle size results in increased plate efficiency as well as nature of separation. HPTLC has an ability to show its performance on graphical representation in the form of chromatogram. Separation can be easily visualized by pictorial representation, which is possible only in case of HPTLC. The procedure used is as follows: silica gel 60 F254 precoated plates (20 × 10 cm) are used with any developed solvent system. Different extracts are to be spotted on precoated HPTLC plates. Spots of different concentration (1 μL) was applied on HPTLC plates to study the exact separation of spots. Saturation time will be 20 min and room temperature 25°C ± 2°C. TLC plates were developed up to 8 cm. After air drying, a plate was heated at 110°C for 2–3 min. In TLC fingerprinting analysis, the information can be stored and recorded using specific highly sophisticated instruments like high performance TLC scanner. It gives information about the chromatogram, retardation factor (Rf) values, the color of the separated bands, their absorption spectra, and λ max. After derivatization and using different visualization reagents, snaps of TLC plates can be obtained and saved for further process. Thus, this represents TLC fingerprint profile of the provided sample. The information so generated has

Plant constituents	Stationary phase	Mobile phase	Detection
Carbohydrates	Silica gel	Ethyl acetate:toluene (1:1)	10% ethanolic sulfuric acid
Alkaloids/phenanthrenes	Silica gel	Toluene:ethyl acetate:diethylamine (7:2:1)	Dragendorff reagent
Flavonoids	Silica gel	Ethyl acetate:formic acid:glacial acetic acid:water (10:1.1:1.1:2.6)	UV 254 nm or 366 nm
Tannins	Silica gel	Ethyl acetate:formic acid:glacial acetic acid:water (7.5:0.3:0.2:2)	Vanillin sulfuric acid reagent
Saponin glycoside	Silica gel	Chloroform:glacial acetic acid:met hanol:water (6.4:3.2:1.2:0.8)	Vanillin sulfuric acid reagent
Specific Mobile phases			
Betasitosterol	Silica gel	Benzene:ethylacetate (9:1)	Vanillin sulfuric acid reagent
Rutin	Silica gel	Ethyl acetate:formic acid:glacial acetic acid:water (10:1.1:1.1:2.6)	UV 254 nm or 366 nm
Curcumin	Silica gel	Chloroform:methanol (9.8:0.2)	Visible light
Gingerol	Silica gel	Toluene:ethylacetate (9.3:0.7)	Vanillin sulfuric acid reagent
Stigmasterol	Silica gel	Petroleum ether:ethyl acetate (7:3)	Vanillin sulfuric acid reagent

Table 1.
TLC mobile phase for important classes of phytoconstituents [15].

a potential application in the identification of an authentic drug when compared with bioactive marker and it helps in maintaining the quality and consistency of the isolates or herbal drugs in natural drug discovery [18].

7.3 Column chromatography (CC)

Column chromatography works on the principle of ion exchange, molecular sieves, and adsorption phenomenon. CC is a most useful technique for separation of active constituents with larger concentration. Sometimes fractions require another step for concentration. Displacement chromatography is a newer method that contains elution of bioactive compounds that have great affinity for the adsorbent. Fractions of elute materials can be more concentrated than the original solution placed in column. The column was prepared using silica for column chromatography. The fraction was dissolved in smallest possible volume of solvent and it was mixed with 2 gms of silica for column chromatography. Wet column or dry column packing can be done. Packing of column plays an important role in good quality separation. The mixture was dried to obtain free flowing powder and it was added to column. Then, the column was eluted with solvent of various proportions. Every eluent was collected in properly cleaned test tube separately for further studies to be carried out.

7.4 High performance liquid chromatography (HPLC)

High performance liquid chromatography (HPLC) plays a mandatory role in isolation of natural products. It is a versatile and widely used technique for the isolation and identification. In the modern era, HPLC technique is becoming popular for studying separation, identification, and fingerprinting study for the quality control of herbal plants. Currently, this technique works as the main choice for research scientists. The multicomponent samples on both an analytical and preparative scale can be separated and studied more easily by HPLC. Thus resolving power of HPLC is ideally used for the rapid processing of herbal extracts. HPLC instruments are designed in modular ways and they contain delivery pump for solvents and manual injection valve along with an auto-sampler. As sample is introduced in autosample, it carries toward the important part or heart of HPLC that is an analytical column, a guard column. Further, a detector, recorder, and printer are used to show a graphical representation on the software based or installed computer device. In every chemical separation, the working and result production differ due to the fact that certain compounds have different migration rates, which can be fulfilled using HPLC by utilizing a particular column and mobile phase as per the requirement for separations. Trial and error concept is applied for developing new mobile phase along with prior knowledge of separation, its structure, and required solvent polarity or nonpolarity. Thus, the extent or degree of separation is based upon the choice of stationary phase or mobile phase. Generally, the identification and separation of phytochemicals can be achieved by using isocratic system that is using single mobile phase. Gradient elution sometimes can be used in which the proportion is altered from organic solvent to water. It also depends on time, and it may be desirable if more than one sample component is studied. Or it also differs from each other significantly in retention of components with column as per the conditions achieved. Identification of compounds by HPLC is a crucial part of HPLC assay. Identification of any bioactive compound by HPLC selection of detector is again the next important step. Once the detector is selected and the setting is done, the assay may be developed by trial and error of solvent system. Once the sharpness of the peak of known sample is obtained, the solvent system can be selected. The important parameters of this assay is that a clean sharp peak of the known sample is observed from the chromatograph. The reasonable retention time of identifying peak should be there. The extraneous peaks at the detection levels should be well separated from the main sharp peak. At maximum time, UV detectors are popularly used in HPLC detection. UV detectors are used among all the detectors because they have high sensitivity and UV absorbance of majority of naturally occurring compounds is possible at low wavelengths of 200–210 nm. If bioactive compound needed to be isolated is only present in small amounts within the sample, then the high sensitivity of UV detection is a bonus in herbal natural drug discovery. Liquid chromatography coupled with mass spectrometry (LC/MS) is also a powerful technique for the analysis of complex botanical extracts. It offers accurate determination of molecular weight of proteins, peptides. Isotopes pattern can also be detected by this technique. A recent advance includes electrospray, thermospray, and ionspray ionization techniques, which offer unique advantages of high detection sensitivity and specificity [19].

HPLC when combined with mass spectrometry (MSn) gives lot of information for structural elucidation of the compounds because its ability of recognition increases and separation with structure identification becomes very easy. Therefore, when a biomarker which is of a pure standard is unavailable, fast and accurate identification of bioactive chemical compounds in medicinal herbs is possible due to the combination of HPLC and MS. In order to count the overall success of natural product in isolation and separation, the most important is processing of raw material further to provide a sample suitable for HPLC analysis. The significant bearing is on the choice of solvent for sample active compounds identification. The source material that is dried powdered herbal plant material should be studied very efficiently in earlier stages and steps: first, its dried form and second to learn about its chemical structural part that is the powder's ability to release the bioactive compound of interest into the solution. In such cases, mobile phase development initially using TLC and having idea about the solvent system before applying to HPLC saves your time. Thus, in normal case of extraction, dried plant material is treated with an organic solvent methanol, chloroform. After extraction, extracts are dried over rotary evaporator and powdered extracts are concentrated and injected into HPLC for separation and analysis. HPLC is useful for compounds that cannot be vaporized or that decompose under high temperature, and it provides a good complement to gas chromatography for detection of compounds.

8. Methods of detection

8.1 Fourier-transform infrared spectroscopy (FTIR)

FTIR has proven to be a valuable tool for the characterization and identification of compounds or functional groups (chemical bonds) present in an unknown mixture of plant extracts. It helps for identification and structure determination of the molecule. In addition, FTIR spectra of bioactive compounds are usually so unique that they are called as a molecular "fingerprint." Once the isolation of bioactive compound is possible, then drying of extract and isolates using rotary evaporator is done. Dried powdered plant extract spectrum can be obtained from FTIR. FTIR software contains library of known compounds, and thus, the spectrum of an unknown compound can be identified by its comparison. Preparation of samples for FTIR analysis can be done in different ways. In earlier years, solid herbal plant extract powder was milled with potassium bromide (KBr) with good trituration techniques and then compressed into a thin pellet, which can be analyzed. Now due to new advancements, only solid or liquid sample is available and you only have to place one drop or one pinch of sample between two plates and the drop or sample forms a thin film between the plates. It is the easiest way for performing FTIR, and graphs and wave number are recorded by using computer-based software. The region in IR spectrum above 1200 cm^{-1} shows spectral bands or peaks due to the vibrations of individual bonds or functional groups under examination. The region below 1200 cm^{-1} is known as the 'fingerprint region.' It indicates bands due to the vibrations of the complete bioactive molecule. Complexity of compounds is seen in fingerprint region. Intensities of the various bands in FTIR are recorded specifically on a simple scale as strong (S), medium (M), or weak (W). And as per new techniques developed, the advanced instruments of company bruker, jasco has made easier by application of one drop or pinch of sample on the instruments and this software will give the results. Lastly, the advantage is that samples can be reused.

8.2 Mass spectrometry (MS)

Mass spectrometry plays a vital role and works as a powerful analytical technique. It is the only technique used for identification of unknown compounds for its molecular weight. Thus, the quantification of known compounds and elucidation of the structure and chemical properties of molecules are possible due to MS. The most powerful MS spectrum gives an idea about the molecular weight of sample, which can be determined. The value of the technique is that it requires only microgram amounts of material and that it can provide an accurate molecular weight and that it may yield a complex fragmentation pattern, which is often characteristic of that particular compound. This technique works successfully for the structural elucidation of herbal extracts and organic compounds, for peptide or oligonucleotide sequencing. MS helps in monitoring the characterization of compounds in complex mixtures with a high specificity by defining both the molecular weight and a diagnostic fragment of the molecule simultaneously. Gas chromatography equipment can be directly coupled with rapid scan mass spectrometer (GCMS) of various types. High resolution analysis can be performed due to coupling of equipment.

Liquid chromatography–mass spectroscopy (LC–MS) offers accurate determination of molecular weight of proteins and peptides. Isotopes pattern can also be detected by this technique. Recent advances include electrospray, thermospray, and ionspray ionization techniques, which offer unique advantages of high detection sensitivity and specificity.

8.3 Nuclear magnetic resonance spectroscopy (NMR)

Nuclear magnetic resonance spectroscopy gives physical, chemical, and biological properties of matter. C^{13} NMR is used to identify the types of carbon present in the compound. H1-NMR is used to find out the types of hydrogen present in the compound and to find out how the hydrogen atoms are connected. Proton NMR spectroscopy basically works on principle by measuring the magnetic moments of its hydrogen atoms and it provides a method for determining the structure of an organic compound. In almost all compounds, hydrogen atoms are present, which are attached to different groups such as -CH2-, -CH-, -CHO, -NH2, -CHOH-, etc. The graphical representation of proton NMR spectrum provides a record of the number of hydrogen atoms in these different situations. It gives information only about the number of hydrogen atoms in the compound but not the number of carbon atoms. However, direct information on the nature of the carbon skeleton of the molecule can only be obtained by carbon 13 NMR spectroscopy. 13C-NMR spectroscopy works hand in hand with proton NMR and thus the combination of the results of two methods provides very useful information for identification of unknown compound. It is a powerful means of structural elucidation for new terpenoids, alkaloids, or flavonoids. It is also useful in the identification or analysis of glycosides, in indicating the linkage between sugar moieties and their configurations. Many proteins or other macromolecules can be identified by both proton and 13C-NMR. For NMR analysis, very small amount of sample is needed for analysis and that sample can be reused for further analysis. For examples, NMR instrument cost much so there are many sophisticated analytical instrumentation technical analysis are available to perform your research work. Scientist handling NMR has good hands on working of NMR. In order to get high resolution, the new technique is liquid chromatography–nuclear magnetic resonance (LC-NMR). It is a combination of chromatographic separation technique for isolation of active fraction and its number of hydrogen or carbon atom identification with NMR spectroscopy. It is one of the most powerful and time-saving method for the separation and structural elucidation of unknown compounds and mixtures, especially for the structure elucidation of herbal plant extracts and their isolates in herbal natural drug discovery.

8.4 Development of new technologies in natural drug discovery research

Nature is a God's gift for finding new herbal drugs for carrying out research scientifically. A new driving force for screening of novel drugs, biologically active metabolites from these products derived from nature which leads to the success of drugs. The chemistry is a branch where the new technologies are emerging in which pharmaceutical chemistry is very important because it deals with the health of common people. Combinatorial chemistry, high-throughput screening, bioinformatics, proteomics, and genomics are newer techniques that have emerged widely in the field of pharmaceutical discovery research. All drug discovery research and technologies have enormous potential to make use of the chemical and natural diversity of products. Newly developed techniques are growing rapidly with good outputs in natural drug discovery [20]. These include molecular diversity, compound-library design, protein 3D structures, NMR-based screening, 3D-QSAR in modern drug design, physicochemical concepts, and computer-aided drug design using different software, its prediction of drug toxicity, and metabolism [21]. New approaches to improve and accelerate the joint drug discovery and development processes are expected to take place mainly from the innovation in drug target elucidation and lead structure discovery. Powerful new technologies are revolutionizing drug discovery. Some software will be useful in performing studies, which are freely available such as Zinc.docking.org. It is used for calculating SWISSADME, drug properties, SMILES formula, drug likeness properties, and many more [8].

Technologies for drug discovery advanced and diversified greatly [22]. NPDD (natural product drug discovery) activities work hand in hand and make use strongly with HTS, combinatorial chemistry, and genomics. New approaches have proved to show improvement and accelerate the joint drug discovery and development processes. New techniques are emerging and take place mainly from the innovation in drug target elucidation. It finally leads to lead structure discovery. Powerful new technologies are revolutionizing natural herbal drug discovery.

8.5 High-throughput screening

High-throughput screening (HTS) is a specially deigned technique in herbal drug discovery that is a standard method for hit discovery based on identification through stored libraries. HTS is relevant to the fields of biology and chemistry and helps for scientific experimentation especially used in drug discovery.

HTS is using data processing and control software and sensitive detectors that help researchers to carry out the research scientifically for designing and developing new structure from herbal drug discovery. It is robotics and allows a researcher to quickly conduct various biochemical, genetic, or phytopharmacological tests. Through HTS, one can rapidly identify bioactive compounds that can be useful in a particular biomolecular pathway in inhibiting the diseased condition. Thus, biomolecular pathway provides information about the mechanism of drug as well as internal way of diseased condition person. The knowledge and the results of these experiments provide starting points for designing a drug and for understanding the interaction or role of a particular biochemical process in biology.

HTS is a relatively recent innovation and it requires high-speed computer technology. It works on the principle of high-throughput screening of large amount of natural compounds using computer-based technology, which is more easy and more time saving. Knowledge can be further utilized for new herbal drug discovery. Interest of research can be generated in natural drug discovery through all these newer techniques. Many well-developed countries have highly specialized and expensive screening labs to run an HTS operation. However, the countries having interest of working in research that cases a small-to-moderately sized research institution will use the existing HTS facility as per their convenience rather than full set up.

9. Conclusion

With growing interest in herbal drug development with minimum side effects, there are better opportunities to explore the medicinal and other biological properties of previously inaccessible natural products. To establish its usefulness, it is mandatory to focus on visualization and identification of unused herbal plants over the world. Then, it is emphasized on extraction, its isolation, and characterization of phytochemicals, which is a gift of nature in a rational and scientific way. There is an unmet need for utilization of the natural products for the benefit of human kind and development of new lead for drug discovery. Once the phytochemical is obtained, this can be used for further exploration through QSAR studies, molecular modeling, and animal studies followed by clinical trial. The success of natural products in drug discovery essentially for pharmaceutical companies and research institutes is essentially related to their ability and benefits to common person that is socio-economic benefits for well-being of common person its health is important for the world rather than all coming come to your hands if health is top priority. Natural products contain complex chemical structures, which differ according to their various species in nature, and when the existing high technology methods that are available are applied, it can lead to new discovery of drugs, benefitting the whole world. Thus, the world is always gifted with nature, and man is gifted with brain, so let us make use of it to discover new entities that will be available to common people in economical rate and we will be happy to lead a life on this earth. Moreover, natural products have been, and will be, important sources of new pharmaceutical compounds. Many years ago life was made possible or was prolonged only due to natural herbs as per the references that can be obtained in literature. In the new era of twenty-first century, no life is possible on earth without herbal drugs or products that are obtained through natural herbal drug discovery. Hats off to it!

Author details

Akshada Amit Koparde[1]*, Rajendra Chandrashekar Doijad[2] and Chandrakant Shripal Magdum[3]

1 Department of Pharmaceutical Chemistry, Dean Academics, KIMSDTU's Krishna Institute of Pharmacy, Malkapur, Karad, India

2 DEAN, KIMSDTU's Krishna Institute of Pharmacy, Malkapur, Karad, India

3 Guide and principal, KES's Rajarambapu College of Pharmacy, Kasegaon, India

*Address all correspondence to: akshadakakade@yahoo.com

References

[1] Sircar NN. Medicinal plants. The Eastern Pharmacist. 1982;**29**(291):49-52

[2] Tariq O, Siddiqi AJ. Vitamin C content of Indian medicinal plants- a literature review. Indian Drugs. 1985;**23**(2):72-83

[3] Panda H. Handbook on Medicinal Herbs With Uses. New Delhi: Asia pacific business press; 2004. p. 564

[4] Kar A. Pharmacognosy and Pharma Biotechnology. New Delhi: New age international Ltd.; 2006. pp. 5-11

[5] Rao AVR, Gurjar MK. Drugs from plant resources: An overview. Pharmatimes. 1990;**22**(5):19-20

[6] Handa SS. Plants as drugs. The Eastern Pharmacist. 1991;**34**(397):79-85

[7] Handa SS. Future trends of plants as drugs. Pharmatimes. 1991;**23**(4):13-23

[8] Farnsworth NR. A computerized data base for medicinal plants. The Eastern Pharmacist. 1985;**28**(326):53-55

[9] Available from: https://pubchem.ncbi.nlm.nih.gov/compound/36314#section=2D-Structure

[10] Mukherjee P. Quality Control of Herbal Drugs – An Approach to Evaluations of Botanicals. 5th ed. 2005. p. 2

[11] Vogel GH. Drug Discovery and Evaluation, Pharmacological Assays. 2003. p. 202

[12] Cragg GM, Newman DJ, Sander KM. Natural products in drug discovery and development. Journal of Natural Products. 1997;**60**:52-60

[13] Hemalatha S, Manda V, Mohan Y. Microwave assisted extraction – An innovative and promising extraction tool for medicinal plant research. Pharmacognosy Reviews. 2007;**1**(1):7-17

[14] Joy PP, Thomas J, Mathew S, Skaria BP. Medicinal Plants. Kerala Agricultural University, Aromatic and Medicinal Plants Research Station; 1998. pp. 3-5

[15] Mukherjee PK. Quality Control of Herbal Drugs. 1st ed. Vol. 2002. Business Horizons Pharmaceutical Publishers. p. 103

[16] Spreeman R, Gaedcke F. Herbal drugs. The Eastern Pharmacist. 2000;**23**(512):29-37

[17] Bhanu PS, Sagar ZR. Herbal drugs. The Indian Pharmacist. 2003;**2**(12):13-16

[18] Samanta MK, Mukherjee PK, Prasad MK, Suresh B. The Eastern Pharmacist. 2000;**23**(512):23-27

[19] Tyagi K, Bhanu PS, Sagar ZR. Failures and successes of herbal medicines. The Indian Pharmacist. 2003;**2**(12):17-23

[20] Gupta AK, Chitme HR. Herbal medicine for health. The Eastern Pharmacist. 2000;**23**(512):41-44

[21] Dobriyal RM, Narayana DBA. Ayurvedic raw material. The Eastern Pharmacist. 1998;**30**(484):31-35

[22] Littleton J. The future of plant drug discovery. Expert Opinion on Drug Discovery. 2007;**2**(5):673-683

Chapter 15

Pharmacognosy: Importance and Drawbacks

Fatai Oladunni Balogun, Anofi Omotayo Tom Ashafa, Saheed Sabiu, Abdulwakeel Ayokun-nun Ajao, Chella Palanisamy Perumal, Mutiu Idowu Kazeem and Ahmed Adebowale Adedeji

Abstract

In many nations of the world, a great number of deaths and morbidity arising from illnesses are witnessed due to lack of basic health care. Phytotherapy has continued to play a significant role in the prevention and treatment of diseases (communicable and noncommunicable). Interestingly, more than 80% of the global populations now adopt phytotherapy as a basic source of maintaining good healthy conditions, owing to the pronounced side effects, nonavailability, and expensive nature of conventional treatment options. While this review looked at the prospects and downsides of phytomedicine as it relates to the national health care system, it established the fact that although a number of medicinal plants had been resourceful (effective) against a range of diseases, with few developed into drugs based on the available phytotherapeutics, quite a large number of them are yet to scale through clinical trials to determine their safety and efficacy. It is believed that until this is done, we hope phytomedicine to be adopted or integrated into the national health care system in many countries.

Keywords: medicinal plants, traditional medicine, secondary metabolites, drug discovery, phytotherapy

1. Introduction

1.1 History of medicinal plant use

The origin of medicinal plants use had been since time immemorial and traced back to Europe, Egypt, etc. many centuries ago [1]. The first records of knowledge documentation were, however, produced by Shen Nung (a Chinese emperor) 2500 BC ago, describing different recipes of drug preparation from more than 300 medicinal plants for the management of numerous human diseases. Records had it that the use of plants (herbs) as medicine started gaining momentum around 500 BC, though prior to this period, their use was not limited to healing but believed to possess spiritual (ritual) power as well until the advent of scientific era particularly around 1960s when much relevance was played on development of synthetic products based on assumption that they are safer and come with little side effects [2]. Despite the aforementioned, the last two decades witnessed a drastic revival in the use and acceptance of phytomedicine by a majority of the people from developing nations (70–90%) as a major source of primary health care. This was also buttressed by WHO's submission, encouraging the discovery and development of lead drugs from plant-based formulations and/or medicines which are believed to be effective and safe [2]. In fact, the development of morphine, quinine, reserpine, ephedrine, etc., from *Papaver somniferum*, *Cinchona* spp., and *Rauwolfia serpentina* as first set of drugs from medicinal plants brought much popularity and attested to their acceptance and potential use across different parts of the globe especially from Europe and Egypt, with records of well over 900 drugs compiled in history by chain of scientists such as Discorides and Galen [3]. Moreover, it suffices to submit that China is the only country with complete catalog of phytomedicine [2].

Mankind relies on plants and/or its extract, an integral part of traditional medicine (TM) which as a matter of fact is the origin for medical medicine. The knowledge of TM particularly in issues relating to the health of both humans and animals has continued to emerge in many nations of the world. Despite the unproven quality, safety, and efficacy, they are becoming the major source of health care for 80% of the entire population in both developed and developing countries (such as USA, China, India) in disease control, prevention, and management [4]. Interestingly, TM or phytotherapy (traditional system of health care) in the last two decades is being adopted by every region based on the specific sociocultural context illustrating the way medicinal plants (MP) or the inherent secondary metabolites are used, as well as their disparity in the approach to health and diseases. This TM varies from one community to another and notable among them are Acupuncture (Chinese), Ayurveda (Indian), Kampo (Japanese), Unani (Arabian), Basotho (among Africans), etc., some or majority of which had been in existence many centuries even before the advent of modern medicine.

Similarly, the reliance on plants by humankind is not only limited to medicine but also to other basic needs such as food, clothing, and shelter, all produced or manufactured from plant matrices (leaves, woods, and fibers) and storage parts (fruits and tubers) [5]. Medicinally, plant harbors chemicals referred to as the secondary metabolites, which are derived biosynthetically from plant primary metabolites (e.g., carbohydrates, amino acids, and lipids) though might not be directly involved in the growth, development, or reproduction of plants [6]. These secondary metabolites can be classified into several groups depending on their chemical classes [7].

2. Plant secondary metabolite and their therapeutic significance

Secondary metabolites are organic compound produced and found in all plant tissues to drive metabolic activities, as well as providing self-defense against herbivore and any form of environmental toxicity [8]. Plant is a well-known source of medicinal product for both traditional and modern medicines for the treatment and management of human illnesses. The usage of the plant in this regard is attributed to the presence of secondary metabolites [9]. Apart from the fact that they are widely used in medicine, they are also employed industrially in the production and manufacturing of dyes, drugs, polymers, waxes, glues, fibers, antibiotics, herbicides, insecticides, cosmetics, etc. [10]. In general, secondary metabolites found in plants can be categorized into three major groups including terpenes (cardiac glycosides, carotenoids, and sterols), phenolics (flavonoids and nonflavonoids), and nitrogen-based compounds (alkaloids and glucosinolates).

Terpenes are the largest and highly diversified class of secondary metabolites derived as a result of polymerization of isoprenoid unit of five carbon compounds [11]. Based on the five carbon compound used as its building block, it can be subdivided into monoterpenes, sesquiterpenes, diterpenes, triterpenes, tetraterpenes, polyterpenes, and steroids whose precursor is triterpenes. The therapeutic significance of terpenoids from different plants has been reported, e.g., terpenes from eucalyptus oil is known for its antidiabetic property [11], ursolic acid from *Rosmarinus officinalis* and β-sesquiphellandrene from *Piper guineense* are known to be psychoprotective [12]. Antibacterial and antifungal potential of terpenoids derived from *Pilgerodendron uviferum*, *Picea abies* and other plant sources have also been reported [13–15]. Furthermore, a steroidal terpenoids called glycyrrhizic acid elicited anti-inflammatory activity [8].

The phenolics are secondary metabolites that are produced in the shikimic acid pathway of plants involving pentose phosphate through phenylpropanoid metabolization of at least one aromatic ring of hydrocarbon attached to one or more hydroxyl groups [10, 16]. Phenolics are generally categorized into two based on their structure, namely, flavonoids and nonflavonoids. Structurally, flavonoids are derived from two aromatic rings linked to a bridge consisting of three carbons (C_6—C_3—C_6) and are sub-divided into six main categories, including flavonols, flavones, flavanones, flavan-3-ols, isoflavones, and anthocyanins. However, the nonflavonoids are subdivided into five main categories, including hydroxybenzoates, hydroxycinnamates, lignans, and stilbenes [17]. Compellingly, wide arrays of pharmacological potentials, such as antidiabetic, antioxidant, antiviral, antimicrobial, anticancer, and anti-inflammatory, have been credited to plant-based phenolic compounds. For example, cyanidin 3-sambubioside and 5-caffeoyl quinic acid derived from the fruit of *Viburnum dilatatum* Thumb. had been found to elicit significant antioxidant and radical scavenging activities while also inhibiting the syndrome-linked complications of postprandial hyperglycemia [16]. Furthermore, plant-based phenolic acids such as garcinone E, kaempferol, resveratrol, syringaresinol, and quercetin are known to be potent anticancer agents [18]. The anti-inflammatory, antiviral, and antibacterial potential of phenolics in the management of skin disorder have also been reported [17, 19–21].

Alkaloids are structurally diversified secondary metabolites derived from nitrogen-based amino acid with nitrogen atom in the heterocyclic ring. Based on the nature of their heterocyclic and building block, alkaloids are classified into different subgroups such as indole, tropane, piperidine, purine, imidazole, pyrrolizidine, pyrrolidine, quinolizidine, and isoquinoline alkaloids [22]. Noteworthy, therapeutic effects have been credited to a wide range of alkaloids from plants. Typical examples from alkaloids are *Callistemon citrinus* and *Vernonia adoensis* reported to elicit antibacterial effects on *Staphylococcus aureus* and *Pseudomonas aeruginosa* [23]. Additionally, alkaloids originating from *Aerva lanata* roots were able to mitigate postprandial hyperglycemia in diabetic rats [24]. The *in vitro* antioxidant activity of *Phoebe declinata* leaves extract has also been attributed to its alkaloid. It was found to inhibit 2,2-diphenyl-1-picrylhydrazyl (DPPH) radical while consequently reducing ferric chloride to ferrous [25]. Furthermore, plant-based alkaloidal compounds such as reserpiline, α-yohimbine, methylaplysinopsin, isoquinoline, physostigmine, and pilocarpine are good psychoprotective agents [12].

3. Medicinal plants as therapeutic agents

Healing with medicinal plants is as old as mankind itself. The link between man and his quest for medicines in nature dates back to ancient times, when there were convincing proofs from written documents, monuments, and even original plant medicines [26]. Specifically, the oldest written evidence of usage of medicinal plants for preparation of drugs was found on a Sumerian clay slab from Nagpur, approximately 5000 years old. It comprised 12 recipes for drug preparation referring to over 250 plants [27]. Awareness of medicinal plants usage is a result of the many years of struggles against illnesses, which has prompted man to seek medicines in leaves, roots, barks, and other parts of plants [28]. The knowledge of the development of ideas related to the usage of medicinal plants, as well as the evolution of awareness, has increased the ability of health providers to respond to the challenges that have emerged with the spreading of professional services in the enhancement of man's life. Until the advent of iatrochemistry in sixteenth century, plants had been the source of treatment and prophylaxis for many diseases [27]. This is well exemplified globally where medicinal plants have always being an integral part of the health care system since time immemorial.

During the last decades, it has become evident that there exists a plethora of plants with medicinal potential, and it is increasingly being accepted that medicinal plants are offering potential lead compounds in the drug discovery process. In fact, the developed world has also witnessed an ascending trend in the utilization of complementary or alternative medicine (CAM) particularly herbal remedies [29]. While over 80% of the population in Sub-Saharan African countries like Nigeria and South Africa use herbal remedies for their primary health care, reports from developed countries such as Canada, Germany, and the US revealed that more than 70% of their populations have tried CAM at least once [29]. The most common traditional medicine in common practice across the globe is the use of medicinal plants. In most of the countries, medicinal plants are the most easily accessible health resource available to the community. In addition, they are most often the preferred option for the patients. For most of these people, traditional healers offer information, counseling, and treatment to patients and their families in a personal manner, as well as having an understanding of their patient's environment [30].

Indeed, modern allopathic medicine has its roots in traditional medicine, and it is likely that many important new remedies will be developed and commercialized in the future from plant biodiversity, as it has been till now, by following the leads provided by traditional knowledge and experiences. The extensive use of traditional medicine, composed mainly of medicinal plants, has been argued to be linked to cultural and economic reasons. This is why the WHO encourages member states to promote and integrate traditional medical practices in their health system [31]. While a good number of plants (with only selected representatives listed here) have elicited significant therapeutic and pharmacological effects against well-known debilitating and degenerating diseases such as diabetes (*Artemisia afra, Chilianthus olearaceus, Vernonia amygdalina* [32], *Dicoma anomala* [33], *Psidium guajava* [34], and *Solanum incanum* [35]), cancer (*Taxus brevifolia, Podophyllum peltatum* [36], and *Catharanthus roseus* [37]), malaria (*Plumbago indica, Garcinia mangostana, Dioscorea membranacea, Artemisia annua, Piper chaba, Myristica fragrans,* and *Kaempferia galangal*) [38], HIV/AIDS (*Geranium phaeum*, *Sambucus racemosa* [39], *Tuberaria lignosa*, and *Sanguisorba minor magnolia* [40]), schizophrenia (*Abrus precatorius*, *Acacia ataxacantha*, *Adansonia digitata*, *Datura innoxia*, *Ficus sycomorus*, *Parkia biglobosa,* and *Ximenia Americana*) [41], tuberculosis (*Adhatoda vasica, Alpinia galangal,* and *Ocimum sanctum*) [42], microvascular and macrovascular disorders (*Anisodus tanguticus*, *Salvia miltiorrhiza* [43], *Camellia sinensis*, *Castanospermum australe, Curcuma longa*, *Ocimum santum* [44], *Stigma maydis* [45], *Spondias mombin* [46], and *Gazania krebsiana* [47]), etc., studies are also in the forefront on the evaluation of plants against the neglected tropical diseases (NTD). **Table 1** presents some of the medicinal plants with reported significant efficacy against the NTDs.

Disease/infection	Selected plants for treatment	Reference(s)
Buruli ulcer	*Acacia nilotica, Ageratum conyzoides, Albizia zygia, Allium sativum, Capsicum annuum, Cassia alata, Chalcas exotica, Carica papaya, Dysphania ambrosioides, Moringa oleifera, Nauclea latifolia, Pergularia daemia, Psidium guajava, Spondias mombin, Zingiber officinale*	[66, 67]
Chagas disease	*Argemone ochroleuca, Capparis spinosa, Commicarpus grandiflorus, Cucumis prophetarum, Euphorbia ammak, Hypoestes forskaolii, Kleinia odora, Marrubium vulgare, Peganum harmala, Psiadia punctulata, Ricinus communis, Solanum villosum, Tribulus macropterus, Withania somnifera*	[68]
Dengue and chikungunya	*Aloysia gratissima, Andrographis paniculata, Artemisia douglasiana, Citrus limon, Cymbopogon citratus, Cleome aculeata, Eupatorium catarium, Heterotheca latifolia, Hyptis mutabilis, Lantana grisebachii, Momordica charantia, Ocimum sanctum, Pelargonium citrosum, Senna angustifolia, Tridax procumbers, Vernonia cinerea*	[69–71]
Dracunculiasis	*Moringa oleifera*	[72]
Echinococcosis	*Azadirachta indica*	[73]
Foodborne trematodiasis	*Artemisia annua*	[74]
Helminthiasis	*Aloe ferox, Cassinopsis ilicifolia, Coddia rudis, Combretum molle, Elephantorrhiza elephantina, Gazania krebsiana, Hypoxis colchicifolia, Leonotis leonurus, Markhamia obtusifolia, Tulbaghia violacea*	[75–81]
Leishmaniasis	*Aloe vera, Chenopodium ambrosioides, Hyptis pectinata, Pfaffia glomerata, Ruta graveolens*	[82]
Leprosy	*Achyranthes aspera, Amaranthus spinosus, Aristolochia indica, Azadirachta indica, Calotropis gigantea, Eclipta alba, Ficus benghalensis, Jasminum grandiflorum, Michelia champaca, Piper betle, Thespesia populnea, Trichodesma indicum*	[83]
Lymphatic filariasis	*Acacia auriculiformis, Aegle marmelos, Centratherum anthelminticum, Ficus racemosa, Hibiscus mutabilis, Mallotus philippensis, Moringa oleifera, Sphaeranthus indicus, Zingiber officinale, Vitex negundo*	[84–90]
Mycetoma	*Acacia nilotica, Acacia nubica, Boswellia papyrifera, Citrullus colocynthis, Cuminum cyminum, Moringa oleifera, Nigella sativa*	[91, 92]
Onchocerciasis	*Annona senegalensis, Anogeissus leiocarpus, Polyalthia suaveolens, Discoglypremna caloneura, Homalium africanum, Khaya senegalensis, Margaritaria discoidea, Parquetina nigrescens*	[93–96]
Rabies	*Amarantheus spinosus, Croton macrostachyus, Phytolacca dodecandra*	[97, 98]
Scabies	*Abelmoschus esculentus, Aegle marmelos, Boerhavia diffusa, Clerodendrum infortunatum, Heliotropium indicum, Pongamia pinnata, Phyllanthus emblica, Schleichera oleosa*	[99, 100]
Schistosomiasis	*Abrus precatorius, Allium sativum, Citrus reticulata, Pterocarpus angolensis, Ozoroa insignis, Vernonia amygdalina*	[101–104]
Snakebite envenoming	*Allium cepa, Areca catechu, Aristolochia shimadai, Byrsonima crassa, Casearia sylvestris, Davilla elliptica, Delonix elata, Eclipta prostrata, Emblica officinalis, Hemidesmus indicus, Schumanniophyton magnificum, Vitis negundo*	[105–107]
Taeniasis	*Capillipedium foetidum, Cymbopogon nardus, Cyperus rotundus, Gardenia lucida, Hedychium coronarium, Hedychium spicatum, Inula racemosa, Litsea chinensis, Pistacia integerrima, Randia dumetorum*	[108–111]
Trachoma	*Abrus precatorius, Aloe marlothii, Calpurnia aurea, Dodonaea viscosa, Erythrina abyssinica, Eucomis pallidiflora, Gethyllis namaquensis, Hypoxis obtusa, Kleinia longiflora, Primula auriculata, Protea caffra, Terfezia claveryi, Tinospora smilacina, Tribulus terrestris, Ziziphus mucronata*	[112–118]

Disease/infection	Selected plants for treatment	Reference(s)
Trypanosomiasis	*Acacia nilotica, Allium sativum, Albizia gummifera, Bombax buonopozense, Heterotis rotundifolia, Morinda lucida, Pterocarpus erinaceus, Securinega virosa, Terminalia avicennioides, Vernonia subuligera, Ximenia americana, Zanthoxylum zanthoxyloides*	[119–125]
Yaws	*Alafia multiflora, Boerhavia diffusa, Commicarpus plubaginieus, Dioscorea hispida, Hibiscus diversifolius, Indigofera hirsuta, Spondias mombin, Strychnos ignatii*	[126]

Table 1.
Some selected medicinal plants used against neglected tropical diseases.

4. Drugs (medicine) discovered from natural sources and development

The development of new drug is a complex, time-consuming, and expensive process (**Figure 1**). The time taken from discovery of a new drug to its reaching the clinic is approximately 12 years, involving more than 1 billion US dollars of investments in today's context [48]. Essentially, the new drug discovery involves the

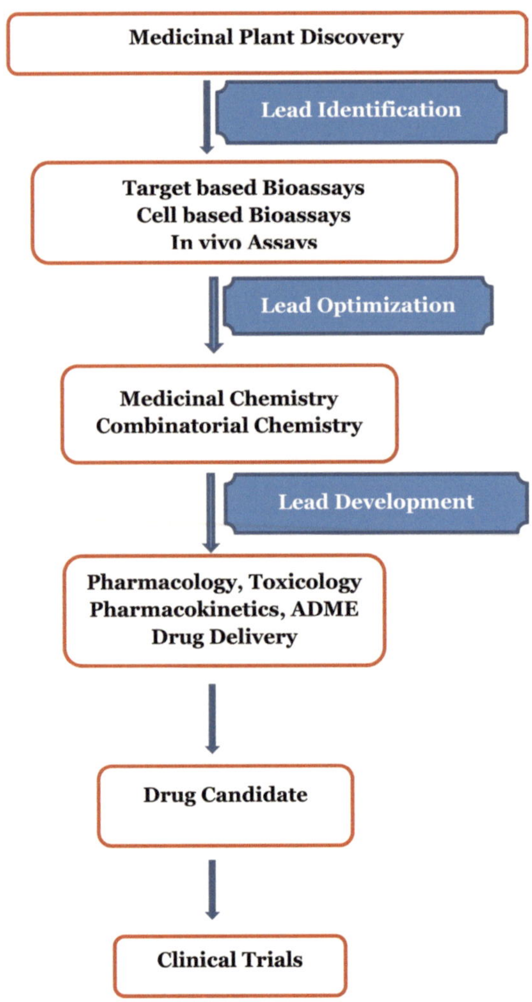

Figure 1.
Modern drug discovery and development processes from the medicinal plant [127].

identification of new chemical entities (NCEs), having the required characteristic of drug ability and medicinal chemistry. These NCEs can be sourced either through chemical synthesis or through isolation from natural products. Initial success stories in new drug discovery came from medicinal chemistry inventions, which led to the need of development of higher number of chemical libraries through combinatorial chemistry. This approach, however, was proven to be less effective in terms of overall success rate. The second source of NCEs for potential use as drug molecules has been the natural products. Before the advent of high throughput screening and the post genomic era, more than 80% of drug substances were purely natural products or were inspired by the molecules derived from natural sources (including semisynthetic analogs) [49]. There are various examples of development of new drugs from the plant sources. Morphine was isolated from opium produced from cut seed pods of the poppy plant (*Papaver somniferum*) approximately 200 years ago [50]. Pharmaceutical research expanded after the Second World War to include massive screening of microorganisms for new antibiotics, inspired by the discovery of penicillin [50]. Few drugs developed from natural sources have undoubtedly revolutionized medicine like antibiotics (e.g., penicillin, tetracycline, erythromycin), antiparasitics (e.g., avermectin), antimalarials (e.g., quinine, artemisinin), lipid control agents (e.g., lovastatin and analogs), immune-suppressants for organ transplants (e.g., cyclosporine, rapamycins), and anticancer drugs (e.g., paclitaxel, irinotecan) [51].

The WHO has estimated that the majority of the populations in Africa, Asia, and Latin America still use TM for their primary health care needs [52]. In industrialized countries, plant-based TM or phytotherapeuticals are often termed complementary or alternative medicine (CAM), and their use has increased steadily over the last 10 years [53]. In the USA alone, the total estimated "herbal" sale for 2005 was $4.4 billion, a significant increase from $2.5 billion in 1995 [54] while also accounting for an estimated 1 billion Malaysia ringgit annually [55]. However, such "botanical dietary supplements" are regulated as foods rather than drugs by the United States Food and Drug Administration (US FDA) [54].

5. Recent developments of plant-derived active compounds in drug development

With the recent interest in molecular modeling, combinatorial chemistry, and other synthetic chemistry techniques by pharmaceutical companies and funding organizations, natural products, and particularly medicinal plants, remains an important source of new drugs, new drug leads, and NCEs [56]. In both 2001 and 2002, approximately one quarter of the bestselling drugs worldwide were natural products or derived from natural products. Some of the plant-derived drugs and their significance are listed in the **Table 2**. Many plant-derived compounds have been used as drugs, either in their original or semisynthetic form. Recent developments in drug discovery from plants, including information on approved drugs and

S/N	Compound	Plant name	Classification	Biological function
1	Aescin	*Aesculus hippocastanum*	saponins	Anti-inflammatory, vasoconstrictor and vasoprotective effects
2	Ajmalicine	*Rauwolfia* spp., *Catharanthus roseus, and Mitragyna speciosa*	alkaloid	Antihypertensive drug used in the treatment of high blood pressure

S/N	Compound	Plant name	Classification	Biological function
3	Berberine	*Berberis vulgaris*	alkaloid	Treatment for bacillary dysentery
4	Colchicine	*Colchicum autumnale*	alkaloid	Antitumor agent
5	Curcumin	*Zingiberaceae*	phenols	dietary supplement
6	Emetine	*Cephaelis ipecacuanha*	alkaloid	Amoebicide, emetic
7	Hesperidin	*Citrus species*	Flavonoid	Treatment for capillary fragility
8	Lapachol	*Handroanthus impetiginosus*	phenols	Anticancer, antitumor
9	Nordihydroguaiaretic acid	*Larrea tridentata*	phenols	Antioxidant activity
10	Quinine	*Cinchona officinalis*	alkaloid	Antimalarial drug

Table 2.
Selected compounds derived from medicinal plants.

plant extracts or compounds now in clinical trials, are available [57]. It is anticipated that in the future, plant-derived compounds will still be an essential aspect of the therapeutic array of medicines available to the physician [57].

6. Importance of phytotherapy (for diseases control) within the global health care system

Phyto (plants in the form of leaves, flowers and roots) therapy (treatment) has continued to reflect a great deal of significance in health care around the world in curing diseases while also ensuring a good state of health and/or conditions is maintained. In fact, a significant proportion of the entire global populace had found solace in phytomedicine, embracing it as a major source for their health care system as maintained by WHO in one of their submissions; hence, presenting the impact or relevance of herbal therapy in this chapter cannot be out of context with regard to medicine or medicinal products emanating from these MPs such as *Papaver somniferum*, *Cinchona*, *Hibiscus sabdariffa*, *Rosmarinus officinalis*, *Nigella sativa*, *Artemisia afra*, *Vatica rassak*, etc., some (about 5000 out over 250,000) had either being developed (as drugs or vaccines) and commercialized (morphine, quinine, ephedrine, etc.) and many others in the final process of drug development [2] for confirmation of safety and efficacy (clinical trials) against avalanches of illnesses including but not limited to hypertension, asthma, malaria, pain, hemorrhage, psychosis, cancer, migraine, etc. [58, 59]. This makes herbal medicine to become a basic health service to people of diverse culture irrespective of their status (poor or rich) and location (remote or urban), and this acceptance (in use either singly or combination with orthodox medicine) has continued to escalate in recent times [60], thereby complementing or reducing the use of modern medicine (despite its availability) probably due to inadequacies in providing holistic healing where behavioral, emotional, and/or spiritual factors are the underlying causes of the diseases [61]. In view of the foregoing, continents such as Asia, Africa, and Latin America with countries such as China, India, etc., had embraced the adoption of the two systems (phytotherapy and modern medicine) for their national health care needs. Although issues of safety, efficacy, and quality of herbal medicines have undermined their integration into national health care policy in some countries, this had not prevented, in any big amount, the popular use by the citizenry. Interestingly too, because MPs are core sources for pharmaceutical manufacturing, they in addition to herbal medicines play an important role in pharmaceutical market (PM). In fact, in a reported submission, in 1995, they occupied 33.1% of the total PMs [55].

7. Shortcomings (if available) of phytomedicine to the conventional or modern medicine

Globally, the high demand of use for herbal medicine for the treatment of illnesses is undisputable, and one begs to ask or wonder whether these products are actually of good quality, safe, and effective. There are assumptions and/or claims that despite general usage, few of them have been attributed to illnesses and fatalities as some of them have reported to cause liver and kidney damage [62–64]. In fact, this was also attributed to why they have not been globally accepted as par with conventional medicine within the national health care policy of many countries. The reason for this was not far-fetched. A lot of people believed that many herbal formulations lacked safety evaluations such as clinical trials as to why they cannot be placed in the same pedigree with modern medicine, but this was somehow disagreed by some researchers and/or policy makers who opined that clinical trials may be conducted only when large batches are intended. Additionally, in clinical practice, the failure to integrate phytotherapy as one of the courses or modules in medical school was seen in some quarters as the reason why it became somehow extremely difficult for medical practitioners to prescribe it, hence, the advantage convention medicine enjoys nowadays. Other problems include but not limited to storage conditions, inexplicit dosage, wrong labeling information, individualization of prescription with numerous active ingredients and other components, lack of information on the industrial use of MPs, little or no fact on the market benefit and business potentials, etc. [65]. It is worthy of mention that despite these limitations, phytotherapy had the potentials in salvaging numerous human diseases.

8. Conclusion

The use of phytotherapy in preventing or curing ill-effects faced by mankind was established by the great roles played by natural products obtained from MP. With continued efforts in research and utilization of HM on daily basis, it is envisioned that it would attain its rightful place and be embraced as efficient system worthy of acceptance within the global health care practice.

Author details

Fatai Oladunni Balogun[1*], Anofi Omotayo Tom Ashafa[1], Saheed Sabiu[2], Abdulwakeel Ayokun-nun Ajao[3], Chella Palanisamy Perumal[1], Mutiu Idowu Kazeem[4] and Ahmed Adebowale Adedeji[5]

1 Department of Plant Sciences, University of the Free State, Qwaqwa, Free State, South Africa

2 Faculty of Applied Sciences, Durban University of Technology, Durban, KwaZulu-Natal, South Africa

3 Department of Botany and Plant Biotechnology, University of Johannesburg, Johannesburg, South Africa

4 Department of Biochemistry, Lagos State University, Lagos, Nigeria

5 Department of Pharmacology, University of Gitwe, Nyanza, Rwanda

*Address all correspondence to: balogunfo@yahoo.co.uk

References

[1] Hassan MA. A short history of the use of plants as medicines from ancient times. Chimia. 2015;**69**:622-623. DOI: 10.2533/chimia.2015.622

[2] Mohamed I, Shuid A, Borhanuddin B, Fozi N. The application of phytomedicine in modern drug development. The Internet Journal of Herbal and Plant Medicine. 2012;**1**(2):1-9

[3] Roberts MF, Wink M. Alkaloids: Biochemistry, Ecology, and Medicinal Applications. New York: Plenum Press; 1998

[4] Balogun FO. Antioxidant, antidiabetic and cardioprotective activities of *Dicoma anomala* (Sond.) used in the Basotho traditional medicine [thesis]. Qwaqwa Free State: University of the Free State; 2017

[5] Perumal PC, Sophia D, Raj CA, Ragavendran P, Starlin T, Gopalakrishnan VK. *In vitro* antioxidant activities and HPTLC analysis of ethanolic extract of *Cayratia trifolia* (L.). Asian Pacific Journal of Tropical Disease. 2012;**2**:S952-S956

[6] Pan SY, Zhou SF, Gao SH, Yu ZL, Zhang SF, Tang MK, et al. New perspectives on how to discover drugs from herbal medicines: CAM's outstanding contribution to modern therapeutics. Evidence-Based Complementary and Alternative Medicine. 2013;**13**:1-25

[7] Fabricant DS, Farnsworth NR. The value of plants used in traditional medicine for drug discovery. Environmental Health Perspectives. 2001;**109**(Suppl 1):69-75

[8] Wink M. Modes of action of herbal medicines and plant secondary metabolites. Medicine. 2015;**2**(3):251-286

[9] Makkar HPS, Norvsambuu T, Lkhagvatseren S, Becker K. Plant secondary metabolites in some medicinal plants of Mongolia used for enhancing animal health and production. Tropicultura. 2009;**27**(3):159-167

[10] Ahmed E, Arshad M, Khan MZ. Secondary metabolites and their multidimensional prospective in plant life. Journal of Pharmacognosy and Phytochemistry. 2017;**6**(2):205-214

[11] Kandi S, Godishala V, Rao P, Ramana KV. Biomedical significance of terpenes: An insight. Biomédica. 2015;**3**(1):8-10

[12] Ajao AA, Alimi AA, Olatunji OA, Balogun FO, Saheed SA. A synopsis of anti-psychotic medicinal plants in Nigeria. Transactions of the Royal Society of South Africa. 2018;**73**(1):33-41

[13] Solís C, Becerra J, Flores C, Robledo J, Silva M. Antibacterial and antifungal terpenes from *Pilgerodendron uviferum* (D. Don) Florin. Journal of the Chilean Chemical Society. 2004;**49**(2):157-161

[14] Kusumoto N, Zhao T, Swedjemark G, Ashitani T, Takahashi K, Borg-Karlson AK. Antifungal properties of terpenoids in *Picea abies* against *Heterobasidion parviporum*. Forest Pathology. 2014;**44**(5):353-361

[15] Ighachane H, Boualy B, Ait Ali M, Sedra MH, El Firdoussi L, Lazrek HB. Catalytic synthesis and antifungal activity of new polychlorinated natural terpenes. Advances in Materials Science and Engineering. 2017;**2017**:7. Article ID 2784303. DOI: 10.1155/2017/2784303

[16] Lin D, Xiao M, Zhao J, Li Z, Xing B, Li X, et al. An overview of plant phenolic compounds and their importance in human nutrition and management of type 2 diabetes. Molecules. 2016;**21**(10):1374

[17] Działo M, Mierziak J, Korzun U, Preisner M, Szopa J, Kulma A. The potential of plant phenolics in prevention and therapy of skin disorders. International Journal of Molecular Sciences. 2016;**17**(2):160

[18] Carocho M, Ferreira CFRI. The role of phenolic compounds in the fight against cancer—A review. Anti-Cancer Agents in Medicinal Chemistry. 2013;**13**(8):1236-1258

[19] Xu Y, Burton S, Kim C, Sismour E. Phenolic compounds, antioxidant, and antibacterial properties of pomace extracts from four Virginia-grown grape varieties. Food Science & Nutrition. 2016;**4**(1):125-133

[20] Ambriz-Pérez DL, Leyva-López N, Gutierrez-Grijalva EP, Heredia JB. Phenolic compounds: Natural alternative in inflammation treatment. A Review. Cogent Food & Agriculture. 2016;**2**(1):1131412

[21] Li R, Narita R, Nishimura H, Marumoto S, Yamamoto SP, Ouda R, et al. Antiviral activity of phenolic derivatives in pyroligneous acid from hardwood, softwood, and bamboo. ACS Sustainable Chemistry & Engineering. 2017;**6**(1):119-126

[22] Kaur RA, Arora SA. Alkaloids-important therapeutic secondary metabolites of plant origin. Journal of Critical Reviews. 2015;**2**(3):1-8

[23] Mabhiza D, Chitemerere T, Mukanganyama S. Antibacterial properties of alkaloid extracts from *Callistemon citrinus* and *Vernonia adoensis* against *Staphylococcus aureus* and *Pseudomonas aeruginosa*. International Journal of Medicinal Chemistry. 2016;**2016**:7. Article ID: 6304163. DOI: 10.1155/2016/6304163

[24] Agrawal R, Sethiya NK, Mishra SH. Antidiabetic activity of alkaloids of *Aerva lanata* roots on streptozotocin-nicotinamide induced type-II diabetes in rats. Pharmaceutical Biology. 2013;**51**(5):635-642

[25] Elya B, Katrin B, Forestrania RC, Sofyan R, Chandra RA. Alkaloid from *Phoebe declinata* Nees leaves. Pharmacognosy Journal. 2017;**9**(6):713-720

[26] Stojanoski N. Development of health culture in Veles and its region from the past to the end of the 20th century. Veles: Society of Science and Art. 1999:13-34

[27] Kelly K. History of Medicine. New York: Facts on file; 2009. pp. 29-50

[28] Biljana BP. Historical review of medicinal plants' usage. Pharmacognosy Reviews. 2012;**6**(11):1-5

[29] Chintamunnee V, Mahomoodally MF. Herbal medicine commonly used against infectious diseases in the tropical island of Mauritius. Journal of Herbal Medicine. 2012;**2**:113-125

[30] Aone M. [Internet]. 2001. Available from: http://www.blackherbals.com/atcNewsletter913.pdf [Accessed: 10-09-2018]

[31] WHO. Fact sheetN◦134 [Internet]. 2008. Available from: http://www.who.int/mediacentre/factsheets/2003/fs134/en/ [Accessed: 11-09-2018]

[32] Erasto P, Adebola PO, Grierson DS, Afolayan AJ. An ethnobotanical study of plants used for the treatment of diabetes in Eastern Cape Province, South Africa. African Journal of Biotechnology. 2005;**4**:1458-1460

[33] Balogun FO, Ashafa AOT. Aqueous root extract of *Dicoma anomala* (Sond.) extenuates postprandial hyperglycaemia *in vitro* and its modulation on the activities of carbohydrate-metabolism enzymes in streptozotocin-induced diabetic Wistar rats. South African Journal of Botany. 2017;**112**:102-112

[34] van de Venter M, Roux S, Bungu LC, Louw J, Crouch NR, Grace OM, et al. Antidiabetic screening and scoring of 11 plants traditionally used in South Africa. Journal of Ethnopharmacology. 2008;**119**:81-86

[35] Sabiu S, Ajani EO, Aladodo RA, Garuba T, Agunbiade MO, Alimi AA, et al. Membrane stabilization and probable mechanisms of hypoglycemic activity of fruit extract of *Solanum incanum* L. (Solanaceae). Comparative Clinical Pathology. 2018;**21**(6):1161-1169

[36] Pezzuto JM. Plant-derived anticancer agents. Biochemical Pharmacology. 1997;**53**:121-133

[37] Solowey E, Lichtenstein M, Sallo S, Paavilainen H, Solowet E, Lorberboum-Galski H. Evaluating medicinal plants for anticancer activity. The Scientific World Journal. 2014;**2014**:1-12

[38] Thiengsusuk A, Chaijaroenkul W, Na-Bangchang K. Antimalarial activities of medicinal plants and herbal formulations used in Thai traditional medicine. Parasitology Research. 2013;**112**(4):1475-1481

[39] Mlinarič A, Kreft S, Umek ŠB. Screening of selected plant extracts for *in vitro* inhibitory activity on HIV-1 reverse transcriptase (HIV-1 RT). Die Pharmazie. 2000;**55**(1):75-77

[40] Bedoya LM, Sanchez-Palomino S, Abad MJ, Bermejo P, Alcami J. Anti-HIV activity of medicinal plant extracts. Journal of Ethnopharmacology. 2001;**77**(1):113-116

[41] Kinda PT, Zerbo P, Prosper T, Guenné S, Compaoré M, Ciobica A, et al. Medicinal plants used for neuropsychiatric disorders treatment in the Hauts Bassins Region of Burkina Faso. Medicine. 2017;**4**:32

[42] Jethva K, Bhatt D, Zaveri M. *In-vitro* anti-tuberculosis activity of selected ethnomedicinal plant. International Journal of Herbal Medicine. 2016;**4**(4):126-128

[43] Behl T, Kaur I. Herbal Plants: A boon in the treatment of diabetic retinopathy. Pharmacologia. 2015;**6**:1-10

[44] Tabassun N, Ahmad F. Role of natural herbs in the treatment of hypertension. Pharmacognosy Reviews. 2011;**5**(9):30-40

[45] Sabiu S, O'Neil FH, Ashafa AOT. Membrane stabilization and detoxification of acetaminophen-mediated oxidative onslaughts in the kidneys of Wistar rats by standardized fraction of *Zea mays* L. (Poaceae), *Stigma maydis*. Evidence-Based Complementary and Alternative Medicine. 2016;**2016**:14. Article ID: 2046298

[46] Sabiu S, Ajani EO, Sunmonu OT, Ashafa AOT. *Spondias mombin* L. (Anacardiaceae) enhances detoxification of hepatic and macromolecular oxidants in acetaminophen-intoxicated rats. Pakistan Journal of Pharmaceutical Sciences. 2017;**30**(6):2109-2117

[47] Balogun FO, Ashafa AOT. Protective action of aqueous leaf extract of *Gazania krebsiana* (Less.) 'Asteraceae' antagonizes isoproterenol-triggered myocardial infarction in *Rattus norvegicus*. Comparative Clinical Pathology. 2018;**27**:461-470

[48] Schuhmacher A, Gassmann O, Hinder M. Changing R&D models in research-based pharmaceutical companies. Journal of Translational Medicine. 2016;**14**:105. DOI: 10.1186/s12967-016-0838-4

[49] Katiyar C, Gupta A, Kanjilal S, Katiyar S. Drug discovery from plant sources: An integrated approach. AYU. 2012;**33**(1):10-19

[50] Jesse W, Li H, Vederas JC. Drug discovery and natural products: End of

an era or an endless frontier? Science. 2009;**325**(5937):161-165. DOI: 10.1126/science.1168243

[51] Kumar S, Shukla YN, Lavania UC, Sharma A, Singh AK. Medicinal and aromatic plants: Prospects for India. J Med Arom Plant Sci. 1997;**19**(2):361-365

[52] Joy PP, Thomas J, Mathew S, Skaria BP. Medicinal plants, Kerala Agricultural University, Aromatic and Medicinal Plants Research Station. 1998

[53] Berdai MA, Labib S, Chetouani K, Harandou M. *Atropa belladonna* intoxication: A case report. The Pan African Medical Journal. 2012;**11**:72

[54] Katiyar C, Gupta A, Kanjilal S, Katiyar S. Drug discovery from plant sources: An integrated approach. AYU. 2015;**33**(1):10-19

[55] WHO. Guidelines for the appropriate use of herbal medicines. In: Essential Medicines and health products information portal. A World Health Organization resource. 1998. Available from: http://apps.who.int/medicinedocs/en/d/Jh2945e/2.1.html#Jh2945e.2.1 [Accessed: 30-08-2018]

[56] Salim AA, Chin YW, Kinghorn AD. Drug discovery from plants. In: Ramawat KG, Mérillon JM, editors. Bioactive Molecules and Medicinal Plants. 1-25. ISBN: 978-3-540-75600-3

[57] Anon. World Health Organization fact sheet No. 134, revised May 2003 [Internet]. 2003. Available from: http://www.who.int/mediacentre/factsheets/fs134/en/ [Accessed: 10-10-2018]

[58] Pithava A, Pithava A. Current prospects of herbal medicines in the World. Research & Reviews: Journal of Pharmacognosy and Phytochemistry. 2016;**4**(4):60-67

[59] Yuan H, Ma Q, Ye L, Piao G. The traditional medicine and modern medicine from natural products. Molecules. 2016;**21**:559. DOI: 10.3390/molecules21050559

[60] Liu Y. Renaissance of marine natural product drug discovery and development. Journal of Marine Science: Research and Development. 2012;**2**:e106

[61] Iwu MM, Gbodossou E. The role of traditional medicine. In: Alternative medicine: Nigeria. The Lancet Perspect. 2000;**s3**:356

[62] Saad B, Azaizeh H, Abu-Hijleh G, Said O. Safety of traditional Arab herbal medicine. Evidence-Based Complementary and Alternative Medicine. 2006;**3**(4):433-439

[63] Debelle FD, Vanherweghem JL, Nortier JL. Aristolochic acid nephropathy: A worldwide problem. Kidney International. 2008;**74**(2):158-169

[64] Park MY, Choi HY, Kim JD, Lee HS, Ku SK. 28 Days repeated oral dose toxicity test of aqueous extracts of mahwangyounpae-tang, a polyherbal formula. Food and Chemical Toxicology. 2010;**48**(8-9):2477-2482

[65] Oladeji O. The characteristics and roles of medicinal plants: Some important medicinal plants in Nigeria. Indian Journal of Natural Products. 2016;**12**(3):102

[66] Addo P, Quartey M, Abbas M, Adu-Addai B, Owusu E, Okang I, et al. *In-vitro* susceptibility of *Mycobacterium ulcerans* to herbal preparations. Internet Journal of Tropical Medicine. 2007;**4**(2007):2

[67] Fokou PV, Nyarko AK, Appiah-Opong R, Yamthe LRT, Addo P, Asante IK, et al. Ethnopharmacological reports on anti-buruli ulcer medicinal plants in three West African countries. Journal of Ethnopharmacology. 2015;**172**:297-311

[68] Vaz NP. Can the cure for Chagas' disease be found in Nature? In: Khater H, Govindarajan M, Benelli G, editors. Natural Remedies in the Fight against Parasites. London, UK: IntechOpen; 2017. DOI: 10.5772/67225. Available from: https://www.intechopen.com/books/naturalremedies-in-the-fight-against-parasites/can-the-cure-for-chagas-disease-be-found-in-nature-

[69] Tang LI, Ling AP, Koh RY, Chye SM, Voon KG. Screening of anti-dengue activity in methanolic extracts of medicinal plants. BMC Complementary and Alternative Medicine. 2012;**12**:3

[70] Rothan HA, Zulqarnain M, Ammar YA, Tan EC, Rahman NA, Yusof R. Screening of antiviral activities in medicinal plants extracts against dengue virus using dengue NS2B-NS3 protease assay. Tropical Biomedicine. 2014;**31**(2):286-296

[71] Frederico ÉHFF, Cardoso ALBD, Moreira-Marconi E, de Sá-Caputo DC, Guimarães CAS, Dionello CF, et al. Anti-viral effects of medicinal plants in the management of dengue: A systematic review. African Journal of Traditional, Complementary, and Alternative Medicines. 2017;**14**(4 Suppl):33-40

[72] Fahey JW. *Moringa oleifera*: A review of the medicinal evidence for its nutritional, therapeutics and prophylactic properties, Part 1. Trees for Life Journal. 2005;**1**(5):1-15

[73] Verma VC, Gond SK, Kumar A, Mishra A, Kharwar RN, Gange AC. Endophytic actinomycetes from *Azadirachta indica* A. Juss.: Isolation, diversity, and anti-microbial activity. Microbial Ecology. 2009;**57**(4):749-756

[74] Keiser J, Utzinger J. Food-borne trematodiasis: Current chemotherapy and advances with artemisinin and synthetic trioxolanes. Trends in Parasitology. 2007;**23**(11):555-562

[75] McGaw LJ, Jäger AK, Van Staden J. Antibacterial, anthelmintic and anti-amoebic activity in South African medicinal plants. Journal of Ethnopharmacology. 2000;**72**:247-263

[76] Ademola IO, Eloff JN. *In vitro* anthelmintic activity of *Combretum molle* (R. Br. ex G. Don) (Combretaceae) against *Haemonchus contortus* ova and larvae. Veterinary Parasitology. 2010;**169**:198-203

[77] Aremu AO, Ndhlala AR, Fawole OA, Light ME, Finnie JF, Van Staden J. *In vitro* pharmacological evaluation and phenolic content of ten South African medicinal plants used as anthelmintics. South African Journal of Botany. 2010;**76**:558-566

[78] Nchu F, Githiori JB, McGaw LJ, Eloff JN. Anthelmintic and cytotoxic activities of extracts of *Markhamia obtusifolia* Sprague (Bignoniaceae). Veterinary Parasitology. 2011;**183**:184-188

[79] Maphosa V, Masika P. *In vivo* validation of *Aloe ferox* (Mill). *Elephantorrhiza elephantina* Bruch. Skeels. and *Leonotis leonurus* (L) R. BR as potential anthelminthics and antiprotozoals against mixed infections of gastrointestinal nematodes in goats. Parasitology Research. 2012;**110**:103-108

[80] Okem A, Finnie JF, Van Staden J. Pharmacological, genotoxic and phytochemical properties of selected South African medicinal plants used in treating stomach-related ailments. Journal of Ethnopharmacology. 2012;**139**:712-720

[81] Tshabalala BD, Alayande KA, Sabiu S, Ashafa AOT. Antimicrobial and anthelmintic potentials of root and leaf extracts of *Gazania krebsiana* Less. subsp. serrulata (DC.) Roessler: An *in vitro* assessment. European Journal of Integrative Medicine. 2016;**8**(4):533-539

[82] De Queiroz AC, Dias TLMF, Da Matta CBB, et al. Antileishmanial activity of medicinal plants used in endemic areas in Northeastern Brazil. Evidence-Based Complementary and Alternative Medicine. 2014;**2014**:9. Article ID 478290. DOI: 10.1155/2014/478290

[83] Johnsy G, Kaviyarasan V. Ethno-medicinal plants used for the treatment of leprosy in tribal peoples of Kanyakumari district. Global Journal of Pharmacology. 2015;**9**(2):190-195

[84] Datta A, Sukul NC. Antifilarial effect of *Zinger officinale* on *dirofilaria immitis*. Journal of Helminthology. 1987;**61**:268-270

[85] Parveen N. Antifilarial activity of *Vitex negundo* L. against *Setaria cervi*. Fitoterapia. 1991;**62**:163

[86] Singhal KC, Sharma S, Mehta BK. Antifilarial activity of *Centratherum anthelminticum* seed extracts on *Setaria cervi*. Indian Journal of Experimental Biology. 1992;**30**(6):546-548

[87] Ghosh M, Babu SP, Sukul NC, Mahato SB. Antifilarial effect of two triterpenoid saponins isolated from *Acacia auriculiformis*. Indian Journal of Experimental Biology. 1993;**31**:604-606

[88] Singh R, Singhal KC, Khan NU. Antifilarial activity of *Mallotus philippensis* Lam. on *Setaria cervi* (Nematoda: Filarioidea) *in vitro*. Indian Journal of Physiology and Pharmacology. 1997;**41**:397-403

[89] Joshi SG. Medicinal Plants. Calcutta: Oxford and IBH Publishing Co Pvt Ltd; 2000. p. 3

[90] Mishra V, Khan NU, Singhal KC. Potential antifilarial activity of fruit extracts of *Ficus racemosa* Linn. against *Setaria cervi in vitro*. Indian Journal of Experimental Biology. 2005;**43**(4):346-350

[91] Ezaldeen EA, Fahal AH, Osman A. Mycetoma herbal treatment: The Mycetoma Research Centre, Sudan experience. PLoS Neglected Tropical Diseases. 2013;7:e2400

[92] Elfadil H, Fahal A, Kloezen W, et al. The *in vitro* antifungal activity of Sudanese medicinal plants against *Madurella mycetomatis*, the eumycetoma major causative agent. PLoS Neglected Tropical Diseases. 2015;**9**:e0003488

[93] Nyasse B, Ngantchou I, Nono JJ, Schneider B. Antifilarial activity *in vitro* of polycarpol and 3-O-acetyl aleuritolic acid from Cameroonian medicinal plants against *Onchocerca gutturosa*. Natural Product Research. 2006;**20**:391-397

[94] Cho-Ngwa F, Abongwa M, Ngemenya MN, Nyongbela KD. Selective activity of extracts of *Margaritaria discoidea* and *Homalium africanum* on *Onchocerca ochengi*. BMC Complementary and Alternative Medicine. 2010;**10**:62

[95] Ndjonka D, Agyare C, Luersen K, Djafsia B, Achukwi D, Nukenine EN, et al. *In vitro* activity of Cameroonian and Ghanaian medicinal plants on parasitic (*Onchocerca ochengi*) and free-living (*Caenorhabditis elegans*) nematodes. Journal of Helminthology. 2011;**85**:304-312

[96] Ndjonka D, Ajonina-Ekoti I, Djafsia B, Luersen K, Abladam E, Liebau E. *Anogeissus leiocarpus* extract on the parasite nematode *Onchocerca ochengi* and on drug resistant mutant strains of the free-living nematode *Caenorhabditis elegans*. Veterinary Parasitology. 2012;**190**:136-142

[97] Admasu P, Deressa A, Mengistu A, Gebrewold G, Fayera T. *In vivo* antirabies activity evaluation of hydroethonolic extract of roots and leaves of *Phytolaccado decandra*. Global Veterinaria. 2014;**12**:12-18

[98] Pagadala VK, Tsegaye B, Kebede N, Elias T, Gemachu G. Significance of traditional medicinal plants used for treatment of rabies at Ambo Town. Medicinal and Aromatic Plants. 2015;**4**:207. DOI: 10.4172/2167-0412.1000207

[99] Xavier TF, Kannan M, Auxilia A. Traditional medicinal plants used in the treatment of different skin diseases. International Journal of Current Microbiology and Applied Sciences. 2015;**4**(5):1043-1053

[100] Topno SC, Sinha MR. Study of medicinal plants used to heal skin diseases by tribes of west Singhbhum district of Jharkhand (India). Journal of Pharmacognosy and Phytochemistry. 2018;**7**(1):371-376

[101] Ndamba J, Nyazema N, Makaza N, Anderson C, Kaondera KC. Traditional herbal remedies used for the treatment of urinary schistosomiasis in Zimbabwe. Journal of Ethnopharmacology. 1994;**42**(2):125-132

[102] Koch HP, Lawson LD. Garlic: The Science and Therapeutic Application of *Allium sativum* L. and Related Species. 2nd ed. Baltimore, MD, USA: Lippincott Williams and Wilkins. p. 329. ISBN-13: 9780683181470

[103] Ogboli AU, Nock IH, Obdurahman EM, Ibrahim NDG. Medicinal application of *Vernonia amygdalina* del leaf extracts in the treatment of schistosomiasis in mice. Nigerian Journal of Natural Products and Medicine. 2000;**4**:73-75

[104] Aly HF, Aly SA. Essential role of *Citrus reticulata* and Mirazid in treatment of *Schistosoma mansoni* infected mice: Biochemical and parasitological studies. Polish Journal of Food and Nutrition Sciences. 2006;**15**:461-467

[105] Martz W. Plants with a reputation against snakebite. Toxicon. 1992;**30**:1131-1142

[106] Houghton PJ, Osibogun IM. Flowering plants used against snakebite. Journal of Ethnopharmacology. 1993;**39**:1-29

[107] Gupta YK, Peshin SS. Do herbal medicines have potential for managing snake bite envenomation? Toxicology International. 2012;**19**(2):89-99

[108] Chung W, Ko B. Treatment of *Taenia saginata* infection with mixture of areca nuts and pumpkin seeds. Chinese Journal of Microbiology and Immunology. 1976;**9**:31-35

[109] Tandon V, Yadav A, Roy B, Das B. Phytochemicals as Cure of Worm Infections in Traditional Medicine Systems. Emerging Trends in Zoology. New Delhi: Narendra Publishing House; 2011. pp. 351-378

[110] Ito A, Li T, Chen X, Long C, et al. Mini review on chemotherapy of taeniasis and cysticercosis due to *Taenia solium* in Asia, and a case report with 20 tapeworms in China. Tropical Biomedicine. 2013;**30**:164-173

[111] Bizhani N. Herbal therapy and treatment of worm infections, Emphasizing *Taenia solium*. Iranian Journal of Public Health. 2015;**44**(11):1555-1556

[112] Li RW, Myers SP, Leach DN, Lin GD, Leach G. A cross-cultural study: Anti-inflammatory activity of Australian and Chinese plants. Journal of Ethnopharmacology. 2003;**85**:25-32

[113] Adedapo AA, Jimoh FO, Koduru S, Afolayan AJ, Masika PJ. Antibacterial and antioxidant properties of the methanol extracts of the leaves and stems of *Calpurnia aurea*. BMC Complementary and Alternative Medicine. 2008;**8**:53

[114] Rani MS, Pippalla RS, Mohan K. *Dodonaea viscosa* Linn.—An overview. Asian Journal of Pharmaceutical

Research and Health Care. 2009;**1**:97-112

[115] Yenesew A, Twinomuhwezi H, Kiremire BT, Mbugua MN, Gitu PM, Heydenreich M, et al. 8-Methoxyneorautenol and radical scavenging flavonoids from *Erythrina abyssinica*. Bulletin of the Chemical Society of Ethiopia. 2009;**23**:205-210

[116] Jaberian H, Piri K, Nazari J. Phytochemical composition and *in vitro* antimicrobial and antioxidant activities of some medicinal plants. Food Chemistry. 2013;**136**:237-244

[117] Semenya SS, Potgieter MJ, Erasmus LJC. Bapedi phytomedicine and their use in the treatment of sexually transmitted infections in Limpopo province, South Africa. African Journal of Pharmacy and Pharmacology. 2013;**7**:250-262

[118] Potroz MG, Cho N. Natural products for the treatment of trachoma and chlamydia trachomatis. Molecules. 2015;**20**:4180-4203

[119] Asuzu IU, Chineme CN. Effects of *Morinda lucida* leaf extracts on *Trypanosoma brucei brucei* infection in mice. Journal of Ethnopharmacology. 1990;**30**:307-313

[120] Freiburghaus F, Ogwal EN, Nkunya MII, Kaminsky R, Brun R. *In vitro* antitrypanosomal activity of African plants used in traditional medicine in Uganda to treat sleeping sickness. Tropical Medicine & International Health. 1996;**1**(6):765-771

[121] Nok AJ, Williams S, Onyenekwe PC. *Allium sativum*-induced death of African trypanosomes. Parasitology Research. 1996;**82**(7):634-637

[122] Abubakar A, Iliyasu B, Yusuf AB, Onyekwelu NA, Igweh AC, Shamaki BU, et al. Antitrypanosomal and hematological effects of selected Nigerian medicinal plants in Wistar rats. Biokemistri. 2005;**17**:95-99

[123] Ibrahim MA, Njoku GC, Sallau AB. *In vivo* activity of stem bark aqueous extract of *Khaya senegalensis* against *Trypanosoma brucei*. African Journal of Biotechnology. 2008;**7**(5):661-663

[124] Maikai VA, Nok JA, Adaudi AO, Alawa CB. *In vitro* antitrypanosomal activity of aqueous and methanolic crude extracts of stem bark of *Ximenia americana* on *Trypanosoma congolense*. Journal of Medicinal Plants Research. 2008;**2**(3):055-058

[125] Abdullahi M, Emmanuel O. Evaluation of medicinal plants from Nupeland for their *in vivo* antitrypanosomal activity. American Journal of Biochemistry. 2012;**2**(1):1-6

[126] Available from: https://herbpathy.com/Herbal-Treatment-for-Yaws-Cid4257 [Accessed: 10-09-2018]

[127] Balunas MJ, Kinghorn AD. Drug discovery from medicinal plants. Life Sciences. 2005;**78**:431-441